Sports Injury Research

Edited by

Evert Verhagen

Willem van Mechelen

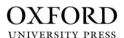

OXFORD

UNIVERSITY PRESS

OXFORD

UNIVERSITY PRESS

Great Clarendon Street, Oxford OX2 6DP

Oxford University Press is a department of the University of Oxford.
It furthers the University's objective of excellence in research, scholarship,
and education by publishing worldwide in

Oxford New York

Auckland Cape Town Dar es Salaam Hong Kong Karachi
Kuala Lumpur Madrid Melbourne Mexico City Nairobi
New Delhi Shanghai Taipei Toronto

With offices in

Argentina Austria Brazil Chile Czech Republic France Greece
Guatemala Hungary Italy Japan Poland Portugal Singapore
South Korea Switzerland Thailand Turkey Ukraine Vietnam

Oxford is a registered trade mark of Oxford University Press
in the UK and in certain other countries

Published in the United States
by Oxford University Press Inc., New York

British Library Cataloguing in Publication Data
Data available

Library of Congress Cataloging in Publication Data
Data available

Typeset in Minion by Cepha Imaging Private Ltd., Banglore, India
Printed in Great Britain
on acid-free paper by the
MPG Books Group, Bodmin and King's Lynn

ISBN 978–0–19–956162–9

10 9 8 7 6 5 4 3 2 1

Sports Injury Research

Preface

A physically active lifestyle and active participation in sports is important, both for adults and for children[1]. Reasons to participate in sports and physical activity are many; pleasure and relaxation, competition, socialization, maintenance, and improvement of fitness and health, etc. However, with the current focus on a physically active lifestyle, an increasing number of sporting and physical activity injuries can be expected. Consequently, sporting and physical activity injuries are becoming a major health problem. Given the unwanted side effects of a healthy activity, successful prevention of sports injuries has great potential health gain: in the short term, the absolute number of sporting injuries falls and, in the longer term, the risk of recurrences of injuries and prolonged periods of impairment will be prevented.

In general, measures to prevent sports injuries do not stand by themselves. They result from a series of four steps that form a sequence of prevention[2]. First, the sports-injury problem must be described in terms of incidence and severity. The second step identifies the aetiological risk factors and mechanisms underlying the occurrence of injury. Based on this information on the underlying risk factors, in the third step preventive measures that are likely to work can be developed and introduced. Finally, the (cost-)effectiveness of the introduced preventive measures should be evaluated by repeating the first step or preferably by performing intervention trials.

With the increasing interest in physical activity and sports for health, comes an increasing interest for safety in physical activity and sports. In the coming years more research efforts within this field can be expected, as well as a higher demand for evidence on injury prevention and treatment. An important problem that will arise is that most individuals involved in sports medicine are not thoroughly trained in epidemiological and methodological rigour. For this reason this book aims to share the current expertise and knowledge of the world's leading researchers within the field of sports-injury research.

This book is intended to be a comprehensive contemporary text on methodology in sports-injury research. It is our intention to provide you, the reader, with a solid and comprehensive background on epidemiological methods employed in sports-injury research, to make you aware of key methodological issues, and to let you recognize the effect of employed methodology on interpretations of study results. In addition, this book will give you—through the division in subsequent sections—a clear and solid outline of the road that leads to sports-injury prevention, i.e. how does one go from an injury problem to successful injury prevention. It should be noted that this book will not provide a comprehensive review of the available literature on sports injuries, prevention, and treatment. It is intended as a thorough epidemiological and methodological background and reference for researchers and professionals in the field of sports medicine.

We expect that the contents of this book will motivate you to conduct well-designed sports-injury studies, and that consequently we will come across your research in future publications.

Evert Verhagen
Willem van Mechelen

References

1. Haskell WL, Lee I, Pate RR et al. (2007). Physical activity and public health: updated recommendation for adults from the American College of Sports Medicine and the American Heart Association. *Circ*; **116**, 1081–93.
2. van Mechelen W, Hlobil H, Kemper HCG (1992). Incidence, severity, aetiology and prevention of sports injuries. *Sports Med*, **14**, 82–99.

Contents

List of contributors *xv*

Part 1 **Key issues in epidemiology and methodology**

1 Defining a research question *3*
Peta White
  Research questions and the research purpose *3*
  Research questions and methodology *4*
    The mechanics of the research question *5*
    Common mistakes and problems when constructing
        questions *6*
    One study, multiple questions *7*
  Conclusion *7*
    References *8*

2 Study designs *9*
James R. Borchers and Thomas Best
  Bias, confounding, and random error *10*
    Bias *10*
    Confounding *10*
    Random error *10*
  Clinical trials *11*
  Cohort studies *14*
  Case-control studies *15*
  Descriptive studies *17*
  Conclusion *17*
    References *18*

3 Basic statistical methods *19*
Jos Twisk
  Dichotomous outcome variables *19*
  95% confidence intervals around the risk difference and
    relative risk *20*
  Testing of the risk difference and the relative risk *22*
  An alternative effect measure: the odds ratio *24*
  Logistic regression analysis *25*
  Adding time at risk to the analysis *28*
  Comparison of two groups: Kaplan–Meier survival curves *29*
  Cox regression analysis *34*

Cox regression analysis with recurrent events *36*

Confounding and effect modification *36*

Conclusion *39*

References *39*

Part 2 **Defining the injury problem**

4 Injury definitions *43*

Colin Fuller

Definition of injury *43*

Definition of a case in injury surveillance studies *44*

Injury severity *46*

Injury classification *49*

Injury causation *50*

Impact of injury definition on the study outcomes *52*

Conclusion *52*

References *52*

5 Research designs for descriptive studies *55*

Jennifer Hootman

Types of descriptive studies *55*

Ecologic studies *55*

Cross-sectional studies *58*

Examples of descriptive sports injury epidemiology studies *60*

Data sources for sports injury descriptive studies *61*

Government databases *61*

Health-care system *62*

Schools/sports organizations *63*

Special studies/registries *64*

Conclusion *65*

References *66*

6 Statistics used in observational studies *69*

Will G. Hopkins

Risk, risk difference, and risk ratio *69*

Odds, odds ratio, and generalized linear modelling *71*

Count and count ratios *74*

Rate and rate ratios *74*

Hazard, time to injury, and their ratios *75*

Severity and burden of injury *77*

Magnitude thresholds for injury outcomes *79*

Acknowledgements *81*

Suggested reading *81*

References *81*

7 Reviews – using the literature to your advantage *83*
  Quinette Louw and Karen Grimmer-Somers
  Definitions and classifications *83*
  Coming to grips with literature *83*
  Function of literature reviews *84*
  Types of literature reviews *84*
  Writing the systematic review protocol and conducting
    the review *85*
  Background information *86*
  Setting an explicit review question *86*
  Review objectives linked to the review question *86*
  Setting inclusion and exclusion criteria *87*
  Search strategies for databases *87*
  A method of selecting eligible papers *88*
  Levels of evidence and a critical appraisal of study
      quality *89*
    Assigning levels of evidence *89*
    Critical appraisal of study quality *91*
  Data extraction and analysis *91*
  Statistical synthesis *94*
  Referring to studies *94*
  Publishing the review *95*
    References *95*

Part 3 **Establishing injury aetiology**

8 The multi-causality of injury – current concepts *99*
  Willem Meeuwisse and Brent Hagel
  Models of injury prevention *99*
  Understanding risk factors and cause *99*
    Origins of causal thinking in epidemiology *99*
    Sport and recreational injuries *101*
  Implications for study design *104*
    Object of study *104*
    Outcome, determinant, and confounder definitions *105*
  Taking action *106*
  Conclusion *107*
    References *107*

9 Investigating injury risk factors and mechanisms *109*
  Tron Krosshaug and Evert Verhagen
  Epidemiological criteria for causation *109*
    Temporality *109*
    Strength *109*

Dose–response relationship *110*

Consistency *110*

Plausibility *111*

Coherence *111*

Consideration of alternate explanations *111*

Experiment *111*

Specificity *111*

Risk factors *111*

Validity *112*

Face validity *112*

Content validity *112*

Construct validity *112*

Criterion validity *112*

Reliability *113*

Joint probability of agreement *113*

Kappa statistics *113*

Correlation coefficients *114*

Intra-class correlation coefficient *115*

Limits of agreement *115*

Mechanisms of injury *115*

Interviews *115*

Clinical studies *117*

Video analysis *117*

Laboratory motion analysis *118*

In vivo strain/force measurements *119*

Injuries during biomechanical experiments *119*

Cadaveric and dummy studies *119*

Mathematical modelling *120*

Conclusion *120*

References *121*

10 Statistics in aetiological studies *125*

Ian Shrier and Russell. J Steele

Do some injuries occur more often than
others? *125*

Injury rates *128*

Choosing covariates in multiple regression *129*

Determining mediating effects through multiple
regression *131*

Conclusion *133*

References *134*

Part 4 **Developing preventive measures**

11 The pragmatic approach *139*
Alex Donaldson
  A 5-step strategic approach to developing sports-injury preventive measures *140*
    Step 1: Tell people about it and get them on board – communication, consultation, co-ordination, and a multi-disciplinary approach *140*
    Step 2: Establish the context – understanding the bigger picture *141*
    Step 3: Identify the safety issues, concerns, and risks *142*
    Step 4: Set priorities – short-term action and long-term planning *144*
    Step 5: Decide what to do – evidenced-informed and theory-based interventions to address identified sports-injury risks *144*
  Time dimension *144*
  Intervention-level dimension *146*
  The direction of the intervention process *150*
  Host–agent–environment relationship *151*
  Conclusion *153*
    References *153*
12 The behavioural approach *157*
Dorine Collard, Amika Singh, and Evert Verhagen
  Intervention mapping: the theory *158*
  Needs assessment *158*
  Preparation of matrices of change objectives *160*
  Selection of theory-based intervention methods and practical strategies *161*
  Production of intervention components and materials *162*
  Adoption, implementation, and sustainability of the intervention *163*
  Generation of an evaluation plan *164*
  Conclusion *165*
    References *166*

Part 5 **Evaluating the efficacy and effectiveness of preventive measures**

13 Research designs for evaluation studies *169*
Carolyn Emery
  Research question *169*
  Research design *170*
  Study population and sampling methods *173*
  Randomization *174*
  Baseline assessment *175*
  Intervention *175*
  Outcome measurement *176*
  Considerations for analysis *177*

Cluster analysis *178*

Conclusion *180*

   References *180*

14 Statistics used in effect studies *183*

Andrew Hayen and Caroline F. Finch

Examples *183*

Incidence rates *185*

Comparison of rates *186*

Difference in rates *187*

Ratio of rates *187*

Hypothesis test for a rate ratio *187*

Confounding *188*

Mantel–Haenszel methods *188*

Poisson regression *190*

Clustering *191*

Robust standard errors *191*

Generalized estimating equations *192*

Multilevel models and random effects models *192*

Intra-cluster correlation coefficient *193*

Implications for sample size *193*

Coefficient of variation *194*

Conclusion *195*

   References *195*

15 Cost-effectiveness studies *197*

Judith Bosmans, Martijn Heymans, Maarten Hupperets,
and Maurits van Tulder

What is an economic evaluation? *197*

Design of an economic evaluation *198*

   Perspective *198*

   Choice of control treatment *198*

Identification, measurement, and valuation of effects *199*

Identification, measurement, and valuation of costs *200*

Statistical analysis *202*

   Analysis of costs *202*

   Incremental cost-effectiveness ratio *203*

   Cost-effectiveness plane *204*

   Uncertainty around ICERs *204*

Decision uncertainty: cost-effectiveness acceptability curves *206*

   Net-benefit approach *206*

   Missing data *207*

   Sensitivity analysis *207*

Critical assessment of economic evaluations *208*

Conclusion *209*

References *210*

16 Implementing studies into real life *213*

Caroline F. Finch

Effectiveness versus efficacy *213*

Intervention implementation study designs *214*

Examples of implementation studies *214*

Towards a theoretical basis for implementation studies *221*

The RE-AIM model *222*

A phased approach towards undertaking an implementation study *227*

Phase 1: Developing the evidence-based intervention package *227*

Phase 2: Refining of the intervention package and development of
a delivery plan *228*

Phase 3: Implementation and evaluation of the intervention package and
its delivery plan *229*

Phase 4: Development and release of a final intervention package *231*

Translation research *231*

References *232*

Index *237*

List of contributors

Thomas Best MD, PhD
Division of Sports Medicine
Department of Family Medicine
The Ohio State University,
Columbus, Ohio, United States of America.

James R. Borchers MD, MPH
Division of Sports Medicine
Department of Family Medicine
The Ohio State University,
Columbus, Ohio,
United States of America.

Judith Bosmans PhD
Section of Health Economics and
Health Technology Assessment,
Department of Health Sciences and
EMGO Institute for Health and Care Research,
Faculty of Earth and Life Sciences,
VU University, Amsterdam,
The Netherlands.

Dorine Collard MSc
Department of Public and
Occupational Health, EMGO Institute
for Health and Care Research,
VU University Medical Center,
Amsterdam, The Netherlands.

Alex Donaldson BHSc
School of Human Movement
and Sport Sciences,
University of Ballarat,
Ballarat, Australia.

Carolyn Emery PT, PhD
Sport Medicine Centre,
Faculty of Kinesiology,
University of Alberta,
Calgary, Canada.

Caroline F. Finch BSc, MSc, PhD, ASTAT
School of Human Movement
and Sport Sciences,
University of Ballarat,
Victoria, Australia.

Colin Fuller BSc, PhD, FRSC
Centre for Sports Medicine, School of
Clinical Sciences, University of
Nottingham, Queen's Medical Centre,
Nottingham, United Kingdom.

Karen Grimmer-Somers PhD
University of South Australia, Division of
Health Sciences, School of Health Sciences,
Adelaide, Australia.

Brent Hagel PhD
Departments of Paediatrics and
Community Health Sciences, Faculty of
Medicine, University of Calgary,
Alberta Children's Hospital,
Calgary, Canada.

Andrew Hayen PhD
The University of Sydney,
Sydney, Australia.

Martijn Heymans PhD
Department of Epidemiology and
Biostatistics, VU University
Medical Center, Amsterdam, The
Netherlands; Section of Methodology
and Applied Biostatistics, Department
of Health Sciences and EMGO Institute
for Health and Care Research,
Faculty of Earth and Life Sciences,
VU University, Amsterdam,
The Netherlands.

Jennifer Hootman PhD, ATC, FACSM
Division of Adult and Community Health,
National Center for Chronic Disease
Prevention and Health Promotion,
Centers for Disease Control and
Prevention, Atlanta,
United States of America.

Will Hopkins PhD, FACSM
Institute of Sport and Recreation Research,
AUT University, Auckland,
New Zealand.

Maarten Hupperets MSc
Department of Public and Occupational
Health, EMGO Institute for Health and Care
Research, VU University Medical Center,
Amsterdam, The Netherlands.

Tron Krosshaug PhD
Oslo Sports Trauma Research Center,
Norwegian School of Sport Sciences,
Oslo, Norway.

Quinette Louw PhD
Stellenbosch University,
Stellenbosch, South Africa.

Willem Meeuwisse MD, PhD
Professor, Sport Medicine Centre,
Faculty of Kinesiology, University of Alberta,
Calgary, Canada.

Ian Shrier MD, PhD
Centre for Clinical Epidemiology
and Community Studies,
SMBD-Jewish General Hospital,
McGill University, Montreal, Canada.

Amika Singh PhD
Department of Public and
Occupational Health, EMGO Institute
for Health and Care Research,
VU University Medical Center,
Amsterdam, The Netherlands.

Russel Steele PhD
Department of Mathematics
and Statistics, McGill University,
Montreal, Canada.

Maurits van Tulder PhD
Professor, Section of Health Economics and
Health Technology Assessment,
Department of Health Sciences and EMGO
Institute for Health and Care Research,
Faculty of Earth and Life Sciences,
VU University, Amsterdam,
The Netherlands.

Jos Twisk PhD
Professor, Department of Health
Sciences, Faculty of Earth and
Life Sciences,
VU University, Amsterdam,
The Netherlands.

Evert Verhagen PhD
Department of Public and Occupational
Health, EMGO Institute for Health
and Care Research, VU University
Medical Center, Amsterdam,
The Netherlands.

Peta White PhD
School of Human Movement and
Sport Sciences, University of Ballarat,
Ballarat, Australia.

Part 1

Key issues in epidemiology and methodology

Chapter 1

Defining a research question

Peta White

Research questions typically begin as general ideas or topics. These ideas may originate from a researcher's interest, an identified problem, or a recognized gap in current knowledge. In the specific area of sports injury, research ideas may be generated in relation to a particular type of injury, sport, or participant population—or a combination of all three. Alternatively, an apparent increase in the incidence of a particular type of injury may spark research attention, as might a lack of knowledge about how to prevent such injury. In any case, it is from an initial research idea that the process towards defining a manageable research question begins.

As in all fields of research, progress in sports-injury research depends on the clear definition of research questions from the outset of projects. Defining a research question requires that a researcher articulate the purpose of the research[1]. In turn, the research question provides the basis on which a researcher can make decisions with regards to methodology and design[2]. Therefore, it follows that a research project with a clearly defined research question will also have a clear purpose, and, perhaps most importantly, an appropriate methodological design. This relationship applies equally to both quantitative and qualitative studies and to clinical, biomechanical, epidemiological, and social behavioural injury research. Unfortunately, there have been a number of methodological limitations in the sports injury studies to date[3]. Encouraging that future studies be undertaken only once the research question has been clearly articulated is one important way of addressing this issue.

Research questions and the research purpose

As stated previously, a clear picture of what the research wants to address is necessary before a specific research question can be constructed. In conceptualizing the purpose of a research project, researchers should be guided by a framework or paradigm that is accepted by their particular research community[4]. This way, it is clear how the research will contribute to progress in the broader research domain.

Arguably the most documented application of a framework to the sports-injury field of research is van Mechelen's four-stage sequence of injury prevention[5]. This was directly adapted from the well-known public health model for preventive research[6]. Recently, Finch [3] has extended the original sequence of prevention [5] in a framework that emphasizes the development of evidence-based interventions and the need to consider—and become informed about—the contextual issues related to the uptake of preventive measures. The Translating Research into Injury Prevention Practice (TRIPP) framework [3] comprises six stages and is presented in Table 1.1. Research based on this framework aims to determine what interventions are likely to work and why, as well as the factors that will facilitate or impede the uptake of recommended preventive measures. This purpose can be translated into research questions around the who, what, when, where, how, and why of sports-injury preventive measures. For example, a researcher might want to know in what particular context a preventive measure will be successful and for whom.

Table 1.1 The six stages in the TRIPP framework[3]

Stage	Description
1	Injury surveillance
2	Establish aetiology and mechanisms of injury
3	Develop preventive measures
4	Scientific evaluation under controlled conditions
5	Describe intervention context of informed implementation strategies
6	Evaluate effectiveness in implementation context

Studies that inform the implementation of preventive measures are currently under-represented in the sports-injury-prevention literature despite the evident need to conduct research in this area[8]. For example, it is clear how research questions that address implementation issues contribute to progress in a research field because they address an acknowledged research problem[9], namely, how to transfer injury prevention success in the controlled environment to success in a real-world setting (e.g. 'What circumstances/conditions would result in recreational distance runners accepting and adopting a low distance/high intensity training program?'). Further, such research questions have the advantage of addressing a practical problem often experienced by sporting clubs and organizations, specifically, how to implement injury prevention measures so that they are adopted willingly by sporting communities. As such, research questions that address implementation issues are most likely to attract support from the general community, including stakeholders, potential funding bodies, and participants for the research.

This is not to suggest that research questions around the aetiology and mechanisms of sports injury should no longer be asked. There will always be scope for this type of research while there is new knowledge to be gained, and inconsistencies to resolve. Further, such information will continue to be critical to the development of effective interventions. The important point is that research questions should allow a field of research to move towards knowledge that creates new insight, instead of producing results that are already well documented[9]. In some cases this will call for completely new research projects, while in others, the replication of previous work will be required. Therefore, research questions need to be constructed on the basis of a sound review of the literature that highlights what is already known, so that there is coherence between the literature review and the question, whereby, the question addresses a clear knowledge gap[4].

For example, if a particular injury remains prevalent despite there being considerable literature regarding the extent and nature of the injury—and scientific evidence for the efficacy of a measure to prevent it—then it is time to ask new questions. The TRIPP framework [3] would suggest that it is time to ask questions about the implementation context and the barriers and facilitators to the uptake of the preventive measure in the real world (e.g. 'What are the barriers and facilitators to recreational distance runners adopting and maintaining a low-distance/high-intensity training programme in order to prevent overuse injury?').

Research questions and methodology

To a large extent, once the research question has been defined, the research methodology has already been determined. There are 'best' study designs and methodologies for answering questions posed at the different stages in both the sequence of prevention [5] and the TRIPP framework[3]. These should be applied, not 'whenever possible', but as standard practice. A list of some examples of the research methodologies and designs required to address questions posed

Table 1.2 Examples of methodological approaches and research designs to address each stage of the TRIPP framework[3]

TRIPP Stage	Purpose of the research	Research method/design
1	Extent of injury problem	Database analysis; surveillance; other data-collection approaches; literature searches
2	Aetiology and mechanisms of injury	Case-control; cohort studies; statistical modelling
3	Develop preventive measures	Case studies; biomechanics; biomedical engineering
4	Intervention effectiveness – scientific evaluation	Clinical testing; randomized controlled studies; non-randomized studies
5	Determine intervention context	Direct observation; focus groups; attitude/behavioural questionnaires; interviews
6	Intervention effectiveness – real-world evaluation	Injury surveillance; direct observation; attitude/behavioural monitoring

at each stage of the TRIPP framework is presented in Table 1.2. These methodologies and designs will be discussed in more detail in the following chapters. Some of these study designs demand higher levels of resources, in terms of time and money, than others. For example, a randomized control study requires more time and money than a database analysis. Therefore, it is essential that consideration is given to methodological issues as part of the process of defining the research question. There is little to be achieved by defining a great research question only to find that the 'best' methodological approach to answer it requires resources above and beyond what are available to the research project. In other words, the only question posed in a research project should be one that can be answered properly with the resources available. Conversely, if the appropriate methodology cannot be applied, then the study should be reframed to ask a different question.

The mechanics of the research question

A research question should be able to be stated in one, clear, unambiguous sentence[2, 10]. Part of the process of defining the research question should involve defining key terms that are being used in the question. Sackett, Strauss, Richardson, Rosenberg, and Haynes [12] propose that a well-structured research question should contain four parts:

1. The problem (including the population of interest)
2. The intervention (not all studies have an intervention, however, this includes variables that predict, impact on, effect, etc.)
3. A comparison or control (if relevant)
4. The outcome (e.g. injury; no injury)

These four components have also been referred to in the literature as the PICO (**P**roblem, **I**nformation, **C**omparison, **O**utcome/s) format [13]. Examples of questions developed for each stage of the TRIPP framework [3] using Sackett, Strauss, Richardson, Rosenberg, and Haynes' [12] four-part model for structuring research questions are presented in Table 1.3.

Framing questions in this way may result in some terms or concepts within the question being refined so that the question and the resulting findings will address exactly what the researcher is interested in[14]. For example, a question such as 'What is the frequency of injuries to long-distance runners?' can be refined to 'What is the frequency of overuse injuries in recreational long-distance runners?'.

Table 1.3 Example questions developed for each stage of the TRIPP framework[3] using the four-part model for structuring research questions from Sackett et al[12].

TRIPP Stage	Problem	Intervention	Comparison	Outcome
1	In recreational distance-runners	what is the frequency and severity of	acute injuries compared to	overuse injuries?
2	In recreational distance-runners	is training distance a better predictor	than training intensity	of overuse injuries?
3	In recreational distance-runners	can a low-distance/high-intensity training programme	when compared to a high-distance/low-intensity training programme (or usual training habits)	reduce the number and/or severity of overuse injuries?
4	In a group of recreational distance-runners	does a controlled delivered low-distance/high-intensity training programme	when compared to high-distance/low-intensity training programme	reduce the number and/or severity of overuse injuries?
5	To a group of recreational distance-runners	would adopting a low-distance/high-intensity training programme	be likely to be accepted/unaccepted and under what circumstances	in order to reduce their chance of sustaining an overuse injury?
6	To what extent in a group of recreational distance-runners	is a low-distance/high-intensity training programme	NA	adopted and maintained as part of their usual training habits?

Common mistakes and problems when constructing questions

In his book, *Research Questions*, Richard Andrews[4] identifies a number of common pitfalls that exist for researchers when they are defining their research question. These pitfalls are also relevant in the context of sports injury research.

First, it is important to frame the research question as a question rather than as a statement[4]. In most cases, a research question should be included in addition to hypotheses; however, hypotheses alone may suffice when the research aims to improve a theory (in which case, the research will be structured around hypotheses based on the theory), or when it aims to replicate previous research (in which case, the research will be structured around hypotheses based on previous findings)[4]. Research questions can be posed when there is little predictability about the likely outcome of the research and can be used to generate hypotheses. On the other hand, hypotheses—being typically more specific than research questions—require a certain degree of acquired knowledge, and as such, do not logically lead to more general research questions being posed[4]. Another important difference between a research question and hypotheses is that, while they do determine the analytical approach taken, hypotheses do not guide the study design and methodology in the same way that a research question does[4].

Second, it is important to distinguish between questions used in interview schedules or questionnaires and research questions[4]. Interview or questionnaire questions will be too specific to be research questions and will usually be framed like a specific question to a respondent rather than as a more general research question[4]. For example, the question 'Do you (i.e. distance runners) do the majority of your training over flat terrain, hilly terrain, or a combination of the two?', on the topic of factors contributing to injuries in distance runners, would be better framed as a specific question to a respondent rather than as a research question. The same question could be converted to a research question with particular rephrasing: 'How does training terrain contribute to injuries in distance runners?'

One study, multiple questions

Until now, the focus of this chapter has been on research projects involving just one research question. However, it is just as likely that a researcher will have more than one question that requires answering in relation to a particular research purpose. In such cases a decision must be made with regards to which question is the main one, which is the subsidiary question(s), and how the questions are hierarchically and/or sequentially related to each other[4].

Subsidiary questions must be considered carefully, and must not take over from the main research question[4]. As a general rule, fewer is better. Each question must be addressed within the research project using the most appropriate methodology, and ideally, the same methodological approach can be used to address all questions. However, since different questions may require different methodology, limiting the number of questions can prevent putting strain on project resources[4]. Further, when more than one aspect of a problem is considered in a single research project, consideration must also be given to how these aspects interact[4]. This is likely to result in a more lengthy and complicated project.

In summary, a researcher may conclude that they have too many research questions when it is no longer clear which is the main question and which are the subsidiary questions; when questions are posed which are more rhetorical in nature and are unlikely to be answered in the course of the study; or when the questions that are being asked extend the boundaries of the research beyond what is achievable given the resources available[4].

Returning to the example used earlier, instead of considering only what recreational distance-runners consider acceptable circumstances under which to adopt a low-distance/high-intensity training programme, a researcher may decide to address that same issue with distance-running coaches as well. Although this may seem a logical inclusion in such a study, it does give rise to some potential complications. For example, it may become unclear whether it is the coaches or the athletes with which the study is most concerned, and the two standpoints may call for quite different methodological approaches. Further, the number of research participants will effectively increase, possibly putting strain on available resources. Finally, additional analysis will be required to address the relationship between what the coaches report and what the athletes report. It would be wise to keep in mind that a single study is not capable of answering all questions relating to a specific topic. Above all, it is better to focus on the quality than on the quantity of study answers.

Conclusion

The sports-injury research field will continue to benefit only from research that answers questions based on a clear research purpose. Researchers in this field are encouraged to define their research questions early so that decisions regarding methodology can be well-informed. The scope of sports-injury research is broad and calls for questions to be asked that move sports-injury prevention forwards and beyond what is already known. Irrespective of what the research question is, it is most important that it can be answered properly with the resources available, in order to contribute quality information to this important research domain.

References

1. Lipowski EE (2008). Developing great research questions. *Am J Health-Sys Pharm*, **65**(1), 1667–70.
2. Moore N (2006). *How to do research: A practical guide to designing and managing research projects.* 3rd rev ed. Facet, London.
3. Finch C (2006). A new framework for research leading to sports injury prevention. *J Sci Med Sport*, **9**, 3–9.
4. Andrews R (2003). *Research questions.* Continuum, London.
5. van Mechelen W, Hlobil H, Kemper HCG (1992). Incidence, severity, aetiology and prevention of sports injuries. *Sports Med*, **14**, 82–99.
6. Robertson LS (1992). *Injury epidemiology.* Oxford University Press, New York.
7. Chalmers DJ (2002). Injury prevention in sport: Not yet part of the game? *Inj Prev*, **8**, 22–5.
8. Finch C, Donaldson A (2009). A sports setting matrix for understanding the implementation context for community sport. *Br J Sports Med*, Online First, published on February 6, 2009 as 10.1136/bjsm.2008.056069.
9. Booth WC, Colomb GG, Williams JM (1995). *The craft of research.* University of Chicago Press, Chicago.
10. Sackett DL, Wennberg JE (1997). Choosing the best research design for each question. *BMJ*, **315**, 1636.
11. Dennis R, Finch C (2008). Sports injuries, in Heggenhougen K, Quah S (eds) *International encyclopedia of public health*, Vol 6, pp. 206–11. San Academic Press, San Diego.
12. Sackett DL, Strauss SE, Richardson WS, Rosenberg W, Haynes RB (2000). *Evidence based medicine: How to practice and teach evidence based Medicine, 2nd edition.* Churchill Livingstone, Edinburgh.
13. Akobeng AK (2005). Principles of evidence based medicine. *Arch. Dis. Child*, **90**, 837–40.
14. Stone P (2002). Deciding upon and refining a research question. *Palliative Med*, **16**, 265–7.

Chapter 2

Study designs

James R. Borchers and Thomas Best

Finding answers to clinical research questions is the foundation of evidence-based medicine. Once a question has been formulated, an appropriate study design is needed to address the specific inquiry. A working knowledge of study design is required to determine the appropriate study design for each research question.

Study designs that help address clinical research questions can be grossly divided into experimental and observational studies (Box 2.1). Experimental studies occur when the investigator controls the allocation of a treatment or exposure to study populations and records outcomes or results. This is very similar to basic laboratory research in that the investigator is in charge of exposure allocation or treatment. The classic experimental design in clinical research is the clinical trial. Observational studies differ from experimental studies in that the investigator has no control over the exposure allocation or intervention. The investigator observes exposures, interventions, and outcomes of study populations and uses various methods to determine associations between exposures, interventions, and outcomes. Such studies are considered 'natural' experiments because the investigator allows nature to take its course. Observational designs in clinical research include cohort studies and case-control studies. An important category of observational studies are descriptive studies which include cross sectional studies, case series, and case reports.

The purpose of this chapter is to describe these study designs and the advantages and disadvantages of each as they pertain to clinical research in sports medicine.

Box 2.1 Study designs

Experimental design

Clinical trial

Observational design

Cohort study

Case-control study

Cross-sectional study

Case series

Case report

Bias, confounding, and random error

The purpose of any study design is to answer a particular question in the most efficient way while maximizing both validity and precision. In this regards, validity refers to the absence of systematic errors in the measurements. In more popular terms the validity questions whether an instrument actually measures what it is intended to measure. In a study design, validity is defined by a limited effect of bias and confounding on the study result[1]. Precision, sometimes referred to as reliability, is defined as the avoidance of random error in study results[1]. A precise measurement is likely to produce the same outcome in a number of trials. One of the main objectives of choosing an appropriate study design is to maximize validity and precision and, thus, to avoid bias, confounding, and random error.

Bias

Bias in a study design is best defined as an error in the design or protocol of the study that leads to erroneous associations between exposures and outcomes[1]. Bias is usually due to investigator ignorance, unavoidable decisions made during a study, or inherent characteristics of a study design[1]. Two main types of bias play a role when designing a study. Selection bias is an error that arises from selecting the study population, creating either differences that were not controlled for between study groups in an experimental design, or a study population not representative for the entire population of interest[2]. To a certain extent selection bias occurs in every study involving human subjects. Potential participants are free in their choice to participate in a given study. Within the field of sports-injury research it is often found that the more serious and motivated athletes are willing to partake in a study. This is in contrast to the more 'amateurish' athlete who might have different injury risk factors or react differently to a given preventive programme. Observation bias is a difference in the way information is obtained on exposures and outcomes between study groups[2]. This can occur in many ways, e.g. participant recall bias, interviewer bias, loss to follow-up, and misclassification of exposures or outcomes. A clear example of observation bias in the field of sports-injury research is recall bias that may occur when registering injuries. Unfortunately it is not always possible to obtain all information with regards to an injury occurrence directly after an incident. Some time will pass between the actual injury occurrence and the injury report. The injured athlete may forget or misreport crucial information due to the time-lag between onset and registration. Differences in such time-lags between participants may create unwanted differences in the quality of data. Considering the potential for bias in any study design is important in order to avoid its effects on the validity of a study.

Confounding

Confounding is defined as a mixing of effects between an exposure, an outcome, and a third variable, called a confounder[3]. A confounder is a variable that can distort an association between the exposure and the outcome. A variable is considered a confounder if it is more or less common in a particular study group and directly related to the outcome in question but is not part of the causal pathway for the outcome. A common confounder in sports-injury research is the presence of a recent previous injury. A previous injury has a strong relationship with current injury risk, and may cloud the results of a study when not accounted for. Controlling for confounding is critical in study design to ensure high validity of study results; different study designs use various methods to limit confounding.

Random error

Random error is defined as a false association between an exposure and an outcome due to chance[1]. A random error occurs by chance and can to a greater extent not be accounted for.

The best method to limit random error is increasing the study sample size. A large sample improves the precision of the study. Hence, a sample-size analysis should always be performed before commencing a study. Such an analysis gives you an indication of the number of participants that is required in order to obtain a given result with statistical precision. Other methods of minimizing random error include repeating the study to validate study results or maximizing study efficiency to obtain all possible information[3]. Despite these strategies, random error can still affect the results of a study but can be addressed in the statistical analyses of various study designs.

Clinical trials

As previously mentioned, a clinical trial is the classic experimental study design for conducting clinical research. The clinical trial study design is defined by the fact that the investigator assigns participants to exposure groups in order to determine the effect of an exposure on a particular outcome. In clinical trials, the investigator actively manipulates the study populations in order to study a specific exposure on a specific outcome. There are four criteria that define any clinical trial[4]. The first is that the study must be prospective in nature. Clinical trials are designed to follow participants forwards in time after allocation to an exposure in order to measure an outcome. The second criterion is that there must be a defined intervention (treatment, medication, device, prevention regimen, etc.) employed in the trial. The third criterion is that there must be a control group for comparison to the intervention group. This is often a group that receives a common or gold standard intervention or a placebo intervention. Such a strategy permits for a comparison between the intervention and control group to determine effects of the intervention being studied. The fourth criterion concerns the ethics of a clinical trial. This has been termed 'clinical equipoise'[5]. This concept suggests that a clinical trial is ethical if there is uncertainty in the medical community as to the benefits and harms from the intervention being studied. This concept also demands that a clinical trial uses a common intervention or gold standard for a control to compare the intervention to and that a placebo should only be used if this does not exist. This concept also demands that proper informed consent is obtained for all participants of a clinical trial.

There are various steps that an investigator must consider when conducting a clinical trial. The first is the formation of a hypothesis based on the intervention being studied. This should be clearly defined so that the expectation of the clinical trial is clear. In developing and defining a hypothesis for a clinical trial, an investigator must make certain that the intervention being studied meets the principle of equipoise. Once the intervention is determined to meet the principle of equipoise, the outcomes of the trial must be clearly defined. An example of this principle is the comparison of non-steroidal anti-inflammatory drugs (NSAIDs) versus placebo or other analgesics in the treatment of acute lateral ankle sprains[6–11]. In these studies the investigators considered a potential benefit of an NSAID in the treatment of an acute ankle sprain but realized there was some doubt to this potential benefit. This permitted the use of the NSAID in the intervention group and justified withholding it from the control group. The principle of equipoise must be met for a clinical trial to be ethical.

It is important to consider various design factors in clinical trials (Box 2.2). Will the intervention be given to individuals or groups? An example in sports medicine would be deciding if individual athletes or groups (i.e. teams, universities, or events) receive the intervention. Is the intervention considered to be preventative or therapeutic? In sports medicine this may mean using an intervention to prevent or treat an injury. Will both study groups receive only one intervention or will there be a crossover in the study design where each group will receive additional

Box 2.2 Design factors for clinical trials

Population: individuals or groups

Intervention: preventative or therapeutic

Intervention allocation: parallel or crossover

Number of interventions: single or multiple

interventions? This is most commonly seen in clinical trials involving medications. Is there only one intervention being studied or are there multiple interventions being studied? Answering these questions helps define the design of the clinical trial.

Next, it is important to identify the study population and determine inclusion/exclusion criteria. Once this has been accomplished it is important to consider issues of compliance for the study group and potential for loss to follow-up. Many clinical trials follow an intention to treat principle which states that all participants in the trial are analysed whether or not they complete or comply with the trial[12]. Using this principle has benefits such as maintaining randomization procedures, limiting bias, and conducting the trial under 'real life' conditions. If an investigator is interested in the true efficacy of the intervention, only the participants that complete the entire study protocol are included in the analyses (per protocol analysis). This eliminates participants that did not maintain compliance throughout the protocol. Using an efficacy principle may limit application of the study results into real-life practice. An investigator must decide what principle to use in the design of a clinical trial because it can affect the required sample size (i.e. drop-out rates, loss to follow up).

It is important to determine in clinical trials how participants will be assigned to the intervention and control groups. Non-random assignment is generally discouraged because of the potential for selection bias. Randomization is commonly used to assign participants to the intervention or control groups. Randomization serves two main purposes in a clinical trial. First, it allows for unbiased assignment of participants to the different groups. Second, it controls for known and unknown confounders among the study population. Randomization strengthens the validity of a clinical trial. Nevertheless, it should be noted that purely by chance once in a while a randomization procedure does not result in equal study groups.

Block-randomization is a method used in clinical trials to ensure a balance among study groups and to avoid secular trends in study-participant enrolment[13]. Block-randomization permits smaller groups of study participants to be randomized to study groups. For example, rather than randomizing all study participants as one large group to an intervention or control, participants may be randomized in smaller blocks (i.e. 4–8 participants) to the study groups (intervention or control). This permits randomization to occur in a balanced fashion while not skewing the allocated number of participants.

Stratification is a strategy that ensures an equal distribution of confounding variables (i.e. age, gender, race, activity level) among study groups. What one actually does when stratifying is introduce multiple levels of randomization, e.g. one randomizes men and women independently into the study groups.

Blinding or masking where participants are unaware if they are receiving the intervention or control is a method to help eliminate bias among participants. Unfortunately, this is difficult to achieve in sports-injury research.

An excellent example of a clinical trial using these methods in sports medicine is the GRONORUN trial[14]. Novice runners were randomized to one of two training groups (training based on 10% rule or standard training programme) in a blocked fashion to determine if the 10% group would have fewer lower-extremity injuries compared to the standard group. Participants were stratified based on gender, activity level, and history of previous injury in order to reduce confounding. In using these methods (randomization, blocking, and stratification), these investigators were able to increase the validity of the study results.

Although clinical trials are considered the best study design for clinical outcomes research, there can be disadvantages to their use (Table 2.1). Clinical trials are expensive and this may prohibit their utilization in various situations. In a sports medicine environment, athletes may not be willing to comply with clinical trial protocols as, within this field of research, clinical trials are characterized by relatively long periods of follow-up. It can therefore be difficult to enrol enough participants to meet adequate sample size and avoid large loss to follow-up rates.

Some clinical trials may not be considered to approximate 'real-life' conditions and their results may be considered inapplicable to those outside the study. There may also be ethical considerations that make a clinical trial impractical. Splenomegaly and the risk of splenic rupture is a chief concern when determining when an athlete with infectious mononucleosis can return to sport. The ideal method for determining when the risk of splenic rupture is minimized would be to randomize individuals with infectious mononucleosis to return to sport at different times following infection. This approach would be considered unethical because of the potential for

Table 2.1 Advantages and disadvantages of various study designs

Clinical trials	Cohort studies	Case-control studies
Advantages		
Investigator allocates study population to intervention	Efficient for studying rare exposures	Efficient for studying rare outcomes
Examines the effect of a specific exposure on a specific outcome	Demonstrate a temporal relationship between exposures and outcomes (prospective)	Appropriate for studying outcomes with long induction or latency periods
Randomization controls confounding and allows for generalization of study results.	Provide good descriptive information about exposures	Generally less expensive and time consuming than cohort studies
	Efficient for studying multiple outcomes associated with a single exposure	
Disadvantages		
Trials may be expensive and inefficient	Inefficient for studying rare outcomes	Inefficient for studying rare exposures
Target population may be reluctant to participate	Inefficient for studying outcomes with long induction or latency periods	Retrospective nature can lead to increased bias
May have difficulty with participant compliance	Can be very time and labour intensive	Retrospective nature can make establishing causation difficult if information on exposures is limited
Trials simulate experiments and not 'real-life' situations	Can be expensive	
Ethical concerns may make trials impractical		

catastrophic consequences following splenic rupture and therefore a clinical trial is impractical in this situation. Fortunately, in this (and other cases) other designs can be employed.

Cohort studies

Cohort studies are observational studies because investigators are not actively involved in the assignment of participants to study groups but only observe what is naturally occurring with participants. Cohort studies compare the occurrence of an outcome such as illness, injury, or death among groups of people that have different exposure status over time. These exposures are random among participants because of choices the participants make (i.e. personal health habits, occupation, activity type) and are not assigned by the investigator. The investigator observes participants over time and allows exposure status to occur naturally. This has lead to cohort studies often being referred to as 'natural experiments'. Within sports-injury research this could include looking at injuries (outcome) occurring during sports participation (exposure).

One of the first decisions an investigator has to make when conducting a cohort study is to define the study population. Populations in cohort studies are usually defined by general or specific criteria depending on the type of exposure and outcome the investigator is interested in. General cohorts are populations usually defined by geographic area or some other broad definition in order to look at a common exposure, e.g. participation in a specific sport. Special cohorts are a more specific population defined to look at a rare exposure and associated outcomes. A clear understanding of the exposure or outcome of interest can help the investigator determine if a general or special cohort study population is appropriate.

Once the study population is identified, a comparison population must be identified as well. The ideal comparison population for a cohort study is one in which the members of the two populations differ only in the exposure of interest. This is often achieved by using an internal control group. These are members of the same cohort as the study cohort but they differ because they do not have the outcome of interest. Women's soccer players have been followed over time to determine the incidence of osteoarthritis of the knee based on whether individuals that had an injury to their anterior cruciate ligament (ACL) had reconstruction or not during their playing career[15]. The study groups are similar except for the outcome of ACL reconstruction following an ACL injury; therefore the group without reconstruction following an ACL injury would be considered an internal control. The use of an internal control limits the effects of confounding and strengthens the study results. If an internal control is unavailable, a control group from a similar population or the general population can be used, but this may introduce confounding variables that can make results of a cohort study difficult to interpret.

Populations in cohort studies are commonly described as either open, fixed, or closed. In an open-cohort study the population is dynamic and individuals may enter and leave the study population at any time during the study period. In an open cohort, being a member of the cohort is defined by some characteristic that changes such as participating in a certain activity, taking a certain medication, or being a member of a certain team. Members of an open cohort can enter and leave the cohort as they choose. A clear example of an open cohort is a fitness club. Members can join and leave the club as they choose and this can affect study results. Fixed cohorts are defined by an event such as a specific injury or a specific medical procedure. Members are followed for period of time beginning from the time of the event and exposures and outcomes are ascertained from the event going forwards. Members of a fixed cohort must have the event to enter the cohort but could leave the cohort and be lost to follow-up. The Multi-Centre Orthopaedics Outcomes Network (MOON) is a large multi-centre cohort study that observes subjects following anterior cruciate ligament (ACL) reconstruction[16]. A person can only become a member of this cohort study once they have had ACL reconstruction. This is an example of a fixed cohort. A closed cohort is similar to a fixed cohort but all members of a closed cohort are followed for a short period of time following a specific event and there is no loss to follow-up. An example of a closed cohort would be all members of a team followed for a short period of time to determine specific exposures that may have caused an acute illness. In 2005 a closed-cohort study was conducted to determine risk factors among American football players associated with methicillin-resistant *Staphylococcus aureus* (MRSA) skin infections[17]. In this study all team members were evaluated for risk factors that may have lead to acquiring a MRSA skin infection over one football season.

Cohort studies are traditionally prospective in nature. An investigator identifies a study population and follows them forwards in time while collecting data on exposures and outcomes as they occur. Cohort studies may also be retrospective in nature. The investigator identifies a study group and then looks retrospectively to collect data on outcomes and exposures. The timing of the cohort study often depends on the research question and variables such as funding and resources for the study. Prospective cohort studies are often preferred to avoid the associated problems with retrospective studies such as observational bias and confounding. Prospective cohort studies are generally expensive and conducting a cohort study in a retrospective manner can decrease the cost of the study. In both prospective and retrospective cohort studies, the common characteristic is that data on exposure status is collected prior to the outcome of interest.

Cohort studies are similar to clinical trials in many ways. Both study designs make comparisons across study groups with different exposures and ascertain outcomes in those groups. Both designs try to make the study groups comparable to each other except for the exposure of interest. It is these similarities that often make the cohort study the design of choice for clinicians when a clinical trial is not possible.

There are differences among the two study designs that an investigator must consider as well. The main difference in the two study designs is the ability of the investigator to assign participants to study groups in a clinical trial but only observe study groups in a cohort study. Clinical trials are always prospective and cohort studies can be prospective or retrospective. Clinical trials can use methods such as randomization and stratification to limit confounding whereas a cohort study depends on careful selection of populations to limit confounding. An investigator should consider these differences when determining if a clinical trial or cohort study is best suited for a particular research question.

Cohort studies have many advantages and disadvantages compared to other study designs (Table 2.1). Cohort studies are generally efficient for studying rare exposures associated with a common outcome. They provide good information on exposures and are efficient for demonstrating a temporal relationship between an exposure and an outcome when the study is prospective. They are also efficient for studying multiple outcomes from a single exposure and can directly measure an outcome incidence or risk over time. In contrast, cohort studies are inefficient for evaluating a rare outcome. They are also inefficient for evaluating outcomes with a long latency or induction period following an exposure. They are often time consuming and can be very expensive and labour intensive. Considering these factors will help the investigator decide if a cohort study design is appropriate for a specific research question.

Case-control studies

Just as with cohort studies, case-control studies are observational studies that have a primary aim of establishing a relationship between exposures and specific outcomes. It is the actual study design and not the aim of the study that makes the case-control study unique from the cohort study. The traditional design of a cohort study moves from exposure to outcome whereas the case-control study moves from outcome to exposures. Some investigators have suggested that because the nature of the case-control study design is retrospective it is inferior to the prospective nature of the cohort design. In fact, when a case-control design is applied to an appropriate research question the results of a case-control study can be as valid and precise as a cohort study.

The basic design of a case-control study begins with identifying a population with a specific outcome (cases). It is important to have a good definition of what defines a case in a case-control study so that cases are clearly identified as having the outcome of interest, and selection bias is minimized. For example, it would be important in a case-control study looking at exercise-induced asthma (EIA) to include those with exercise-induced shortness of breath. If that were the only criteria used to define EIA, then some subjects without reported exercise-induced shortness of breath with EIA may not be included within the case population and some subjects with exercise-induced shortness of breath for a reason other than EIA would be misclassified in the case population. Having a more rigorous case definition that is restrictive is preferable to make certain that those subjects identified as cases in a case-control study are truly cases and not misclassified[18].

Once a clear and precise definition of the case population is defined, a control population must be selected for comparison purposes. The goal is to try and select a control group that is as similar to the case population as possible with the only difference being the outcome of interest. The control population should represent the same source population as the cases and should not differ in major characteristics from the case population. In a case-control study design it is important that if a member of the control population had the outcome of interest that they would become a member of the case population. If this 'would' criterion is met, it ensures that the cases and controls are similar with respect to important characteristics except the outcome of interest. Following this method of control-population selection can minimize selection bias in the case-control design.

Following the accurate definition of case and control populations, the investigator must decide how to obtain exposure information of interest. Such information can be obtained through direct interviews with study participants, participant questionnaires, reviewing participant records, or using biomarkers. All of these methods have the potential for information bias that an investigator needs to consider. Limiting recall and interviewer bias can be difficult with direct interviews. Questions should be standardized and asked similarly of both cases and controls, e.g. by means of a (semi-)structured interview. They should be easy for the study participant to understand. Interviewers can be masked as to whether a participant is a case or control to limit the potential for interviewer bias. Data from records must be complete and accurate and similar among both study populations. The use of biomarkers requires that they are similarly collected in a standard fashion among both cases and controls. Considering how to obtain exposure data in the initial study design will decrease the potential for information bias in the case-control study.

Limiting confounding in a case-control study design is crucial. As previously mentioned, strict definitions for case and control populations will help to limit confounding. Another common way to limit certain confounding variables in a case-control study is through the method of matching. Matching allows the investigator to decide on specific characteristics that are important to exclude in the study as potential confounders. These may include characteristics such as age, gender, race, environmental exposure, or activity level in athletes. Participants in both the case and control populations are then matched according to these characteristics so that they are similar in both populations. This eliminates the possibility of confounding due to these characteristics and can increase the validity of the study results. For example, if a case-control study is interested in comparing activity exposure amongst athletes with and without ACL tears, the investigator could decide to match on age and gender in order to eliminate these variables as confounders between the two study groups. Both age and gender might contribute to the risk of an ACL tear and could confound any relationship between activity exposure and ACL tear identified in the study. It is preferable that the investigator determines what characteristics may affect the results of the study and match on the basis of those characteristics in both study groups to avoid any predictable confounding effect.

Case-control studies have advantages and disadvantages when compared to other study designs (Table 2.1). They are preferred for studying outcomes that are rare or where little is known about the outcome in question. In contrast to cohort studies, case-control studies are more suitable for studying outcomes associated with a long induction or latency period. They are generally less expensive and time consuming than cohort studies. Case-control studies are inefficient for studying rare exposures. They are also limited by their retrospective nature and can be prone to bias. Because case-control studies move from outcome to exposure, it can be difficult to infer causation if there is poor information on exposures and differences between case and control populations.

Descriptive studies

Descriptive studies are a category of observational studies that typically are used to report on a specific outcome in a certain population or on an outcome which little is known about. These studies are generally considered less rigorous than the cohort and case-control study designs for determining causation between an exposure and an outcome. They are considered helpful in suggesting what exposures and outcomes need further study.

The cross-sectional study design is specifically used to evaluate the relationship between an outcome and exposures or variables of interest in a certain population at one specific point in time. Cross-sectional study designs are commonly used to establish the point prevalence of an outcome and specific associations between exposures or variables and the outcome of interest. The results of a cross-sectional study are generally applicable to the population studied but are not applicable to other populations. Because cross-sectional study designs are limited to data at one time point, they are unable to establish causality between exposures or variables and the outcome of interest. The cross-sectional study design only shows associations between exposures or variables and the outcome because of the lack of temporality in the study design. Cross-sectional study designs are common because they are easily accomplished in an efficient manner and are generally completed at a lower cost than other study designs. They are generally considered good 'hypothesis-generating' studies. It is common for the results of a cross-sectional study to generate new and more focused questions that are then often studied using a more advanced methodology.

Case series and case reports are true descriptive studies in that their primary purpose is to describe specific outcomes and associated exposures or variables. There is commonly descriptive analyses that arise from these studies and their primary purpose is to introduce an outcome about which little is known or to report on an outcome in a specific population. These studies have no ability to establish causation or temporality and their benefits are limited to description only. Their results are usually only applicable to the population studied. They are valuable in alerting clinicians to potentially new or less common outcomes of interest and can lead to more rigorous study of a specific outcome. An excellent example of this in sports medicine is the initial reports of MRSA infection in high school wrestlers[19]. This case series lead to further reports of similar infections in other athletes and more rigorous study of MRSA skin infections in athletes to determine exposures associated with MRSA skin infections and the development of prevention and treatment recommendations.

Conclusion

A general understanding of clinical study designs is essential to efficiently and appropriately answer clinical research questions. Determining the appropriate study design for a specific research question requires knowledge of the advantages and disadvantages of each type of study design and which specific approach is best suited to answer a specific research question.

References

1. Aschengrau A, Seage GR (2003). *Essentials of epidemiology in public health*, 1st edn. Jones and Bartlett, Sudbury, MA.
2. Last JM (1995). *A dictionary of epidemiology*, 3rd edn. Oxford University Press, New York.
3. Rothman KJ, Greenland S (1998). *Modern epidemiology*, 2nd edn. Lippincott-Raven, Philadelphia.
4. Friedman LM, Furberg CD, DeMets DL (1998). *Fundamentals of clinical trials*, 3rd edn. Springer Science + Business Media, New York.
5. Freedman B (1987). Equipoise and the ethics of clinical research. *N Engl J Med*, **317**(3), 141–5.
6. Moran M (1991). Double-blind comparison of diclofenac potassium, ibuprofen and placebo in the treatment of ankle sprains. *J Int Med Res*, **19**(2), 121–30.
7. Slatyer MA, Hensley MA, Lopert R (1997). A randomized controlled trial of piroxicam in the management of acute ankle sprain in Australian Regular Army recruits. The Kapooka Ankle Sprain Study. *Am J Sports Med*, **25**(4), 544–53.
8. Ekman EF, Ruoff G, Kuehl K, Rakph L, Hormbrey P, Fiechtner J, Berger MF (2006). The Cox-2 specific inhibitor valdecoxib versus tramadol in acute ankle sprain: a multicenter randomized, controlled trial. *Am J Sport Med*, **34**(6), 945–55.
9. Petrella R, Ekman EF, Schuller R, Fort J (2004). Efficacy of celecoxib, a Cox-2-specific inhibitor, and naproxen in the management of acute ankle sprain. *Clin J Sport Med*, **14**(4), 225–31.
10. Cukiernik VA, Lim R, Warren D, Seabrook JA, Matsui D, Rieder MJ (2007). Naproxen versus acetaminophen for therapy of soft tissue injuries to the ankle in children. *Ann Pharmacother*, **41**(9), 1368–74.
11. Kayali C, Agus H, Surer L, Turgut A (2007). The efficacy of paracetamol in the treatment of ankle sprains in comparison with diclofenac sodium. *Saudi Med J*, **28**(12), 1836–9.
12. Newell DJ (1992). Intention-to-treat analysis: implications for quantitative and qualitative research. *Int J Epidemiol*, **21**(5), 837–41.
13. Meinert CL (1996). *Clinical trials dictionary, terminology and usage recommendations*. The Johns Hopkins Center for Clinical Trials, Baltimore, MD.
14. Buist I, Bredeweg SW, van Mechelen W, Lemmink KA, Pepping GJ, Dierks RL (2008). No effect of a graded training program on the number of running-related injuries in novice runners: a randomized controlled trial. *Am J Sports Med*, **36**(1), 33–9.
15. Lohmander LS, Ostenberg A, Englund M, Roos H (2004). High prevalence of knee osteoarthritis, pain and functional limitations in female soccer players twelve years after anterior cruciate ligament injury. *Arthritis Rheum*, **50**(10), 3145–52.
16. Wright RW, Dunn W, Amendola A, Andrish JT, Bergfeld J, Kaeding CC, Marx RG, McCarty EC, Parker RD, Wolcott M, Wolf BR, Spindler KP (2007). Risk of tearing the intact anterior cruciate ligament in the contralateral knee and rupturing the anterior cruciate ligament graft during the first two years after anterior cruciate ligament reconstruction. *Am J Sports Med*, **35**(7), 1131–4.
17. Kazakova SV, Hageman JC, Matava M, Srinivasan A, Phelan L, Garfinkel B, Boo T, McAllister A, Anderson J, Jensen B, Dodson D, Lonsway D, McDougal LK, Arduino M, Fraser VJ, Killgore G, Tenover FC, Cody S, Jernigan DB (2005). A clone of methicillin-resistant Staphylococcus aureus among professional football players. *N Engl J Med*, **352**(5), 468–75.
18. Lasky T, Stolley PD (1994). Selection of cases and controls. *Epidemiol Rev*, **16**(1), 6–17.
19. Lindenmayer JM, Schoenfeld S, O'Grady R, Carney JK (1998). Methicillin-resistant Staphylococcus aureus in a high school wrestling team and the surrounding community. *Arch Intern Med*, **158**(8), 895–9.

Chapter 3

Basic statistical methods

Jos Twisk

In the first two chapters of this book, the importance of defining a proper research question and the advantages and disadvantages of several study designs are extensively discussed. In this chapter, it is assumed that a proper research question is formulated and that a suitable study design is chosen. When the study is performed and the data are stored, the next step in the process of a performing a scientific study must be taken. In that step, statistical analyses come into play. This chapter explains some general statistical approaches to analyse data from sports-injury research.

To do so, an example will be used. In this example an intervention study is performed in which the effectiveness of preventive ankle taping with regards to an ankle injury is investigated. For that purpose, 225 soccer players were selected at the beginning of the season. From the 225, 110 soccer players were in the intervention group; i.e. preventive ankle taping before each training session and each match. The other 115 soccer players were in the control group; i.e. no preventive ankle taping. The main research question of the study was whether preventive ankle taping was effective in reducing the number of ankle injuries. The intervention continued for a whole season (40 weeks).

In the discussion of the different statistical techniques, the statistical computer software of SPSS (Statistical Package for the Social Sciences) will be used, and the output of this programme will be given to illustrate what we can we do with the results of the different statistical techniques.

Dichotomous outcome variables

Sports injury research is mostly characterized by an outcome variable that is dichotomous. Subjects are injured or subjects are not injured, or the other way round; subjects are recovered from injury or subjects are not recovered from injury. In addition, in our example the outcome variable is dichotomous. Besides this, the main determinant (intervention yes or no) is dichotomous. The results of a study with a dichotomous outcome variable and a dichotomous determinant can be nicely depicted in a so-called 2×2 table. Output 3.1 shows the results of the exemplary study.

From Output 3.1, it can be seen that of the 115 soccer players in the control group, 45 sustained an injury and 70 did not. The intervention group did slightly better; of the 110 soccer players in this group, only 25 sustained injured, while 85 players did not not sustain an injury. Although we can see directly from the 2×2 table that the intervention group did better in avoiding injuries, we would need to know how much better? In fact, we are looking for an effect measure. There are several possibilities to estimate this effect. First of all, we can see that in the intervention group $25/110 = 23\%$ were injured, while in the control group $45/115 = 39\%$ were injured. The difference between these two percentages (i.e. $39\% - 23\% = 16\%$) can be seen as a measure of the effect of the intervention. This measure of effect is called the risk difference (RD). Another, often used, possibility is to estimate the ratio between the two percentages (i.e. $23\%/39\%) = 0.59$.

Output 3.1 Results of the exemplary intervention study to evaluate the effectiveness of preventive ankle taping in soccer players

studygroup * did you get an injury? Crosstabulation

Count

		Did you get an injury?		Total
		no	yes	
studygroup	control	70	45	115
	intervention	85	25	110
Total		155	70	225

This measure of effect is called the relative risk (RR), which can be interpreted as follows: in the intervention group, the probability of sustaining an injury is 0.59 times as high as the probability of sustaining an injury in the control group. The other way round, a soccer player in the control group has a 1/0.59 = 1.69-times higher probability of sustaining an ankle injury compared to the probability of a soccer player in the intervention group. The conclusion therefore is that the intervention works!

Up to now, we have not used many statistics. However, one of the problems of this study (or of a scientific study in general) is that it is based on a relatively small sample of soccer players and the question arises whether we would have obtained a comparable result in another sample or whether or not the intervention also works on other soccer players. To answer that question we have to quantify the uncertainty of the observed results. Within statistics, there are two possibilities to estimate the uncertainty of a study result. The first and definitely best option is to estimate a 95% confidence interval (CI) around the effect measure and the second option is to use statistical testing in order to estimate a p-value for the observed result.

95% confidence intervals around the risk difference and relative risk

The uncertainty of a study result depends on two issues: (i) the sample size, and (ii) the heterogeneity (or standard deviation) in the study. To obtain an estimate of the uncertainty, first we have to estimate the standard deviation of a percentage (because the effect measure of the study deals with percentages). Formula 3.1 depicts the way to estimate the standard deviation of a percentage, where $sd(p)$ = standard deviation of a percentage, and p = the percentage.

Formula 3.1: $$sd(p) = \sqrt{p(1-p)}$$

The uncertainty (i.e. standard error) is then given by the standard deviation divided by the square root of the number of observations (Formula 3.2), where $se(p)$ = standard error of the percentage; p = the percentage and n = the number of observations.

Formula 3.2: $$se(p) = \sqrt{\frac{p(1-p)}{n}}$$

In the example, however, the separate percentages in both groups are not the most important, but the difference between the percentages is. The standard error of this difference can be estimated with Formula 3.3, where p_1 and p_2 = percentages of a certain outcome in both groups and n_1 and n_2 = the number of subjects in both groups.

Formula 3.3:
$$se(p_1 - p_2) = \sqrt{\frac{p_1(1-p_1)}{n_1} + \frac{p_2(1-p_2)}{n_2}}$$

When we fill in the numbers given in Output 3.1, we get a standard error of the risk difference of 0.059.

$$se(p_1 - p_2) = \sqrt{\frac{0.23(1-0.23)}{110} + \frac{0.39(1-0.39)}{125}} = 0.059$$

The 95% confidence interval can then be estimated with Formula 3.4, where $p_1 - p_2$ = risk difference and $se(p_1 - p_2)$ = the standard error of the risk difference.

Formula 3.4:
$$p_1 - p_2 \pm 1.96 \times se(p_1 - p_2)$$

When we fill in the numbers, we will obtain a 95% confidence interval around the risk difference which ranges between 0.04 and 0.28. The interpretation of the 95% confidence interval is that with 95% certainty, we know that the 'real' risk difference lies somewhere between 0.04% and 0.28%, $0.16 \pm 1.96 \times 0.059 = [0.04 - 0.28]$

As mentioned earlier, another effect measure that is often used in these situations is the relative risk. Also around a relative risk, we can estimate a 95% confidence interval. This is slightly more complicated and therefore we will not depict the formulae to estimate this confidence interval. Furthermore, the computer software will give you an estimation of this 95% confidence interval. Output 3.2 shows the relative risk and the 95% confidence interval from the example study.

The output is slightly difficult to understand. In fact the software provides two relative risks. One (0.788) for the cohort: did you get an injury? = no, and another (1.722) for the cohort: did you get an injury? = yes. Of course we are interested in the last one, because the outcome variable of the study is whether or not a soccer player sustains an injury. The relative risk shown in Output 3.2 is calculated from [45/115]/[23/110] and is therefore the same as we have calculated before; in the control group the probability of sustaining an injury is 1.722 times higher than in the intervention group (the difference between 1.722 and 1.69 is due to rounding errors). The 95% confidence interval around this relative risk goes from 1.14 to 2.60, or in other words, with 95% certainty we can say that the 'real' relative risk is somewhere between 1.14 and 2.60.

Output 3.2 Relative risk estimate and 95% confidence interval of the exemplary intervention study evaluating the effectiveness of preventive ankle taping in soccer players

	Risk estimate		
	Value	**95% Confidence interval**	
		Lower	**Upper**
For cohort did you get an injury? = no	0.788	0.659	0.941
For cohort did you get an injury? = yes	1.722	1.139	2.603
N of valid cases	225		

Testing of the risk difference and the relative risk

As mentioned above, with statistical testing we are able to obtain a *p*-value of the estimated risk difference or relative risk. The general idea behind statistical testing is that the observed result is tested against a certain hypothesis, which is called the null-hypothesis. This null-hypothesis is always something which assumes there is no effect or there is no difference. In light of our example, the null-hypothesis is that the risk difference equals zero or the relative risk equals 1. In all statistical tests, the observed result is compared to the results which would have been obtained if the null-hypothesis was true. The obtained *p*-value can be interpreted as the probability of the obtaining the observed result (or more extreme away from the null-hypothesis) when the null-hypothesis is actually true.

In light of our example, the observed 2×2 table is compared to a 2×2 table obtained when the null-hypothesis would have been true. To obtain the second 2×2 table, we have to calculate the number of subjects expected to sustain an injury when there is no effect of our preventive ankle taping. To calculate this number, we can use a rule that goes with independence of probabilities. When two probabilities are independent, the two probabilities can be multiplied with each other. When for instance a dice is thrown twice, the probability of getting a 6 twice is 1 out of 6 (for the first dice) multiplied with 1 out of 6 (for the second dice). Because the two probabilities are independent of each other, the overall probability is 1/36. The same rule can be used with the 2×2 table, because when the null-hypothesis is true the probability of being in the intervention or control group is independent of the probability of obtaining the outcome. This will be illustrated with a very simple example (Table 3.1).

The probabilty of being in the upper-left cell when the null-hypothesis is true is equal to the probability of being in the upper row (i.e. 40/100) multiplied by the probability of being in the first column (i.e. 30/100). In other words, the probability of being in the upper-left cell when the null-hypothesis is true is 12%. Thus, the expected number of subjects in the upper-left cell is 12 (12% multiplied by the number of subjects in the sample). We can use the same calculations for the other cells in the 2×2 table (Table 3.2).

Assume that the 2×2 table depicted in Table 3.3 is found in a certain study. To calculate the probability of obtaining the observed 2×2 table (or more extreme away from the null-hypothesis) for each cell, we have to compare the expected number of subjects with the observed number of subjects. It is obvious that the greater the difference between the expected number of subjects when the null-hypothesis is true and the observed number of subjects, the more unlikely the null-hypothesis is. This corresponds then with a low *p*-value. To calculate the *p*-value of the 2×2 table, we have to use the so-called chi-square test. Chi-square refers to the probability distribution used to estimate the *p*-value and the test statistic. The test statistic of the chi-square test can be calculated as follows (Formula 3.4), where X^2 = test statistic; O = observed number of subjects, and E = expected number if subjects when the null-hypothesis is true.

Formula 3.5:
$$X^2 = \sum \left[\frac{(O-E)^2}{E} \right]$$

Table 3.1 Example of a 2 × 2 table

	Outcome +ve	Outcome –ve	Total
Determinant +ve			40
Determinant –ve			60
Total	30	70	100

Table 3.2 Expected 2 × 2 table, when the null-hypothesis is true

	Outcome +ve	Outcome –ve	Total
Determinant +ve	12	28	40
Determinant –ve	18	42	60
Total	30	70	100

The test statistic calculated in this way follows a chi-square distribution with one degree of freedom. The chi-square distribution is a probability distribution that can be used to get a *p*-value. That we have one degree of freedom can be illustrated easily by taking an empty 2×2 table with only the total numbers of the rows and columns present. When one arbitrary number is filled in, the other numbers are fixed; so we have one degree of freedom.

When we return to the example, we can estimate the *p*-value of the observed 2×2 table in the same way (Output 3.3)

In Output 3.3 we can see that the *p*-value of the (Pearson) chi-square test is 0.008. So, the probability of obtaining the observed 2×2 table (or more extreme away from the null-hypothesis), assuming the null-hypothesis is true, is 0.8%. This is very low and because this *p*-value is below the arbitrary cut-point of 5%, we can say that the effect of the intervention is statistically significant. Please bear in mind that the cut-off point of 5% is arbitrary; the importance of finding a significant result is not so great as often suggested.

In the second line of the output we see the result of the so-called Fisher exact test. Actually, the chi-square test is an approximation, which is easy to compute, but which has some limitations. In fact, the rule of thumb is that the chi-square test can only be applied when the expected number of subjects in >80% of the cells is >5 and in all cells the expected number of subjects is >1. This is, again, a rule of thumb and not a very strict rule. When this assumption is not met, the Fisher exact test can be used. With the Fisher exact test, the exact *p*-value can be computed. The chi-square test was developed because in earlier days it was rather difficult to calculate by hand the exact *p*-value with the Fisher exact test. However, with the statistical software available at present it is possible to estimate the exact *p*-value even for large 2×2 tables, so it is a bit strange that we still use the approximation of the chi-square test. It should be noted that the *p*-value of the chi-square test is always a bit lower than the exact *p*-value estimated with the Fisher exact test. The larger the expected numbers in the different cells of the 2×2 table, the more the two *p*-values are alike. In the example (Output 3.3) we can see that the *p*-value estimated with the Fisher exact test is only slightly higher than the *p*-value estimated with the chi-square test (0.009 vs. 0.008).

The estimated *p*-value pertains to the 2×2 table, so it pertainss to both the relative risk and the risk difference. There are two different measures of effect, one statistical test, and therefore one *p*-value.

Table 3.3 Example of a 2 × 2 table observed in a certain study

	Outcome +ve	Outcome –ve	Total
Determinant +ve	20	20	40
Determinant –ve	10	80	60
Total	30	70	100

Output 3.3 Part of the result of a chi-square test regarding the exemplary intervention study evaluating the effectiveness of preventive ankle taping in soccer players

Chi-square tests

	Value	df	Asymp. sig. (2-sided)	Exact sig. (2-sided)	Exact sig. (1-sided)
Pearson chi-square	7.058**b**	1	0.008		
Fisher's exact test				0.009	0.006
N of valid cases	225				

b. 0 cells (0%) have expected count less than 5. The minimum expected count is 34,22.

An alternative effect measure: the odds ratio

In the first paragraphs of this chapter, the risk difference and the relative risk were introduced as effect measures that can be calculated from a 2×2 table. These measures of effect can only be calculated in prospective cohort studies. In all other study designs we cannot calculate absolute probabilities of the outcome and therefore relative probabilities of the outcome must be used. These relative probabilities are known as the odds. The odds is defined as the probability divided by 1 minus that probability (Formula 3.6), where $P(Y=1)$ = the probability to get the outcome.

Formula 3.6:
$$odds = \frac{P(Y=1)}{1 - P(Y=1)}$$

So, instead of the relative risk, which was defined as the ratio between the probability of sustaining an injury in the two groups, we can calculate the odds ratio (OR), i.e. the ratio between the odds of getting an injury in the intervention group and the odds of getting an injury in the control group. If we go back to the 2×2 table of our example (Output 3.1) we can calculate the odds ratio in the following way.

$$OR = \frac{(25/110)/(85/110)}{(45/115)/(70/115)} = 0.46$$

In other words, the odds of sustaining an injury while in the intervention group is 0.46 times as high as in the control group. In addition, a 95% confidence interval can be estimated around the odds ratio (Output 3.4).

When we want to calculate the corresponding p-value, we can apply the same chi-sqaure test we performed to calculate the p-value of the relative risk and the risk difference. The p-value of the odds ratio is calculated from the same 2×2 table, so the p-value is 0.008.

Output 3.4 Odds ratio and 95% confidence interval of the exemplary intervention study evaluating the effectiveness of preventive ankle taping in soccer players

Risk estimate

	Value	95% Confidence interval	
		Lower	Upper
Odds Ratio for studygroup (intervention/control)	0.458	0.256	0.819
N of valid cases	225		

Although the odds ratio is the measure of effect that should be used in cross-sectional or retro-spective studies, it is often also used in prospective studies. The reason for this is that the odds ratio is the measure of effect that is estimated from a logistic regression analysis (see next para-graph). In prospective studies, the odds ratio is often interpreted as a relative risk; however, one should be careful in doing so. The odds ratio is not the same as the relative risk! If we compare the odds ratio with the relative risk in our example we can see that the odds ratio is lower (i.e. 0.46 vs. 0.58). The effect of the intervention estimated with the odds ratio is a bit stronger (i.e. further away from 1) than that estimated with the relative risk. This is always the case, and the difference between the two will become larger when the prevalence of the outcome becomes higher. In our example the prevalence of the outcome (i.e. getting an injury) is 31%, which leads to a rather 'big' difference between the two effect measures. It is sometimes said that the two are comparable when the prevalence of the outcome is below 5%. However, this is again a rather arbitrary cut-off value.

Logistic regression analysis

Until now, we have analysed the effect of the intervention in a rather simple way. We created a 2×2 table and calculated either the relative risk, the risk difference, or the odds ratio and the corresponding 95% confidence intervals. To obtain the corresponding p-value, we performed the chi-square test (or even better, the Fisher exact test). However, in sports-injury research (and also in other research) there is more than just the so-called crude effect measure. In most research situations the effect has to be adjusted for several covariates and/or we are interested in the ques-tion whether the effect of the intervention is, for instance, different for males and females. Stated in epidemiological terminology we have to adjust for possible confounders and/or we have to investigate possible effect modification. To do so, a chi-square test is not enough. We have to use a more general statistical technique which is known as regression. In light of the dichotomous outcome variable, we have to use logistic regression analysis. Before explaining what the logistic regression analysis is, we need to understand something about linear regression analysis. Linear regression analysis is used to analyse, for instance, the relationship between two continuous vari-ables. Say, e.g. we are interested in the relationship between systolic blood pressure and age. The first step in analysing that relationship is to make a scatterplot in which all observations are plotted (Output 3.5).

The next step in a linear regression analysis is to draw a straight line through the points. The characteristic of the line is that the distance between the observations and the line is as small as possible. The regression line is characterized by two parameters: b0 and b1: diastolic blood pressure = b0 + b1* age.

The interpretation of the two parameters is as follows: the b0, which is also known as the intercept or the constant is the value of the outcome variable when the determinant (the X-variable) is zero. The b1 says something about the relationship between the two variables. It indicates the difference in outcome variable which corresponds with a difference in one unit in the X-variable. When a linear regression analysis is applied for the scatterplot shown in Output 3.5, we will get the following regression equation: diastolic blood pressure = 60.5 + 1* age

The interpretation of this equation is that diastolic blood pressure at age 0 is equal to 60.5 mmHg, while a difference of 1 year in age corresponds with a difference of 1 mmHg in diastolic blood pressure. Suppose the determinant is not continuous but, for instance, a dichotomous variable, such as intervention versus control. Then the regression coefficient for the intervention variable can be interpreted as the difference in outcome variables between the two groups. Because this is a very convenient way of analysing the relationship between a continuous outcome variable and

Output 3.5 Relationship between diastolic blood pressure and age

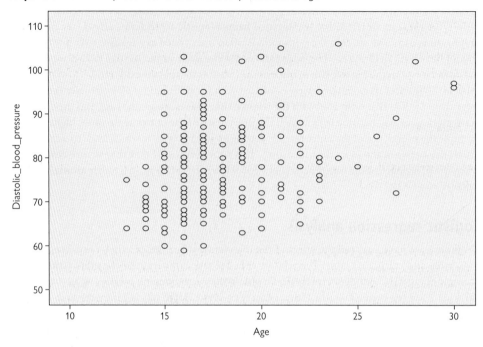

other variables, statisticians were trying to create a comparable regression analysis for dichotomous outcome variables. The result from that search was logistic regression analysis. Without going into much detail, logistic regression analysis is the same as linear regression analysis; the only difference between the two is that the outcome variable looks a bit different (Formula 3.7), where $P(Y_{dichotomous})$ = probability of getting the outcome.

Formula 3.7:
$$\ln\left(\frac{P(Y_{dichotomous})}{1 - P(Y_{dichotomous})}\right) = b_0 + b_1 X$$

The outcome variable of a logistic regression is the natural log of the probability of getting the outcome divided by 1 minus that probability. So following the interpretation of the regression coefficients in a linear regression analysis, the b0 is the value of the outcome variable (i.e. the natural log of the probability of getting the outcome divided by 1 minus that probability) when the X-variable is zero. The b1 is the difference in outcome variable (i.e. the natural log of the probability of getting the outcome divided by 1 minus that probability) which corresponds with a difference of one unit in the X-variable. Although this looks quite complicated, we will see that this leads to a very nice interpretation. Suppose that, as in our example, we are dealing with a dichotomous determinant (i.e. intervention versus control). In that situation the interpretation of the regression coefficient is the difference in outcome variable between the intervention and the control group.

Formula 3.8a:
$$b_1 = \ln\left(\frac{P(Y=1)}{1 - P(Y=1)}\right)_{intervention} - \ln\left(\frac{P(Y=1)}{1 - P(Y=1)}\right)_{control}$$

This formula can also be written as:

Formula 3.8b: $b_1 = \ln\left(odds(Y=1)\right)_{intervention} - \ln\left(odds(Y=1)\right)_{control}$

One of the nicest characteristics of logarithms is that a difference between two logarithms of the same kind is equal to the logarithm of the ratio of the two corresponding numbers. So Formula 3.8b can be simplified in the following way:

Formula 3.8c: $b_1 = \ln\left(\dfrac{odds(Y=1)_{intervention}}{odds(Y=1)_{control}}\right)$

The regression coefficient is therefore equal to the natural log of the odds ratio. To get rid of the natural log we can raise both sides to the e-power.

Formula 3.8d: $EXP(b_1) = \dfrac{odds(Y=1)_{intervention}}{odds(Y=1)_{control}}$

So, when we raise the regression coefficient to the e-power we will end up with the odds ratio.

Let us go back to the example in which we wanted to evaluate the effect of the intervention. We have seen that there was a significant intervention effect and we have calculated three different effect measures; the relative risk, the risk difference, and the odds ratio. We now can apply a logistic regression analysis. Output 3.6 shows the results.

A lot of information is given in the output. First of all, we see the values of the regression coefficients (b1 equals −0.782 and b0 equals −0.442) and the corresponding standard errors. As has been mentioned before, the standard errors are needed for statistical testing as well as for the calculation of a 95% confidence interval. For the first purpose the so-called Wald statistic is calculated.

Formula 3.9: $Wald = \left(\dfrac{b}{se(b)}\right)^2$

From the output we can see that the Wald statistic for the intervention variable is 6.972. To obtain the corresponding p-value we have to know that the Wald statistic follows a chi-square distribution with one degree of freedom. From the output we can see that the p-value equals 0.008. Note that this is exactly the same p-value we obtained from the chi-square test performed earlier. The next column in the output shows the value of the odds ratio (EXP(B)). Of course, we have seen this value (0.458) before. In the last two columns of the output we see the values of the 95% confidence interval. The values of the 95% confidence interval are estimated as follows, where b = regression coefficient and se(b) = standard error of the regression coefficient.

Formula 3.10: $EXP\left[b \pm 1.96 \times se(b)\right]$

Output 3.6 Results of a logistic regression analysis to evaluate the effectiveness of preventive ankle taping in soccer players

			Variables in the equation				95% C.I. for EXP(B)	
	B	S.E.	Wald	df	Sig.	Exp(B)	Lower	Upper
Intervention	−0.782	0.297	6.927	1	0.008	0.458	0.256	0.819
Constant	−0.442	0.191	5.347	1	0.021	0.643		

In fact, all the results we obtained from the logistic regression analysis were already know from the calculation of the odds ratio and the chi-square test. However, the use of logistic regression is important the moment we want to adjust for particular covariates and/or we want to investigate possible effect modification or in general when there is more than one X-variable. Furthermore, the use of logistic regression analysis is necessary when we want to compare a dichotomous outcome between more than two groups or when we want to relate the dichotomous outcome variable with a continuous determinant. Another nice aspect of logistic regression analysis is that, based on the results we can compute the probability of getting the outcome given the values of the determinants (Formula 3.11).

Formula 3.11:
$$P(Y = 1) = \frac{1}{1 + EXP^{[-(b_0 + b_1 X_1 + ...)]}}$$

Adding time at risk to the analysis

One of the problems in sports-injury research is that subjects are not always at risk to get the outcome. When you do not sport, you will never get a sports injury. In other words, the prevalence (or cumulative incidence) of injuries (as been analysed with 2×2 tables and logistic regression analysis) is may not be sufficient for sports-injury research. If possible, it would be better to add the time at risk to the analysis; in other words, it would be better to analyse incidence densities instead of prevalences or cumulative incidences. The statistical technique that adds the time at risk to the analysis is known as 'survival' analysis. The reason for this terminology is that these techniques were first used to analyse death and time to death. To illustrate how this works, Fig. 3.1 shows the results of a very small study in which soccer players are followed for 10 months and in which we were interested whether or not the players got injured and when the players got injured.

   With this kind of data, two situations can occur during the follow-up period. The first situation is that the subject reaches the outcome; in other words, the soccer player got injured and the other situation is that the subject did not reach the outcome; in other words, the soccer player did not get injured. The last situation can occur at the end of the study or can occur somewhere during the follow-up period when the particular subject is not part of the study anymore. Within the survival analysis terminology, when subjects do not reach the outcome, the subjects are censored.

   In Fig. 3.1 we can see that five out of 10 soccer players got injured and that the other five soccer players were censored. From Fig. 3.1 it is quite easy to calculate the incidence density. To do so,

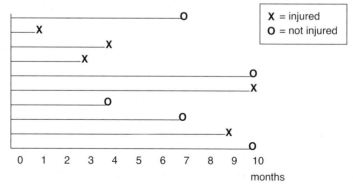

Fig. 3.1 Example of a simple study in which 10 soccer players are followed-up over a period of 10 months.

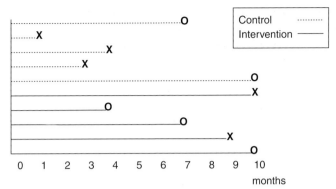

Fig. 3.2 Example of a simple study in which 10 soccer players divided across two study groups (intervention and control) are followed-up over a period of 10 months.

we have to calculate the total time, the subjects were at risk. From the figure, we can see that the first subject was 7 months at risk, the second subject 1 month, etc. The total population was 65 months at risk. The incidence density was therefore 5/65 months; i.e. 0.077 injury per person-month.

Although the incidence density of a certain group can provide interesting information, it is much more interesting when we compare different groups with each other. In Fig. 3.2 we divided the group of soccer players into an intervention group and a control group.

Based on Fig. 3.2 we can calculate the incidence density for both groups. For the control group, the incidence density is three injuries per 25 months, i.e. 0.12 injury per person-month, while for the intervention group the incidence density is two injuries per 40 months, i.e. 0.05 injury per person-month. From these two incidence densities we can calculate two measures of effect. Comparable to the risk difference and the relative risk, we can calculate the incidence density difference and the incidence density ratio. In the small example, the incidence density difference is equal to 0.12 – 0.05; i.e. 0.07 injuries per person-month. The incidence density ratio is equal to 0.12/0.05 = 2.4. The latter is often interpreted as a relative risk, but it is not the same. With a relative risk only the numbers who get the outcome are compared to each other, while in the incidence density ratio also the time at risk is taken into account. In fact, the relative risk in the small example is only 1.5 (0.6/0.4). This is much lower than the incidence density ratio of 2.4. The difference between the relative risk and the incidence density ratio gives an indication how important the time at risk is in the calculation of the effect measure. One should realize that the classical survival analysis is a bit strange in sports-injury research. The most important limitation is that subjects are not always at risk to get a sports injury. So, actually, we should measure the 'real' time at risk and calculate the incidence densities with these real times. In order to make the explanation not too complicated, in the next paragraphs – where we explain all the features of using 'survival' analysis, we will use the total time as time at risk. Again, this is a simplification and not the same as the actual time at risk for getting a sports injury.

Comparison of two groups: Kaplan–Meier survival curves

Another way to describe 'survival' data is with a survival curve or Kaplan–Meier curve. The Kaplan–Meier curve is a graphical display of survival over time. To create a Kaplan–Meier curve, the follow-up time is divided into small periods and for each period the probability of survival is calculated given the probability to reach that period without having the outcome. Formula 3.12 shows how these probabilities can be calculated, where $S(t)$ = probability to survive in period t, given the probability to reach that period without getting the outcome.

Formula 3.12: $$S(t) = S(t-1) \times survival\ fraction$$

The way the Kaplan–Meier curve is constructed will be illustrated with the small example shown in Fig. 3.1. The first probability not to sustain injury is 1, because all soccer players are not injured at the beginning of the study.

After 1 month, one player is injured. The 'survival' probability is equal to 1 time the survival fraction (1 time 0.9) = 0.9. At month 2, nothing happens, while at month 3 another player was injured. The probability not to sustain injury after 3 months is therefore 0.9 times 8/9 (the 'survival' probability over the third month) = 0.8, etc. Table 3.4 shows the 'survival' probabilities over the whole follow-up period of 10 months.

It is common to display the 'survival' probabilities as has been given in Table 3.4 graphically by means of a Kaplan–Meier curve. Output 3.7 shows the Kaplan–Meier curve for the data from Fig. 3.1 and Table 3.4.

As mentioned earlier, it is much more interesting to compare different survival curves between groups. Based on Fig. 3.2 we can calculate the survival probabilities at different time-points for the two groups (Table 3.5) and we display the Kaplan–Meier curves for both groups (Output 3.8).

When we compare the two curves with each other, we can see that the intervention group performs better than the control group. The question is then: How much better is the intervention group compared to the control group? From 2×2 tables (when only the number of injured people are compared to each other) we could estimate three measures of effect, but from a Kaplan–Meier analysis (which is in fact the same as a 2×2 table including the time to the injury) we cannot calculate any effect measure. Therefore, we need a regression approach (see paragraph 3.8). However, we can estimate a p-value based on the Kaplan–Meier curves. The test that can be used for this is called the log rank test.

The principle of the log rank test is quite simple and is comparable to the chi-square test discussed earlier. The difference between the two is that with the log rank test, the comparison between observed number of people with the outcome and the expected number of people with

Table 3.4 Calculation of the survival probabilities over the different time-periods of example shown in Fig. 3.1

S(0)	=	1		
S(1)	=	1 * 9/10	=	0.9
S(2)	=	0.9		
S(3)	=	0.9 * 8/9	=	0.8
S(4)	=	0.8 * 7/8	=	0.7
S(5)	=	0.7 * 6/6	=	0.7
S(6)	=	0.7		
S(7)	=	0.7		
S(8)	=	0.7 * 4/4	=	0.7
S(9)	=	0.7 * 3/4	=	0.53
S(10)	=	0.53 * 2/3	=	0.35

Output 3.7 Kaplan–Meier survival curve based on the data of Fig. 3.1 and Table 3.4

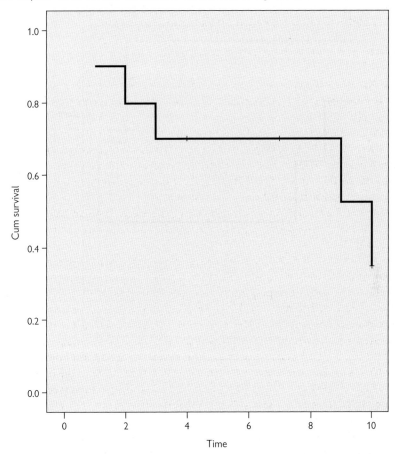

Table 3.5 Calculation of the 'survival' curves based on the data of Fig. 3.2

Control group					Intervention group				
S(0)	=	1			S(0)	=	1	=	
S(1)	=	1 * 4/5	=	0.8	S(1)	=	1	=	
S(2)	=	0.8			S(2)	=	1	=	
S(3)	=	0.8 * 3/4	=	0.6	S(3)	=	1	=	
S(4)	=	0.6 * 2/3	=	0.4	S(4)	=	1	=	
S(5)	=	0.4			S(5)	=	1 * 4/4	=	1
S(6)	=	0.4			S(6)	=	1	=	
S(7)	=	0.4			S(7)	=	1	=	
S(8)	=	0.4 * 1/1	=	0.4	S(8)	=	1 * 3/3	=	1
S(9)	=	0.4			S(9)	=	1 * 2/3	=	0.67
S(10)	=	0.4			S(10)	=	0.67 * 1/2	=	0.335

Output 3.8 Kaplan–Meier survival curves for the intervention (dotted line) and control group (straight line) based on the data shown in Fig. 3.2 and Table 3.5

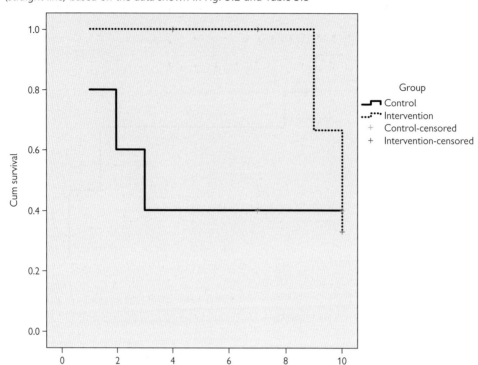

the outcome when the null-hypothesis is true is done at each time point. How the log rank test works can be best explained by Table 3.6.

In Table 3.6 we see the 10 time-points of the study and we see six columns. In these columns, first the observed injuries are given (O1–O2), second the numbers at risk in both groups (n1–n2), and last the expected number of injuries when the null-hypothesis is true (E1–E2). 'When the null-hypothesis is true' means in this situation that the probability of sustaining injuries in both groups is equal. In Fig. 3.2 we can see that at time 1, one person gets injured; so the observed number of injuries is 1. In both groups, five people are at risk of being injured and because when the null-hypothesis is true, the probability to get injured in both groups is 50%, we expect 0.5 injury in the intervention group and 0.5 injury in the control group. At time 2, there is also one observed injury and again this injury is observed in the control group. The difference with the first time-point is that the numbers at risk in both groups are not equal anymore. In the control group, we only have four subjects at risk, while in the intervention group there are still five subjects at risk. This ratio of subjects at risk has to be taken into account in the estimation of the expected number of injuries in both groups. For the control group this number is 4/9 times 1 (the observed injury), which is equal to 0.44 injuries. In the intervention group this number is 0.56 injuries (5/9 times 1). This principle can be followed across all time-points (Table 3.6).

The next step in the log rank test is to add all the expected numbers for both groups. For the control group the total number of expected injuries is 1.895 and for the intervention group this

Table 3.6 Principle of the log-rank test based on the data of Table 3.5 and Fig. 3.2

	Control	Intervention	Control	Intervention	Control	Intervention
Time	O_1	O_2	n_1	N_2	E_1	E_2
1	1	0	5	5	0.50	0.50
2	-	-	-	-	-	-
3	1	0	4	5	0.44	0.56
4	1	C	3	5	0.375	0.625
5	-	-	-	-		
6	-	-	-	-		
7	C	C	2	4		
8	-	-	-	-		
9	0	1	1	3	0.25	0.75
10	C	1C	1	2	0.33	0.67
Total	3	2			1.895	3.105

number is 3.105. With Formula 3.13, the test statistic of the log rank rest can be calculated, where G = number of groups to compare; O = observed number, and E = expected number (given the null-hypothesis).

Formula 3.13:
$$X^2 = \sum_{g=1}^{G} \frac{(O-E)^2}{E}$$

When we enter the values of Table 3.6 into Formula 3.13, we obtain a test statistic of 1.04.

$$X^2 = \frac{(3-1.895)^2}{1.895} + \frac{(2-3.105)^2}{3.105} = 1.04$$

This test statistic follows a chi-square distribution and the number of degrees of freedom for this chi-square distribution is the number of groups that are compared to each other −1.

If we go back to the real example that is used in this chapter, we can also create Kaplan–Meier curves for the intervention and control groups and we can perform the log rank test to derive a p-value for the difference in Kaplan–Meier curves between the groups (Output 3.9 and 3.10).

From Output 3.9 it can be seen that the intervention group performs better than the control group. Not only is the number of injuries in the intervention group lower than in the control group (this can be seen at the end of the Kaplan–Meier curves where the intervention group is higher than the control group), but also the duration to sustain an injury is shorter in the control group than in the intervention group. The curve for the intervention group stays at 1 for about 15 weeks, where the curve for the control group goes down immediately after the commencement of the study. From the result of the log rank test (Output 3.10) we can further see that the p-value is 0.003. This indicates that the probability of obtaining the curves we have found in our study (or more extreme away from the null-hypothesis), when actually the null-hypothesis is true, is only 0.003. This is lower than the arbitrary cut-off point of 0.05, so we can say the two curves are significantly different from each other. Again, from the Kaplan–Meier analysis we only obtain a p-value. To get an estimate of effect we have to perform a regression analysis.

Output 3.9 Kaplan–Meier curves for the intervention group (dotted line) and the control group (straight line) for the exemplary evaluation on the effectiveness of preventive ankle taping in soccer players

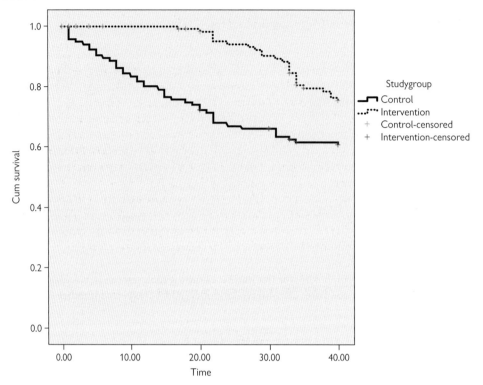

Cox regression analysis

Comparable to the situation with continuous outcome variables (linear regression analysis) and dichotomous outcome variables (logistic regression analysis), also for 'survival data' a regression technique is available; i.e. the Cox regression analysis. As with logistic regression analysis, the general idea of the Cox regression analysis is to transform the outcome variable in such a way that a linear regression analysis can be performed. With survival data this procedure is a bit simpler than for logistic regression analysis, because the natural log of the hazard can be described by a linear function. We will not go into much detail, because it is mathematically quite complicated[1]. There is a difference among the Cox regression analysis and the other two regression techniques; with Cox regression, there is no intercept reported. This has to do with the fact that the intercept can be seen as a baseline hazard, which is not reflected by one number, but by a function over time.

Output 3.10 Result of the log rank test for the exemplary evaluation on the effectiveness of preventive ankle taping in soccer players

Overall comparisons			
	Chi-square	df	Sig.
Log rank (Mantel–Cox)	8.963	1	0.003

Test of equality of survival distributions for the different levels of studygroup

Formula 3.14 shows the general formula for a Cox regression analysis, where Y = dichotomous outcome; $\ln[ht0]$ = 'baseline hazard'; $b1$ = regression coefficient for the independent variable $X1$ and $b2$ = regression coefficient for the independent variable $X2$.

Formula 3.14:
$$\ln\left[hazard(Y)\right] = \ln\left[h_{t0}\right] + b_1 X_1 + b_2 X_2 + \ldots$$

Let us go back to the example study in which the effectiveness of preventive ankle taping is soccer players was investigated. In paragraph 3.7 it was show (by the log rank test) that the intervention group performed significantly better than the control group. The same comparison can also be analysed with the Cox regression analysis. Output 3.11 shows the result of that analysis.

In Output 3.11 we can see that the regression coefficient for the intervention equals −0.727. The interpretation of this number is comparable to the interpretation of a regression coefficient in the other two regression techniques, i.e. the difference in outcome variable between the intervention group and the control group. Because the outcome variable in a Cox regression analysis is the natural log of the hazard to get injured, this means that the difference in natural log of the hazard to get injured between the two groups is −0.727. To get a better interpretation of this number, we can (as in logistic regression analysis) use the characteristic of logarithms, i.e. the difference between two logarithms of the same kind is the same as that logarithm of the ratio of the two numbers (so $\ln(a) - \ln(b) = \ln(a/b)$). The next step is to raise that number to e-power to get rid of the natural log (Formula 3.14).

Formula 3.15a:
$$b_1 = \ln\left[hazard(injury)\right]_{int} - \ln\left[hazard(injury)\right]_{cont}$$

Formula 3.15b:
$$b_1 = \ln\left[\frac{hazard(injury)_{int}}{hazard(injury)_{cont}}\right]$$

Formula 3.15c:
$$EXP(b_1) = \frac{hazard(injury)_{int}}{hazard(injury)_{cont}}$$

The regression coefficient raised to the e-power can therefore be interpreted as a hazard ratio, which is the same as an incidence density ratio. In Output 3.12 we have seen that the regression coefficient was −0.727, which leads to a hazard ratio of 0.438. In the output this number is shown as Exp(B). The hazard ratio is a combination of two effects: (1) the difference in number of soccer players that get injured in the two groups and (2) the difference in the 'time to injury' in both groups. The first part of the hazard ratio is therefore exactly the same as the relative risk. The difference between the relative risk and the hazard ratio is the difference in 'time to injury' between the two groups. The most frequently used interpretation of the hazard ratio is a relative risk at each time-point or a sort of average relative risk over time. In our example where a hazard ratio

Output 3.11 Result of a Cox regression analysis for the exemplary evaluation on the effectiveness of preventive ankle taping in soccer players

	B	S.E.	Wald	df	Sig.	Exp(B)	95C.I. for EXP(B)	
							Lower	**Upper**
Intervention	−0.727	0.250	8.478	1	0.004	0.483	0.296	0.788

Variables in the equation

of 0.438 was found, it means that the risk to get injured in the intervention group at each time-point is 0.438 times as high as the risk to get injured in the control group at each time-point. When we compare the hazard ratio with the relative risk which was calculated in paragraph 3.2 (i.e. 0.59), we see that the hazard ratio is a bit lower, which means that the effect estimated with the hazard ratio is a bit stronger than that estimated with the relative risk. This difference reflects the difference in 'time to injury' which was already seen in the Kaplan–Meier curves (Output 3.8). Because the hazard ratio is a sort of average relative risk over time, it is obvious that this is only a good estimate when the relative risk is more or less stable over time. Within survival terminology this means that the hazard ratio must be proportional over time. Therefore, the Cox regression analysis is also known as the Cox proportional hazards regression. In the statistical literature, there are several ways to evaluate whether the hazard ratio is proportional over time[1]. However, this goes beyond the scope of this chapter.

In Output 3.11 we see, besides the regression coefficient and the hazard ratio, the standard error of the regression coefficient (0.250) and the Wald statistic. As with logistic regression analysis, the Wald statistic can be calculated by dividing the regression coefficient by its standard error, squared (Formula 3.16), where Wald = Wald-statistic; b = regression coefficient en se(b) = standard error of the regression coefficient.

Formula 3.16:
$$Wald = \left(\frac{b}{se(b)} \right)^2$$

The Wald statistic in the example is 8.478 and on a chi-square distribution with 1 degree of freedom the corresponding p-value equals 0.004. The standard error can also be used to calculate the 95% confidence interval around the hazard ratio. To do so (again as in logistic regression analysis) we have to calculate the 95% confidence interval around the regression coefficient first and raise the two borders to the e-power (Formula 3.17), where b = regression coefficient and se(b) = standard error of the regression coefficient.

Formula 3.17:
$$EXP\left[b \pm 1.96 \times se(b) \right]$$

This leads to a 95% confidence interval around the hazard ratio which goes from 0.296 to 0.788. The interpretation of this confidence interval is the same as ever; with 95% certainty we can say that the 'real' hazard ratio lies somewhere between 0.296 and 0.788.

Cox regression analysis with recurrent events

Besides the assumption of proportional hazard, a big drawback with the use of the classical Cox regression analysis is that the events cannot be recurrent. In injury research, this not represents the real-life situation. In our example for instance, after injury (depending on the severity), a soccer player recovers, starts playing again, and is therefore again at risk of being injured. So, in fact, injury research deals with recurrent events. Within statistics there are several possibilities to take those recurrences into account in the analyses. One technique that can be used is an extension of the classical Cox regression analysis, and this is known as Cox regression analysis for recurrent events. This method not only takes into account that subjects can suffer from recurrent events, but also that subjects after an injury are probably at a higher risk to sustain another injury[2].

Confounding and effect modification

With the use of regression techniques it is also possible to adjust for possible confounders and to investigate possible effect modification. This holds for all regression techniques, so also for

Output 3.12 Result of a logistic regression analysis for the exemplary evaluation on the effectiveness of preventive ankle taping in soccer players

Variables in the equation

	B	S.E.	Wald	df	Sig.	EXP(B)
Intervention	−0.782	0.297	6.927	1	0.008	0.458
Constant	−0.442	0.191	5.347	1	0.021	0.643

logistic regression analysis and Cox regression analysis. Confounding means that the observed effect could maybe caused by something else, the possible confounder. Let us go back to the logistic regression analysis explained earlier. Output 3.12 shows again the result of the logistic regression analysis to evaluate the effectiveness of preventive ankle taping in soccer players.

Assuming we want to adjust for gender to see whether or not the intervention effect observed in the so-called 'crude' analysis is (partly) caused by age differences between the intervention and control groups, we can perform a second logistic regression analysis in which both the intervention variable and age are analysed together (Output 3.13). The interpretation of the intervention effect has changed now in such a way, that the intervention effect is estimated independent of age. When we compare both results with each other, then we can see that the intervention effect hardly changed when age was put into the logistic regression analysis (−0.782 vs. −0.786). In other words, age is not a confounder in this analysis. There is an arbitrary rule of thumb which says that when the regression coefficient of interest changes with more than 10%, there is relevant confounding.

Another issue is effect modification. Effect modification means that the effect of interest is different for different groups of the possible effect modifier. In the example we could, for instance, investigate whether the effect of the intervention is different for soccer players with a former ankle injury or not. To investigate this, we have to add an interaction term to the logistic regression analysis. The interaction term is a multiplication of the variable in which we are interested and the possible effect modifier. Output 3.14 shows the results of the analysis with an interaction term.

By adding an interaction term to the logistic regression analysis, we create four groups and we can calculate the outcome variable for each of the four groups. To understand the meaning of the different regression coefficients in Output 3.14, the regression equation should be written down.

$$\ln\left(\frac{P(injury)}{1 - p(injury)}\right) = -0.223 - 1.135 \times intvervention - 0.421 \times former + 0.640$$
$$\times intervention \times former$$

Output 3.13 Result of a logistic regression analysis to investigate the possible confounding influence of age in the exemplary evaluation on the effectiveness of preventive ankle taping in soccer players

Variables in the equation

	B	S.E.	Wald	df	Sig.	EXP(B)
Intervention	−0.786	0.297	6.983	1	0.008	0.456
Age	−0.025	0.051	0.236	1	0.627	0.976
Constant	0.005	0.938	0.000	1	0.996	1.005

Output 3.14 Result of a logistic regression analysis to investigate the possible effect of modification of former injuries in the exemplary evaluation on the effectiveness of preventive ankle taping in soccer players

Variables in the equation

	B	S.E.	Wald	df	Sig.	EXP(B)
Intervention	−1.135	0.463	6.009	1	0.014	0.321
Former	−0.421	0.384	1.202	1	0.273	0.656
Former by intervention	0.640	0.608	1.107	1	0.293	1.896
Constant	−0.223	0.274	0.664	1	0.415	0.800

The intervention effect for the group without former injury can be estimated by filling in 0 for the variable former (former is coded 0 for 'no former injury'). For the control group (intervention = 0), the outcome variable equals:

$$\ln\left(\frac{P(injury)}{1-p(injury)}\right)_{control} = -0.223 - 1.135 \times 0 - 0.421 \times 0 + 0.640 \times 0 \times 0 = -0.233$$

For the intervention group the outcome variable equals:

$$\ln\left(\frac{P(injury)}{1-p(injury)}\right)_{intervention} = -0.223 - 1.135 \times 1 - 0.421 \times 0 + 0.640 \times 1 \times 0 = -0.233 - 1.135$$

The difference between the intervention group and the control group for soccer players without a former injury equals −1.135, i.e. the regression coefficient for the intervention variable in Output 3.15. The odds ratio is then equal to EXP[−1.135] = 0.321.

In the same way, the intervention effect for soccer players with a former injury (former coded 1) can be estimated.

$$\ln\left(\frac{P(injury)}{1-p(injury)}\right)_{control} = -0.223 - 1.135 \times 0 - 0.421 \times 1 + 0.640 \times 0 \times 1 = -0.233 - 0.421$$

$$\ln\left(\frac{P(injury)}{1-p(injury)}\right)_{intervention} = -0.223 - 1.135 \times 1 - 0.421 \times 1 + 0.640 \times 1 \times 1$$

$$= -0.223 - 1.135 - 0.421 + 0.640$$

The difference between the intervention group and the control group for the soccer players with a former injury is therefore −1.135 + 0.640 = −0.495. The odds ratio for the soccer players with a former injury is EXP[−0.495] = 0.61.

In other words, the intervention effect for the soccer players with a former injury equals the sum of the regression coefficient for the intervention variable (i.e. −1.135) and the regression coefficient for the interaction term (i.e. 0.640).

So there is quite a big difference in the intervention effect between the soccer players with a former injury and the soccer players without a former injury; for the latter the intervention seems to have a larger effect. The question then is whether this difference is important. In the logistic regression output, the difference in effect between the two groups (with and without former injury) is reflected in the regression coefficient for the interaction term. From Output 3.15 we can see that this regression coefficient is not statistically significant different from zero (the corresponding p-value is 0.293). So, even though the difference in effect seems to be quite large, this difference is not statistically significant.

For Cox regression, exactly the same procedure can be followed. Confounding is evaluated by investing the change in regression coefficient of the variable of interest in an analysis without the possible confounder and with the possible confounder. Again, a change of more than 10% is (arbitrarily) seen as relevant. Effect modification is investigated by adding an interaction term to the model. This interaction term is a multiplication of the variable of interest and the possible effect modifier. When the regression coefficient of the interaction term is significant, there is a significant difference in effect. When this is the case, we should report different measures of effect for the different groups of the possible effect modifier.

Conclusion

In this chapter we discussed some basic statistical approaches to analyse data from sports-injury research. In some of the next chapters, this basic information will be used to explain more complicated techniques.

References

1. Kleinbaum, D.C. (1996). *Survival analysis. A self learning text. Statistics in the Health Sciences.* Springer Verlag, New York.
2. Twisk, J.W.R., N. Smidt, W. de Vente (2005). Applied analysis of recurrent events: a practical overview. *J Epidemiol Commun H*, **59**, 706–10.

Part 2

Defining the injury problem

Chapter 4

Injury definitions

Colin Fuller

A fundamental question that must be addressed in research studies investigating the incidence, nature, causation, treatment, and prevention of injuries sustained during sport and exercise is 'what constitutes an injury?'. To many people, discussion about the definition of an injury is an unnecessary, over-complex, theoretical debate about what is essentially a simple issue. At first sight this may appear to be true, as most people, when asked, intuitively feel they can define an injury. Unfortunately, as the issue is examined in more detail, it becomes apparent that defining an injury for research purposes is not quite so simple. Importantly, the severity, nature, and causes of injuries reported in research studies depend directly on the injury-definition adopted[1]. Resolving the complexities associated with defining an injury for the purpose of sports epidemiology and reaching a consensus agreement about the definition is, therefore, a crucial matter; otherwise differences between studies will create anomalies when attempting to benchmark levels of injury risk, identify the nature and causes of injury, and develop and evaluate injury prevention, treatment, and rehabilitation strategies. Without a general agreement on the definition of an injury, research studies will continue to produce inconsistent results and conflicting conclusions[2].

Although the problems caused by a lack of agreement on injury definitions in injury-surveillance studies have been recognized and discussed in the sports medicine literature for many years, it is only since 2005 that positive attempts have been made to develop an international consensus on the definition of a sports injury. Although these efforts have remained largely sport-specific (cricket [3], football [4], rugby union [5], and rugby league [6]), there is a convergence towards the injury definition proposed for football. Factors that impact on the definition of injury are discussed in this chapter and the effect that variations in injury definition can have on the reported values of incidence, severity, nature, and causes of sports injury are illustrated using data from a large injury-surveillance study.

Definition of injury

Definitions of injury can be discussed in both theoretical and operational terms. Langley and Brenner[7] stressed the difficulties of producing a theoretical definition that differentiated between an injury and a disease on the grounds that there were no clear scientific distinctions between the two conditions. However, the view that an injury relates to physical damage to the body's tissues as a consequence of energy transfer and develops over a short period of time while a disease relates to pathologies that develop over longer periods of time has achieved a level of acceptance. This theoretical definition of injury does, however, leave a number of questions. Osteoarthritis and other chronic conditions – which are common pathological sequelae of injury amongst athletes and develop over several years – would be excluded from the 'injury' category on the basis of the time to appear. In addition, psychological damage would be excluded on the grounds that it does not manifest itself as a physical complaint even though the condition may be a sequelae of a severe traumatic injury. Other conditions – such as hypothermia and hypoxia – which arguably result from the absence rather than the transfer of energy, would also be excluded, even though the conditions are important in some sport and leisure activities. Despite these concerns, a physical complaint caused by a transfer of energy that exceeds the body's ability to maintain its structural and/or functional integrity and which manifests itself within a short period of time following an adverse event remains the best theoretical definition available at the present time for sports-injury research.

For most researchers in sport and exercise medicine, defining an injury is not a matter of theoretical discussions about the differences between injuries, diseases, syndromes, etc., but a matter of defining simple, pragmatic, consistent, operational criteria that describe an injury and that can be applied across a range of sports medicine research topics. For example, it is essential that the incidence and severity of injuries are reported consistently by all researchers involved with injury surveillance, prevention, treatment, and rehabilitation. Similarly, when inter-study comparisons of techniques for the treatment and rehabilitation of injuries are made, the results relate to similar injuries with similar severities. Unfortunately, many operational injury-reporting systems avoid the difficult issue of defining an injury and rely on providing a list of categories that describe the nature, location, and cause of conditions. This is the approach adopted in both the International Classification of Diseases[8] and the Occupational Injury and Illness Classification[9] systems.

An effective operational definition of injury for sports medicine research requires setting criteria that describe (i) what conditions should be counted as a case (or injury), (ii) how the severity of the injury should be measured, (iii) how the injury should be classified in terms of location and pathology, and (iv) what the underlying cause of the injury was.

Definition of a case in injury surveillance studies

The injury definition articulated in the consensus statement for football[4] received general acceptance in the subsequent statements produced for other sports; namely, rugby union[5], rugby league[6], and the Olympic Games[10]. The following definition of injury is therefore proposed as being appropriate for application within most sport and exercise activities:

> Any physical complaint (caused by a transfer of energy that exceeds the body's ability to maintain its structural and/or functional integrity) sustained by an athlete during competition or training directly related to the sport or exercise activity investigated, irrespective of the need for medical attention or time-loss from athletic activity.

As an operational definition, it is debatable whether the qualifying phrase 'caused by a transfer of energy that exceeds the body's ability to maintain its structural and/or functional integrity' should be included because the person recording the injury is unlikely to know whether a transfer of energy had actually taken place. The matter of whether energy transfer took place is even arguably superfluous because damage can only take place when there is a transfer of energy. In the definition proposed, 'medical attention' refers to an assessment conducted by a medical practitioner, these injuries may therefore range from onsite first aid to hospitalization. Not every physical complaint meeting the criteria described in the definition will, however, be included within every injury-surveillance study. The definition is intended to be comprehensive and to include a wide range of injuries from minimal tissue damage at one end to a fatality at the other end of the injury spectrum. Whilst it may be necessary to investigate very minor injuries in some specific studies, the inclusion of every injury would impose unacceptable workloads on medical practitioners and researchers, which would inevitably lead to poor compliance. The baseline definition of injury should therefore be qualified by defining the minimum severity of injury that should be recorded in the study (Box 4.1). Injuries to athletes that are not directly related to the sport environment being investigated should not be counted.

Box 4.1 The effect of the case definition for injury severity on the reported number and incidence of injuries

This example shows how variations in the case definition of injury severity (i.e. time loss, missed match, required surgery) affect the reported incidence of injury.

Case definition of injury severity	Number of injuries included in study	Incidence of injury*	95% confidence interval
>1 days' absence	2184	88.7	85.1–92.5
≥1 match absence	986	40.0	37.6–42.6
Required surgery	120	4.9	4.1–5.9

*injuries/1000 player hours

By using the missed-match definition of injury for an injury case, the incidence of injury would be reduced to <50% of the value obtained using the time loss definition and by using injuries requiring surgery as the case definition the incidence would be reduced even further to ~5% of the time loss value.

For some research studies, further clarification of the baseline-injury definition may be required in order to differentiate between 'new' and 'recurrent' injuries[4]. For example, an index injury is recognized as a major risk factor for subsequent injuries of the same type at the same site. When differentiating between index and recurrent injuries, it is essential that the primary definition of injury described above be adopted but with the additional criterion that a recurrent injury is:

> An injury of the same type and at the same site as an index injury that occurs after an athlete's return to full participation in training and/or competition from the index injury.

The time elapsed since an athlete's return to competition or training following an index injury to the time of the recurrent injury should be recorded, as this time provides a subjective indicator of whether the recurrence is likely to be a consequence of incomplete rehabilitation from the index injury. Recurrences occurring within 2 months of an athlete's return to competition or training are referred to as 'early recurrences'[4]. In some studies, a recurrence has been defined as a second injury of the same type and at the same site as an index injury and which occurred in the same year, the same season, or within 12 months of the index injury. This additional limitation on the definition of a recurrence creates anomalies and should be avoided because the more severe an index injury is the less likely it will be that an athlete would recover within the time-scale specified and this would reduce the possibility that an athlete could experience a further injury within the specified time period. If this definition is used, severe injuries therefore appear less likely to result in recurrences than if the preferred definition is used (Box 4.2).

It is important to emphasize that an injury should only be recorded as a recurrence if the second injury occurs at the same site rather than just at the same general body location (e.g. lower limb or thigh). Even with this requirement, it is not always possible to confirm that the second injury occurred at exactly the same point in a structure as the index injury, so there will always be some doubt as to whether an injury of this nature is actually a recurrence or is in fact a new, index injury. Reliance on athletes self-reporting previous injuries should be avoided as this raises the issue of recall bias. Injuries such as contusions and lacerations – which are more likely to occur at

Box 4.2 The effect of the case definitions of injury severity and recurrence on the reported proportion of recurrent injuries

This example examines the combined effects of variations in the case definitions of severity and recurrent injury (i.e. clinical judgement, same site/same type/recorded in same season as the index injury).

Case definition of injury severity	Proportion of injuries reported as a recurrence (%)	
	Clinical judgement	Injured in same season
>1 days' absence	14.9	9.6
≥1 match absence	6.9	4.5
Required surgery	1.0	0.6

By restricting the criteria for a recurrent injury to an injury that occurred in the same season as the index injury reduced the proportion of injuries reported as recurrences by ~1/3, irrespective of the case definition of severity used in the study.

a particular site solely by chance mechanisms rather than as a consequence of the index injury – should not normally be recorded as recurrent injuries. It should be noted that an injured athlete's recovery from an index injury is defined pragmatically by the athlete's return to training and competition rather than by a clinical judgement of when the injury is fully recovered. This pragmatic approach is particularly necessary in the context of elite sport in order to avoid wide variations in the interpretation and recording of when an injury is fully recovered, as elite athletes often return to training and competition before they are completely pain free.

Because an index injury is closed when the injured athlete returns to full training or competition, any subsequent period of absence caused by an injury of the same type at the same site would be recorded as a new, recurrent injury. However, as discussed above, there are often circumstances when athletes return to training or competition before they are fully recovered and subsequent injuries of the same type at the same site could be an exacerbation of the original index injury rather than a new injury. To accommodate this common scenario, Fuller et al.[11] proposed that when an injury-surveillance study is focussed on studying risk factors for recurrent injuries or the effectiveness of treatment and rehabilitation strategies, recurrences should be subdivided into 're-injuries' (i.e. injuries occurring after the index injury had fully recovered) and 'exacerbations' (i.e. injuries occurring when the index injury had not fully recovered). In this situation, fully recovered is determined by the clinical judgement of an appropriate medical professional.

Injury severity

The second facet of injury-definition relates to the severity of the injury and this can be sub-divided into two subsidiary issues. The first issue being the minimum severity of injury that should be recorded and, the second issue being the 'return to fitness' criteria, which determines when an injury is considered closed. A hierarchy of injury severities has been adopted in epidemiological studies; namely, in increasing level of severity – tissue damage, time loss, match loss, hospitalization, catastrophic, and fatal; the severity criteria adopted to define a case significantly affects the mean and median severities of injury reported in a study (Box 4.3). If recorded injuries include superficial

Box 4.3 The effect of the case definition of injury severity on the reported mean and median severity of injury

The case definition of injury severity used in a study has a profound impact on the mean and median severities of injuries reported when reported as the number of days lost from training and competition.

Case definition of injury severity	Injury severity (days)	
	Mean	Median
>1 days' absence	18.2	7
≥1 match absence	33.6	20
Required surgery	102.4	97

In addition to the gross differences observed in the reported mean and median severity values, the median severity value approaches the mean value as the case definition of severity for injuries included in the study increases.

tissue injuries, such as abrasions and bruises, the number of injuries recorded will be very high, mean and median severity values will be lower, and the distribution of injury types will be biased towards muscle injuries. If, on the other hand, the definition focusses on injuries treated within a hospital, minor injuries will already have been filtered out so that only the more severe injuries will be recorded; in this case, the number of injuries will be smaller, mean, and median severity values will be higher, and injury distributions will be biased towards joint and bone injuries (Box 4.4).

Box 4.4 The effect of the case definition of injury severity on the reported distribution of injury types

This example demonstrates how the nature of injuries reported is dependent on the case definition of injury severity used in the study.

Structure injured	Case definition of injury severity (% of injuries)		
	>1 days' absence	≥1 match absence	Required surgery
Bone	4.7	9.1	25.2
Joint (non-bone), ligament	38.0	42.4	53.9
Muscle, tendon	46.0	36.9	15.7
Skin	1.4	0.8	1.7
Central and peripheral nervous system	9.9	10.8	3.5

These results highlight that if surgery is the entry requirement for a case, joint (non-bone)/ligament represents the major type of injury followed by bone injuries, whereas if the time loss definition is used muscle/tendon injuries represent the major type followed by joint (non-bone)/ligament injuries.

It should be recognized that no injury-surveillance study is capable of recording every injury covered by the injury definition presented above. Some surveillance studies may be specifically interested in recording 'medical attention' injuries if the main research interest is, e.g. an examination of the impact of minor injuries on long-term sequelae such as osteoarthritis. Most injury-surveillance studies, however, are more concerned about injuries that have an immediate impact on the ability of an athlete to continue training and playing or assessing the personal, social, or financial implications of injury[12]. For this reason, most injury-surveillance studies qualify the definition of injury to cover those injuries resulting in an athlete being unable to take part in training or competition on the day following the event. In these studies, injury severity is defined as:

> The number of days elapsed from the date of injury to the date of the athlete's return to full participation in training and availability for competition.

The day on which an athlete sustains the injury and the day he/she returns to training or competition are not included when counting the number of days' absence. Sometimes, a single injury event may result in more than one injury; on these occasions, it is essential to differentiate between the overall severity of the injury event (determined by the most severe injury) and the severity of the other, less severe, injuries. Although the definition of injury severity provides a very pragmatic determinant of severity, it is still subject to a number of confounding factors. Pain tolerance varies between athletes significantly and this impacts on when an athlete feels ready to return to training and competition. Physicians, similarly, have different views on what constitutes an acceptable level of pain for athletes to experience when returning from injury. At the professional level, particularly with team sports, return to training and competition may also be influenced by squad size, the importance of upcoming games, and decisions on whether to delay the treatment of chronic complaints until the end of the season. Different athletes have access to different levels of medical support, which impacts on the quality of the treatment and rehabilitation received and consequently the time taken for athletes to return to full fitness. Additionally, some physicians advocate the use of medication, such as local anaesthetics, to allow an athlete to return to sport at an earlier date[13,14]. These factors all contribute to the observed variation in the number of days that different athletes require to recover from apparently identical injuries.

There are three categories of injury that do not fit easily within the time-loss definition of severity; namely, career ending, non-fatal catastrophic, and fatal injuries. These injuries present problems because it is not sensible to record the time loss in these cases as the remainder of the athlete's expected sporting career or as their anticipated life span because this would grossly distort the mean injury-severity value in a study; there would, however, be little impact on the median injury-severity value reported for the study. Rare injuries of this type are, therefore, counted but normally reported separately from the other time-loss injuries within an epidemiological study. Careful consideration should be given to what constitutes a 'career-ending injury', as the level of athlete participation in a study is often a major contributory factor. For example, in football, a broken fibula combined with a dislocated ankle would almost certainly be categorized as a career-ending injury for most amateur players, whereas for a professional player, although it would represent a very severe injury, it would not be career ending as the player would most probably have access to the appropriate medical support. Non-fatal catastrophic injuries were defined in the rugby union consensus statement[5] as:

> A brain or spinal cord injury that resulted in permanent (>12 months) severe functional disability.

In this context, the World Health Organization's[8] definition of severe functional disability (i.e. loss of more than 50% of the capability of a structure) was adopted.

Although it is preferable to record injuries based on a time-loss definition, it has been argued that this is not always practicable and that a better option is to record only those injuries resulting in an athlete missing competitive activities[15]. While injury severity based on missed competition does provide a simpler methodology, it limits the utility of the data collected[16]. If severity is recorded solely as the number of matches missed, minor injuries resulting in <7 days absence will be lost to the study and this will result in (i) a lower incidence of injury being reported, (ii) little discrimination between injuries lasting from 7 to 13 days, (iii) mean and median injury-severity values being inflated compared to studies using a lost-time definition, and (iv) lack of sensitivity for investigations of the efficacy of injury-prevention and rehabilitation strategies, as it will be more difficult to quantify reductions in injury severity. The use of the missed-match definition of severity also creates large discrepancies in the number of injuries recorded within individual, same-sport, and cross-sport studies. The basic assumption made in the argument for using missed-match injuries is convenience and that the time between competitive activities is constant. A fixed time between competitive activities may be true in some circumstances but it cannot be relied on to provide the consistency required for an effective injury-surveillance protocol. For example, in Europe the national football and rugby union seasons involve league, cup, and European matches and there are weeks set aside for international matches; additionally, the days on which individual games are played are frequently determined by television companies. Therefore, depending on the time of the season, television requirements, and the player's individual and club performances, some players could be involved in either none or up to three games in a single week; this means the case definition is inconsistent within the study, as the severity criteria could vary from 2 to 14 days. If the missed-match definition were extended into other sports, such as athletics, sailing, tennis, and golf, even larger discrepancies could arise because an athlete may wait several weeks between competitive meetings by which time an injury is more likely to have recovered and therefore not be recorded as an injury case.

In some studies it may be appropriate to group time-loss injuries into general categories such as '1 to 3 days', '4 to 7 days', '1 to 4 weeks', '1 to 3 months', 'greater than 3 months', 'career-ending', and 'catastrophic' injuries. Although this approach is useful when it is not possible to record the exact number of days' absence, it restricts the application of the information in studies related to the risk of injury and injury prevention[17] because it is not possible to calculate the mean or median number of days' lost through injury.

Injury classification

The third facet of injury definition is the ability to classify each injury in terms of the body region affected, the structure involved, and the exact nature of the injury sustained. Established protocols for classifying injuries exist, including the International Classification of Diseases (ICD) system developed by the World Health Organization[8] and the Occupational Injury and Illness Classification (OIIC) system developed by the US Department of Labor[9]. These systems, however, have limited application in sports medicine because of their lack of relevant, sport-specific detail; e.g. an anterior cruciate ligament injury would be categorized in the OIIC system[9] simply as a 'knee' 'traumatic ligament injury'. Langley and Brenner[7] discussed a number of limitations associated with the widely used ICD system while Rae et al.[18] and Finch and Boufous[19] highlighted shortcomings in the system in the context of its specific application to sports medicine. It is generally accepted that sport-specific injury-classification systems, such as the alpha-numeric coding systems developed in Australia by Orchard[20] and in Canada by Meeuwisse and Wiley[21], are preferable for sports medicine research.

Table 4.1 Recommended injured body regions and OSICS classification codes[4,5]

Body region injured		OSICS Version 8
Main group	Sub-group	
Head, neck	Head, face	H
	Neck, cervical spine	N
Upper limb	Shoulder, clavicle	S
	Upper arm	U
	Elbow	E
	Forearm	R
	Wrist	W
	Hand, fingers	P
Trunk	Sternum, ribs, upper back	C, D
	Abdomen	O
	Lower back, pelvis, sacrum	B, L
Lower limb	Hip, groin	G
	Thigh	T
	Knee,	K
	Lower leg, Achilles tendon	Q, A
	Ankle,	A
	Foot, toe	F

The Orchard Sports Injury Classification System (OSICS) is currently available either as a 3-character (OSICS v8)[20] or a 4-character (OSICS v10)[22] coding system. The first character (coded A–Z) in the 3-character system identifies the anatomical location, the second character (coded A–Z) the injury pathology, while the third character (coded 1–9 and A–Z) provides a more detailed pathology. With the 4-character system, the first character (A–Z) again identifies the anatomical location and the second character (A–Z) the pathology with the third and fourth characters (A–Z) providing an even more detailed subdivision of the injury diagnosis. A comparison between the ICD-10 and OSICS (v8) systems for recording sports injuries indicated that the OSICS sports-specific system was more appropriate and easier to use for sports physicians. [18] The Sports Medicine Diagnostic Coding System (SMDCS)[21] also uses a 3-character coding system; however, with SMDCS each character comprises double digits, which provides the possibility of greater specificity than either the OSICS 3-character (v8) or 4-character (v10) single-digit systems. With SMDCS, the first pair of digits (AA–ZZ) identifies the body region, the second pair of digits (00–99) the type of structure, and the third pair of digits (00–99) the diagnosis code. The recommended body region and structure groupings used in injury-surveillance studies[4,5] are shown in Tables 4.1 and 4.2, respectively, with the corresponding OSICS (v8) codes included for comparison.

Injury causation

Finally, injuries should be defined in terms of whether they are traumatic (i.e. caused by a single, specific, and identifiable event) or gradual-onset (i.e. caused by repeated micro-trauma without

Table 4.2 Recommended injury structures and OSICS classification codes[4,5]

Structure injured		OSICS Version 8
Main group	**Sub-group**	
Bone	Fracture	F
	Other bone injuries	G, Q, S
Joint (non-bone), ligament	Dislocation, subluxation	D, U
	Sprain, ligament injury	J, L
	Lesion of meniscus, cartilage, disc	C
Muscle, tendon	Muscle rupture, tear, strain, cramps	M, Y
	Tendon injury, rupture, tendinopathy, bursitis	T, R
	Haematoma, contusion, bruise	H
Skin	Abrasion	K
	Laceration	K
Central and peripheral nervous systems	Concussion	N
	Structural brain injury	
	Spinal cord compression, transection	N
	Nerve injury	N
Other	Dental injury	G
	Visceral injury	O
	Other injuries	

evidence of a single, identifiable event) injuries (Box 4.5). Gradual-onset injuries are sometimes referred to as 'overuse' injuries but there is debate about the efficacy of using this term to define this type of injury. It has been argued that injuries classified as 'overuse' in sports clinics may be influenced by the fact that sports physicians are more likely to deal with athletes who train and compete extensively; the injuries may be equally prevalent in less active athletes[23]. It is also argued that there is little evidence of a relationship between the level of an athlete's activity and

Box 4.5 The effect of the case definition of injury severity on reported injury causation

The final example shows that the case definition of injury severity adopted in a study has less effect on the reported causation of injuries than it has on the other outcome factors discussed above.

Case definition of injury severity	Injury causation, %	
	Acute	**Gradual onset**
>1 days' absence	90.4	9.6
≥1 match absence	90.1	9.9
Required surgery	84.2	15.8

overuse injuries and importantly a level of activity above which an overuse injury manifests itself. Without this evidence, it could be argued that an overuse injury is simply related to the athlete's level of exposure in the same way that a traumatic injury is[23]. An argument has also been postulated that if the term overuse is used to define an injury, there should be a category referred to as an 'underuse' injury which occurs when an athlete is injured as a consequence of being under-trained or under-prepared[24].

Impact of injury definition on the study outcomes

The examples, which are referred to in the textboxes, are based on data from a 6-year study of match injuries sustained by professional rugby union players during Premier league matches in England. In total, 2184 match injuries resulted in players losing time from competition and or training, of which 986 injuries caused the player to miss one or more subsequent matches and 120 required surgery, and 24 634 player-hours of match exposure were recorded. Injuries were classified according to the Orchard Sports Injury Classification System (v8).

Conclusion

The discussion presented has identified a number of injury-definition issues that must be considered when establishing an injury-surveillance study. Criteria based on established, published consensus statements that should be integrated into an operational injury-definition are presented. The examples described demonstrate the importance of using consistent injury-definitions and they highlight the magnitude of the differences that could be observed in reported values if definitions are varied from study to study. It is not possible to eliminate all sources of operational inconsistency related to injury-definition in injury-surveillance studies; grey areas associated with the interpretation and implementation of the definitions will always remain. However, the adoption of consistent criteria for defining injuries will undoubtedly increase the level of consistency achievable.

References

1. Meeuwisse WH, Love EJ (1997). Athletic injury reporting. Development of universal systems. *Sports Med*, **24**, 184–204.
2. Brooks JHM, Fuller CW (2006). The influence of methodological issues on the results and conclusions from epidemiological studies of sports injuries: illustrative examples. *Sports Med*, **36**, 459–72.
3. Orchard JW, Newman D, Stretch R, Frost W, Mansingh A, Leipus A (2005). Methods for injury surveillance in international cricket. *Br J Sports Med*, **39**, e22.
4. Fuller CW, Ekstrand J, Junge A, Andersen TE, Bahr R, Dvorak J, Hägglund M, McCrory P, Meeuwisse WH (2006). Consensus statement on injury definitions and data collection procedures in studies of football (soccer) injuries. *Clin J Sport Med*, **16**, 97–106.
5. Fuller CW, Molloy MG, Bagate C, Bahr R, Brooks JHM, Donson H, Kemp SPT, McCrory P, McIntosh AS, Meeuwisse WH, Quarrie KL, Raftery M, Wiley P (2007). Consensus statement on injury definitions and data collection procedures for studies of injuries in rugby union. *Clin J Sport Med*, **17**, 177–81.
6. King DA, Gabbett TJ, Gissane C, Hodgson L (2009). Epidemiological studies of injuries in rugby league: Suggestions for definitions, data collection and reporting methods. *J Sci Med Sport*, **12**, 12–19.
7. Langley J, Brenner R (2004) What is an injury? *Inj Prev*, **10**, 69–71.
8. World Health Organization (2001). *International Classification of Functioning, Disability and Health System (ICF)*. World Health Organization: Geneva.
9. Bureau of Labor Statistics (2007). *Occupational injury and illness classification manual*. US Department of Labor; Washington. www.bls.gov/iif/osh_oiics_1.pdf (Accessed on 1 February 2009)

10. Junge A, Engebretsen L, Alonso JM, Renström P, Mountjoy M, Aubry M, Dvorak J (2008). Injury surveillance in multi-sport events: the International Olympic Committee approach. *Br. J. Sports Med,* **42,** 413–21.

11. Fuller CW, Bahr R, Dick RW, Meeuwisse WH (2007). A framework for recording recurrences, reinjuries, and exacerbations in injury surveillance. *Clin J Sport Med,* **17,** 197–200.

12. van Mechelen W (1997). The severity of sports injuries. *Sports Med,* **24,** 176–80.

13. Orchard JW (2002). Benefits and risks of using local anaesthetic for pain relief to allow early return to play in professional football. *Br J Sports Med,* **36,** 209–13.

14. Orchard J (2004). Missed time through injury and injury management at an NRL club. *Sport Health,* **22,** 11–19.

15. Orchard J, Hoskins W (2007). For debate: consensus injury definitions in team sports should focus on missed playing time. *Clin J Sport Med,* **17,** 192–6.

16. Hodgson L, Gissane C, Gabbett TJ, King DA (2007). For Debate: Consensus injury definitions in team sports should focus on encompassing all injuries. *Clin J Sport Med,* **17,** 188–91.

17. Fuller CW (2007). Managing the risk of injury in sport. *Clin J Sport Med,* **17,** 182–7.

18. Rae K, Britt H, Orchard J, Finch C (2005). Classifying sports medicine diagnoses: a comparison of the International Classification of Diseases 10 – Australian Modification (ICD-10-AM) and the Orchard Sports Injury Classification System (OSICS – 8). *Br J Sports Med,* **39,** 907–11.

19. Finch CF, Boufous S (2008). Do inadequacies in ICD-10-AM activity coded data lead to underestimates of the population frequency of sports/leisure injuries? *Inj Prev,* **14,** 202–4.

20. Orchard J (1993). Orchard sports injury classification system (OSICS). *Sport Health,* **11,** 39–41.

21. Meeuwisse WH, Wiley JP (2007). The sports medicine diagnostic coding system. *Clin J Sport Med,* **17,** 205–7.

22. Rae K, Orchard J (2007). The Orchard sports injury classification system (OSICS) version 10. *Clin J Sport Med 2007,* **17,** 201–4.

23. Gregory PL (2002). "Overuse" – an overused term? *Br J Sports Med,* **36,** 82–3.

24. Stovitz SD, Johnson RJ (2006). "Underuse" as a cause for musculoskeletal injuries: is it time that we started reframing our message? *Br J Sports Med,* **40,** 738–9.

Chapter 5

Research designs for descriptive studies

Jennifer Hootman

As briefly introduced in Chapter 2, a descriptive study is one in which the primary purpose is to describe current or past phenomena such as disease or injury. These types of studies can describe characteristics or experiences, reveal patterns, generate hypotheses, and assist in needs assessment and resource allocation. Descriptive studies are typically the first step in investigating a research question but also serve as primary sources of data for displaying and tracking the prevalence or incidence and impact of a variety of health conditions including sports injuries[1, 2].

Often, descriptive studies paint a picture of sports injuries by answering questions such as how big is the problem, who is affected (person), where does it occur (place), and when does it occur (time) (Figs. 5.1, 5.2, and 5.3). However, the 'description' of injury can be presented in many ways. For example, injuries may be described by severity, the place of occurrence, a specific sub-population, the type of injury, the site of injury, the activity or sport, the level of play, the mechanism, and many other categories[2].

Descriptive studies emphasize the estimation of injury occurrence and related characteristics rather than test hypotheses. Examples of things that can be estimated include prevalence and incidence of injuries; characteristics associated with prevalence/incidence; indicators of impact (e.g. health-care utilization) of injuries in the population or a subgroup; injury patterns over time – natural history of an injury; resources required to treat/respond; and knowledge, attitudes, and behaviours.

Types of descriptive studies

Arguably the two most common types of descriptive study designs used in sports-injury research are ecologic and cross-sectional studies. Other study designs can be used descriptively, but the focus of this chapter will be to provide examples and data sources for the most commonly used descriptive designs. The pros and cons of ecologic and cross-sectional study designs are listed in Table 5.1.

Ecologic studies

Ecologic study designs compare data that are aggregated at the group level. Since data is only available at the group level – and not for individuals within the group – ecologic studies often are considered low in terms of strength of evidence. In addition, they cannot be used to determine causal relationships because the temporal sequence between exposures and outcomes cannot be ascertained. However, these studies can be useful for assessing the initial relationships between variables of interest, especially variables that represent contextual measures at the macro-societal level[3].

Disclaimer: "The findings and conclusions in this chapter are those of the author and do not necessarily represent the official position of the Centers for Disease Control and Prevention."

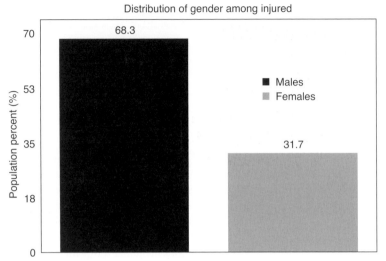

Fig. 5.1 Data describing person characteristics of sports- and recreational-injury episodes in the United States.
Adapted from Conn et al.[8]

They can be done relatively inexpensively and easily because they (i) often use data already collected for other purposes (birth and death records, registries, population health surveys, etc.), and (ii) do not require direct contact with subjects for data collection. Together, these qualities can reduce the complexity of human subjects and confidentiality-protection processes involved in research.

To understand the usefulness and some of the potential biases that arise from ecologic study designs, lets consider the following example. Fig. 5.4 shows data from National Federation of State High School Associations and the National Electronic Injury Surveillance System (NEISS).

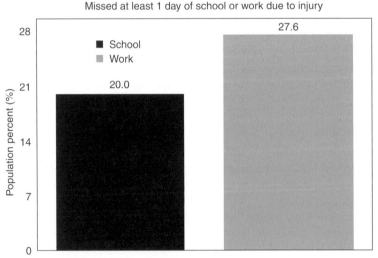

Fig. 5.2 Data describing place characteristics of sports- and recreational-injury episodes in the United States.
Adapted from Conn et al.[8]

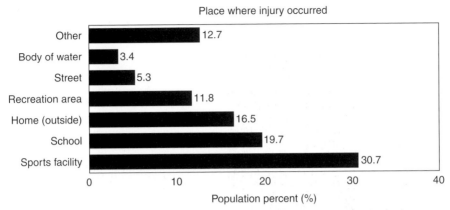

Fig. 5.3 Data describing time characteristics of sports- and recreational-injury episodes in the United States.
Adapted from Conn et al.[8]

We are interested in the possible association between increased participation (exposure) in a sport and the sport-related injuries (outcome). We would suspect that as the participation increases so would the incidence of injuries because more people are being exposed to potential injury. We have group level data on the number of high school students participating in soccer over a 10-year period. We also have estimates of soccer-related injuries seen in emergency rooms over the same time period.

Looking at the graph we see that as the number of youth participating in high school soccer goes up so does the number of emergency department visits for soccer-related injuries amongst youth in the age group 14–18 years. This relationship makes sense, but does not tell the whole story. First, the data on participation (exposure) and injury (outcome) come from two different sources. Therefore, we cannot say for sure that the injuries seen in the emergency department came directly from the population of high school soccer players. For example, a 16-year-old may have been injured and treated in an emergency department while playing soccer on a community-based soccer league or in their backyard and not while playing for their high school team. This level of detailed information is not available in the NEISS database. In addition, the source of data on participation may exclude a significant part of the high school population (e.g. private high schools are not included). This could be a source of bias if private schools offer soccer more often than public schools. Second, these data do not account for the within-area variation in participation and injury patterns that may occur across schools and communities. Participation in soccer at the high school level varies widely from community-to-community. Some high schools and even entire school districts do not offer soccer as an interscholastic sport. So, in communities where soccer is not offered at high schools, there should very low rates of soccer-related emergency department visits.

Ecologic fallacy – falsely inferring that associations between exposures and outcomes at the group level apply to individuals within that group – is the specific bias associated with ecologic study designs[4, 5]. Although ecological studies are prone to most all types of bias (See Chapter 2), the two most common sources are misclassification bias and specification bias[3, 5]. In ecologic sports-injury studies, misclassification bias related to exposure measurement is likely a large contributor to bias. In the above example, the exposure (numbers of high school soccer participants) is a crude measure of actual exposure to the risk of injury because among high school soccer participants the range of exposure to injury is large. For instance, exposure to potential injury events would vary for junior varsity versus varsity players, first string versus reserve, etc.

Table 5.1 Types, characteristics, and select examples of descriptive-injury research-study designs

Study type	Characteristics	
	Pros	**Cons**
Ecologic	Assess initial relationships between an outcome and a broad continuum of exposures	Group aggregated data, cannot assess exposure/outcome status of individuals
	Use existing data; relatively inexpensive to do	Seasonal (e.g. migration of population) and other local or regional events (e.g. natural disasters) may severely affect validity and interpretation of results
	Macro-societal level associations between exposures and outcomes	'Loss of information' when using aggregated summary measures; may obscure relationships; aggregate data are often based on administrative or political units and are poor contextual measures
	Best when variance occurs at the group level	
	Newer advanced statistical techniques allow for a combination of data from ecologic and individual sources (multilevel analysis)	May need information from external secondary sources to aid interpretation
	Stratification of exposure data may improve potential bias; Limited by the availability of sufficient details in the dataset, typically information on only 1 or 2 potential confounding variables are available	Relationships can be very sensitive to the grouping definition
		Changes in relationships based on different assumptions are rarely done
		Cannot determine cause and effect
		Direction of non-differential misclassification bias is not always predictable; may be highly sensitive to error in exposure measurement
Cross-sectional and surveillance	Measures injury burden and impact (e.g. prevalence)	Study design not based on case or exposure status
	Provides distributions of exposures, outcomes and characteristics in the population	Cannot determine cause and effect due to lack of temporal sequencing of exposure and outcome
	Describe person, place and time	
	Hypothesis generating	Potentially unreliable estimates for rare conditions due to small sample sizes
	Identify potential risk/preventive factors	
	Assess resource needs and allocation	Outcome and exposures are often self-reported and may not be verified
	Monitor trends over time	
	Evaluate effectiveness of interventions	Surveys can have low response rates and subsequent poor generalizability
	Relatively easy, quick, and lower cost (cost-efficient)	Over-represents prevalence in conditions with long duration and under-represents prevalence in conditions with short duration
	Population samples do not rely on individuals accessing the medical care system	
		Less sensitive to conditions that re-occur or are seasonal

Despite these drawbacks, ecologic studies can be useful sources of information on sports injuries at the population level when done with methodological rigour, particularly by incorporating newer, more sophisticated, multilevel analysis techniques[3, 4].

Cross-sectional studies

In cross-sectional studies, exposures and outcomes are measured at one point in time, and are often called a 'snapshots' or 'slices' of the population[1, 6]. The 'snapshot' time period can range

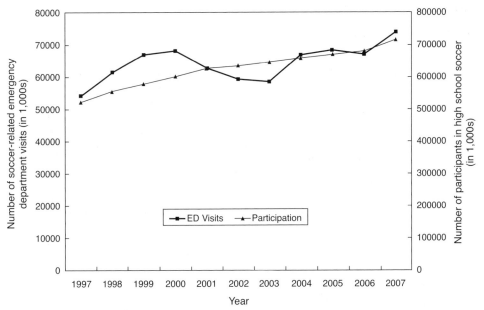

Fig. 5.4 Example of an ecologic study using group-level exposure* and outcome** data.
* Exposure data source: National Federation of State High School Associations sport participation statistics available at: http://www.nfhs.org/custom/participation_figures/default.aspx.
** Outcome data source: National Electronic Injury Surveillance System (NEISS) online query system available at https://www.cpsc.gov/cgibin/NEISSQuery/home.aspx. Search limited to age range 14–18 years and product code 1267 (Soccer Activity, Apparel Or Equipment).

from minutes or days, to months or years. These studies capture prevalent cases of disease or injury, cases that are existing at a single moment of time.

Cross-sectional studies are useful for assessing the overall burden (e.g. prevalence) and impact (disability, health-care utilization, etc.) of sports injuries in a population. They provide valuable information on the distribution of exposures, outcomes, and their associated characteristics. They can be used to (i) generate hypotheses; (ii) assess the need for and allocation of resources; (iii) monitor changes over time in population health states; and (iv) assess the effectiveness of interventions[6]. Measures of association between an exposure and an outcome can be calculated based on the ratio of events in those exposed and unexposed (also see Chapter 6). This information can help identify potential risk or preventive factors that can be further verified in longitudinal studies. The drawback of cross-sectional studies is the lack of temporal sequencing and therefore cannot be used to determine cause and effect. Because exposures and outcomes are measured simultaneously, the true timing of the exposure before the outcome is unknown.

Cross-sectional data is most commonly gathered from surveys, but can also come from interviews or examinations of persons in the population. Surveys can be done using the telephone, in-person interviews, or self-reported instruments. Survey research has a specific defined set of methods and a detailed description of how to go about conducting a survey research study is out of the scope of this text. However, survey research usually involves the following general steps[7]:

♦ Identification of the population of interest and topic area

♦ Developing, testing, and validating the survey instrument

♦ Identifying a sampling frame, sample size, and taking a sample of the population

- Administering the survey
- Collecting, entering, and cleaning data
- Analysing data

Examples of descriptive sports injury epidemiology studies

Two types of approaches are common with cross-sectional data – describing the population (descriptive) with measures of injury occurrence and quantifying the relationship between exposure and outcomes (analytic) using measures of association. To illustrate the differences in the these types of cross-sectional analyses we can use data from the National Health Interview Survey (NHIS), an annual in-person interview health survey conducted annually in the United States (US). The NHIS samples households from the US population, selects children and adults from each household, and administers a standardized survey on a variety of health topics, including information on injury episodes and their causes experienced in the past 3 months. Each year, over 30 000 adults are interviewed and are statistically weighted to represent all civilian, non-institutionalized US residents.

Conn et al.[8] reported the number, population rates, and characteristics of sports- and recreation-injury (SRI) episodes requiring medical attention using the NHIS data. From these data we can describe SRI events in the US population (Fig. 5.1), by answering some questions.

- How many persons experience a SRI per year?
  7 million; 26 SRIs per 1000 people

- Who was most commonly injured?
  64% aged 5–24, 68% males

- Where did SRIs occur?
  31% at sports facilities, 20% at school

- What was the impact?
  20% missed school, 28% missed work

This information can be used to evaluate potential risk factors (e.g. age) in prospective studies as well as to target specific population subgroups for interventions. For example, these data suggest that school-age children have higher population rates of SRI, many of which occur at school facilities and result in one of five children missing at least 1 day of school. Injury-prevention campaigns and interventions can be effectively targeted at schools and parents of school-age children to reduce SRIs in this subgroup.

This descriptive information is important and has many uses, but we cannot assess the relationship between the level of exposure (frequency or hours of participation in physical activity) and the outcome (injury) because there is no information on how often a person may be exposed to a potential injury situation. Some people do not participate in physical activity at all and thus have no real opportunity to be injured. Others participate daily in physical activity and subsequently have many cumulative opportunities to be injured. Carlson et al.[9] used NHIS data to investigate the association between participation in leisure-time physical activity and injury. These data show that the rate of SRIs increase with increasing levels of leisure-time physical activity as expected, but rates of non-SR injuries (e.g. motor vehicle-related) were highest among those reporting no leisure-time physical activity (Fig. 5.5). For instance, persons meeting physical activity recommendations are 53% (odds ratio 1.53, 95% confidence interval 1.19–1.98) more likely to report a sports/leisure injury than inactive persons. On the other hand, active persons were 17–19%

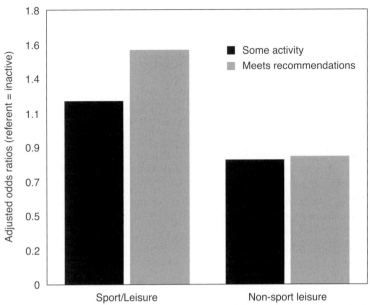

Fig. 5.5 Adjusted odds ratios of sport/leisure and non-sport/leisure injuries by level of leisure-time physical activity.
Adapted from Carlson et al.[9]

less likely to report a non-sport or leisure injury suggesting being physically active confers some protection against non-sport injuries. By breaking down the exposure and injury information into different levels we gain considerable insight into the associations between exposures and outcomes. However, due to the cross-sectional study design we still cannot be sure of the cause-and-effect relationship between leisure-time physical activity and injury.

Data sources for sports injury descriptive studies

Most published data on sports injuries come from four general sources: government databanks, health-care-system records or administrative databases, school or sports organization surveillance or medical record systems, and special studies done by academic or other research institutions. In some databases, data on sports injuries are collected as part of existing, ongoing record keeping (e.g. insurance claims), while others are designed to collect data specifically on the topic of sports injuries in a defined population (e.g. National Collegiate Athletic Association Injury Surveillance System [10]). Horan and Mallonee[11] published a comprehensive review of data sources used for general injury surveillance, some of which can be used for descriptive studies of sports injuries.

Government databases

Governmental organizations often collect health information on the population annually for a variety of reasons. Vital statistic systems record births and deaths as well as associated causes of death. Deaths from injuries can be counted, although at the current time it is difficult to define fatal injuries related to sports and recreation using existing coding systems such as the International

Classification of Disease, tenth Revision (ICD-10) external cause of injury codes. While ICD-10 does have optional activity codes that can identify injuries while 'engaged in sport', however, the specificity of codes and lack of coding guidance limits their use and utility[12]. The ICD-10-AM (Australian Modification) provides more detailed specificity in mapping of ICD-10 codes to specific sports and recreation activities[13].

Governments in many countries collect health information at the population level using health surveys. The NHIS, mentioned above, collects information on medically attended-injury episodes, including sports and recreation injuries. However, the exposure information in the NHIS is limited to self-reported frequency, intensity, and duration of leisure-time physical activity. The Youth Risk Behavior Survey is another large survey of students in grades 9–12 in the US which asks information about physical activity, injury-related behaviours (e.g. wearing bike helmets), and injuries occurring during sports or exercise[14].

Injury data can also be obtained from national surveys done in physician offices and hospitals. The National Ambulatory Medical Care Survey and the National Hospital Ambulatory Medical Care Survey capture patient visits to physician offices, hospital outpatient clinics, and emergency departments and the National Hospital Discharge Survey captures data on patients admitted and discharged from non-federal hospitals[15]. The National Electronic Injury Surveillance System (NEISS) – conducted by the US Consumer Product Safety Commission – is an annual survey of injuries seen in hospital emergency departments that were caused by or associated with a consumer product. In 2000, in partnership with the Centers for Disease Control and Prevention, NEISS was expanded to capture all non-product related injuries[16, 17].

In most governmental surveys, injury cases can be identified using ICD diagnostic and procedure codes, although as noted above, sports and recreation injuries are difficult to ascertain using this coding system. In addition, in both the NHIS and the ambulatory medical care surveys, there is a limited ability to define injury cases using a verbatim text variable. This text variable describes the injury event and circumstances surrounding the event in the patient's own words. Keywords such as 'basketball' or 'cheer-leading' can be identified in the verbatim text and used to define cases of sports and recreation activities. Some information on mechanism of injury (fall, tackle, rebound, etc.) can also be coded from the verbatim text description.

A drawback of these government-subsidized surveys is that exposure data are rarely collected. Participation data from other sources such as sports organizations (National Federation of State High School Associations) or commercial professional groups (e.g. Sporting Goods Manufactures Association) can be used to calculate sports-injury rates[18], but may be a source of bias as discussed above in regards to ecologic studies. However, by adding a few simple questions to these government surveys it is feasible to obtain general measures of exposures, however, adding questions to these large surveys can be expensive. For example, walking is a popular activity widely promoted for health. Asking simple questions about the frequency of walking for exercise or transportation per week and asking about any injuries that happened during a walking episode could provide important information about the prevalence of walking-related injuries in the population.

Health-care system

In addition to the governmental surveys done annually in physician offices and hospital emergency departments described above, other parts of the health-care system can be a source of sports-injury data[11]. Trip or 'run' logs from the emergency medical system, such as ambulance and/or paramedic calls, can capture data on sports injuries, particularly information about the scene or place where the injury occurred – information often not captured in emergency department or other health-care-records databases. For example, in a Swedish study, 8% of ambulance responses were for injuries occurring in sports areas, the fourth most common site[19]. Billing, administrative, or insurance data is another source of sports-injury data and may best be used for describing the costs of sports injuries[20]. Specialty clinics, such as sports medicine centres, can abstract information from patient medical records, providing a local or regional description of sports injuries[21]. Clinic or medical records are good sources for case studies or series studies, particularly describing rare sport-related injuries[22] as well as unusual presentations or complications of sports injuries[23].

Schools/sports organizations

The most commonly cited source of sports-injury data (see Box 5.1) come from the ongoing or periodic collection of injury-surveillance data by sports-related organizations (National Collegiate Athletic Association, NCAA), local schools or school districts, community-based organizations (e.g. Little League Baseball), and professional sports (National Football League, National Basketball Association, etc.). University-based researchers also conduct ongoing injury-surveillance studies such as the High School Reporting Information Online (RIO™) study conducted by the Center for Injury Research and Policy of The Research Institute at Nationwide Children's Hospital.

The NCAA Injury Surveillance System (ISS) is probably the largest collection of sports injury data in the world. Data from this system has helped improve the safety of collegiate US sports for

Box 5.1 Sports injury surveillance: Data for action

The term, "surveillance," as used in the public health field, refers to the ongoing and systematic collection, analysis, interpretation and dissemination of health information. Surveillance systems historically have focused on identification and control of infectious diseases. Since the 1980's, methods for surveillance of causes of mortality and morbidity due to injury have been adapted from the infectious disease field. The primary role of surveillance is to provide information for data-driven decision making. Usually, surveillance activities monitor high priority events (high prevalence, severe, costly) which have at least a minimum ability to be prevented or controlled. [34] For example, the identification of gender-disparities in the incidence of non-contact anterior cruciate ligament injuries in soccer and basketball using the NCAA injury Surveillance System (NCAA ISS) data [25] paved the way for the development and evaluation of injury prevention programs. [35]

The longest running surveillance system for sports injuries is the NCAA ISS. Data have been collected on injuries and exposures occurring in a sample of collegiate athletes since 1982. In 2007, a surveillance summary capturing 16 years of data for 15 male and female sports using the NCAA ISS was published. [10] These data reported exposure-based injury rates by sport and type of injury (describing the burden), identified high rates of specific, highly preventable, injuries and potential risk factors by sport (e.g. head, and facial injuries in field hockey), explored time trends (increasing rates of concussions), and evaluated the effectiveness of rule/policy changes on injury rates (e.g. spring practice guidelines in football). These data have also been used to inform resource needs (e.g. medical coverage of contact and collision sports) and have initiated further study of risk factors for specific injuries in prospective studies (e.g. gender differences in rates of non-contact anterior cruciate ligament injuries). The NCAA ISS not only provides annual cross-sectional 'snapshots' in time but over time has been providing critical information for evidence-based decisions regarding sports safety.

over 25 years as well as contributed to safety decisions by other sports organizations (e.g. USA Lacrosse)[24]. The gender-disparity in non-contact, anterior cruciate ligament injuries was first identified using NCAA data[25]. This landmark descriptive epidemiology report, laid the foundation for a decade of risk factor and prevention research related to anterior cruciate ligament injuries in female athletes. The NCAA ISS data have also been used to stimulate descriptive studies investigating gender differences in injury patterns among professional athletes in the National Basketball Association and the Women's National Basketball Association[26].

Many subsequent sports-injury studies have been modelled after the NCAA ISS, including the High School RIO™ study. Because injury cases and exposure definitions and data-collection methods are almost identical in the NCAA ISS and High School RIO™, injury rates can be compared to provide a high-level view of the injury patterns in high school and collegiate sports and how they differ. For example, overall injury rates in the sport of football are twice as high in college athletes (8.61 injuries per 1000 athlete-exposures) compared to high school athletes (4.36 injuries per 1000 athlete exposures). But, patterns of specific types of injuries differed. Fractures and concussions accounted for a higher proportion of all injuries among high school football players than among college players[27].

The NCAA ISS, High School RIO™ and other periodic sports-injury-surveillance studies[28] have provided a minimal body of literature. However, little information is known about the occurrence and patterns of sports and recreation injury in other settings and contexts. There is a critical need for injury-surveillance data on youths and adults participating in community-based sports, leisure-time physical activity, and formal exercise programmes outside of interscholastic and intercollegiate sports.

Special studies/registries

Registries

Cases of disease or injury meeting a strict set of defined criteria are often collected in registries. Registries attempt to capture all cases within a defined geographic area and gather detailed demographic and disease diagnosis and outcome data. Registries are useful for estimating the incidence, prognosis, and outcomes of care and are particularly useful for conditions that occur rarely[11].

Since sports and recreation injuries are rarely fatal, registries that record all known deaths due to sports and recreation in a selected area (community, state, country, etc.) are an example of how registries can be used to describe sports-injury mortality. The vital statistics system mentioned above is a very large registry of all deaths in the US each year. Although not subsidized by the federal government, there are several examples of sports-injury registries in the US including the National Center for Catastrophic Sport Injury Research, which has collected data since 1965 on deaths and disability from brain and/or spinal cord injury attributed to sports participation[29] and the National Registry of Sudden Death in Athletes which tabulates deaths and cardiac resuscitation incidents among young competitive athletes[30].

State- or hospital-based trauma registries exist in almost every state. These systems primarily were developed for the purpose of monitoring outcomes of trauma care, but have also been used for sports-injury surveillance[31]. Because trauma registries often only capture data from trauma centres or large hospitals, they often only include the most severe cases of injuries and may exclude some causes of injuries altogether, subsequently, they may not be the most representative source of descriptive data on sports injuries[11]. However, some trauma registries do link with other surveillance systems such as emergency medical services and administrative databases mentioned above which can contribute important information to provide a comprehensive 'snapshot' of the burden of sports injuries in a community or population.

Special studies

Descriptive information on sports injuries can also be found in special studies conducted by academic or other research organizations. A noted above, one of the major limitations of many governmental health surveys is the lack of information on exposure, information necessary to be able to calculate exposure-based injury rates of sports and activity-related injuries. Also, because physical activity is recommended for a variety of health benefits by many governments and health organizations, there was an identified need for information on injuries that occurred outside of organized sports activities and across the life span. In response, the Centers for Disease Control and Prevention designed and conducted a special study to estimate the prevalence of injuries associated with common moderate-intensity physical activities often recommended for health benefits. The Injury Control and Risk Study (ICARIS), a national telephone survey of over 5000 American adults, collected information on participation in select physical activities in the prior 30 days and injuries occurring during these activities (walking, bicycling, gardening, weightlifting, and aerobic dance)[32]. Findings indicate injury rates in these activities were relatively low, but because many adults participate in these activities, the number of people injured was large. In 2001–03, a second survey (ICARIS-2) was completed which also captured minimal information on injuries sustained during sports and recreation activities.

Ongoing, longitudinal studies can also be a source of descriptive information on sports-and activity-related injuries. The main purpose of Aerobics Center Longitudinal Study, a large cohort study started in the 1970s, is to investigate the health effects of cardiorespiratory fitness and physical activity. After a baseline health examination, including objective measures of fitness, the participants are followed approximately every 5 years using standardized surveys. Detailed information on participation in various activities such as walking, running, biking, aerobics, strength training, and other conditioning exercises are collected on every follow-up survey and data on activity-related injuries were collected on several of the follow-up surveys. Cross-sectional analysis of these data provided some of the first descriptive information on activity-related injuries in a large sample of community-dwelling adults[33]. These data described the distribution of activity-related and injuries by gender, age, body mass index, activity type, and body site injured. Although exposure-based rates of injuries were not calculated, these data were the first to suggest that even physically inactive persons can experience activity-related injuries (16% of sedentary adults reported an activity-related injury in the previous 12 months). A finding particularly relevant given the high population rates of physical inactivity in many countries.

Conclusion

Descriptive studies of sports- and activity-related injuries are important for establishing the extent of the problem, identifying potential risk and protective factors, and evaluating the effectiveness of intervention strategies. Ecologic and cross-sectional study designs are the most common in descriptive epidemiology and have inherent strengths and weaknesses. Sources of data for descriptive injury studies come from governmental surveys, health-care systems, school and sport organizations, registries, and special studies. Currently, exposure data is rarely collected in many data systems and therefore there is a critical need for integrated and linked injury data systems which can eventually track an injury from the sports field to the hospital and through outpatient rehabilitation.

References

1. Gordis L (1996). *Epidemiology*. W.B. Saunders Company, Philadelphia.

2. Robertson LS (1992). *Injury Epidemiology*. Oxford University Press, New York.

3. Greenland S (2001). Ecologic versus individual-level sources of bias in ecologic estimates of contextual health effects. *Int J of Epidemiol*, **30**, 1343–50.

4. Lancaster GA, Green M, Lane S (2006). Reducing bias in ecological studies: an evaluation of different methodologies. *J R Statist Soc A*, **169**, 681–700.

5. Wakefield J (2008). Ecologic studies revisited. *Ann Rev Public Health*, **29**, 75–90.

6. Timmreck TC (1994). *An introduction to epidemiology*. Jones and Bartlett Publishers, Boston, MA.

7. Rea LM, Parker RA (1997). *Designing and conducting survey sesearch: A comprehensive guide*. 2nd edition, John Wiley & Sons, Inc., San Francisco, CA.

8. Conn JM, Annest JL, Gilchrist J (2003). Sports and recreation related injury episodes in the US population, 1977–99. *Inj Prev*, **9**, 117–23.

9. Carlson SA, Hootman JM, Powell KE, Macera CA, Heath GW, Gilchrist J, Kimsey CD, Kohl HW (2006). Self-reported injury and physical activity levels: United States 2000 to 2002. *Ann Epidemiol*, **16**, 712–19.

10. Hootman JM, Dick R, Agel J (2007). Epidemiology of collegiate injuries for 15 sports: Summary and recommendations for injury prevention initiatives. *J Athl Train*, **42**(2), 311–19.

11. Horan JM, Mallonee S (2003). Injury Surveillance. *Epidemiol Rev*, **25**, 24–42.

12. Langley JD, Chalmers DJ (1999). Coding the circumstances of injury: ICD-10 a step forward or backwards? *Inj Prev*, **5**, 247–53.

13. Finch CF, Boufous S (2008). Do inadequacies in ICD-10 activity coded data lead to underestimates of the population frequency of sports/leisure injuries? *Inj Prev*, **14**(3), 202–4.

14. Eaton DK, Kann L, Kinchon S, Chanklin SROss J, Hawkins J, et al. (2008). Youth Risk Behavior Surveillance – United States, 2007; *MMWR Surveill Summ*, **57**(4), 1–131.

15. Burt CW, Overpeck MD (2001). Emergency visits for sports-related injuries. *Ann Emerg Med*, **37**(3), 301–8.

16. Centers for Disease Control and Prevention (2002). Nonfatal sports- and recreation-related injuries treated in emergency departments – United States, July 2000 to June 2001. *Morb Mort Weekly Rep*, **51**(33), 736–40.

17. Centers for Disease Control and Prevention (2007). Nonfatal traumatic brain injuries from sports and recreation activities – United States, 2001–2005. *Morb Mort Weekly Rep*, **56**(29), 733–7.

18. Kyle SB, Nance ML, Rutherford GW, Winston FK (2002). Skateboard-associated injuries: participation-based estimates and injury characteristics. *J Trauma*, **53**(4), 686–90.

19. Backe SN, Andersson R (2008). Monitoring the "tip of the iceberg": ambulance records as a source of injury surveillance. *Scand J Public Health*, **36**(3), 250–7.

20. Marshall SW, Mueller FO, Kirby DP, Yang J (2003). Evaluation of safety balls and faceguards for prevention of injuries in youth baseball. *JAMA*, **289**(5), 568–74.

21. Iwamoto J, Takeda T, Sato Y, Matsumoto H (2008). Retrospective case evaluation of gender differences in sports injuries in a Japanese sports medicine clinic. *Gend Med*, **5**(4), 405–14.

22. Echlin PS, Plomaritis ST, Peck DM, Skopelja EN (2006). Subscapularis avulasion fractures in 2 pediatric ice hockey players. *Am J Orthop*, **35**(6), 281–4.

23. Imade S, Takao M, Miyamoto W, Nishi H, Uchio Y (2009). Leg anterior compartment syndrome following ankle arthroscopy after Maisonnueve fracture. *Arthroscopy*, **25**(2), 215–18.

24. Dick R, Agel J, Marshall SW (2007). National Collegiate Athletic Association Injury Surveillance System commentaries: introduction and methods. *J Athl Train*, **42**(2), 173–82.

25. Arendt E, Dick R (1995). Knee injury patterns among men and women in collegiate basketball and soccer. NCAA data and review of the literature. *Am J Sports Med*, **23**(6), 694–701.

26. Dietch JR, Starkey C, Walters SL, Moseley JB (2006). Injury risk in professional basketball players: A comparison of Women's National Basketball Association and National Basketball Association athletes. *Am J Sports Med*, **34**(7), 1077–83.

27. Shankar PR, Fields SK, Collins CL, Dick RW, Comstock RD (2007). Epidemiology of high school and collegiate football injuries in the United States, 2005–2006. *Am J Sports Med*, **35**(8), 1295–303.

28. Powell JW, Barber-Foss KD (1999). Injury patterns in selected high school sports: A review of the 1995–1997 seasons. *J Athl Train*, **34**(3), 277–84.

29. Boden BP, Tacchetti RL, Cantu RC, Knowles SB, Mueller FO (2007). Catastrophic head injuries in high school and college football players. *Am J Sports Med*, **35**(7), 1075–81.

30. Maron BJ, Doerer JJ, Haas TS, Tierney DM, Mueller FO (2009). Sudden deaths in young competitive athletes. Analysis of 1866 deaths in the United States, 1980–2006. *Circulation*, **119**, 1085–92.

31. Wan J, Corvino TF, Grenfield SP, DiScala C (2003). Kidney and testicle injuries in team and individual sports: Data from the National Pediatric Trauma Registry. *J Urol*, **170**, 1531–2.

32. Powell KE, Heath GW, Kresnow MJ, Sacks JJ, Branche CM (1998). Injury rates from walking, gardening, weightlifting, outdoor bicycling, and aerobics. *Med Sci Sports Exerc*, **30**(8), 1246–9.

33. Hootman JM, Macera CA, Ainsworth BE, Addy CL, Martin M, Blair SN (2002). Epidemiology of musculoskeletal injuries among sedentary and physically active adults. *Med Sci Sports Exerc*, **34**(5), 838–44.

34. Teutsch SM, Churchill RE (1994). *Principles and Practice of Public Health Surveillance*. Oxford University Press, New York.

35. Gilchrist J, Mandelbaum BR, Melancon H, Ryan GW, Silvers HJ, Griffin LY, et al. (2008). A randomized controlled trial to prevent noncontact anterior cruciate ligament injury in female collegiate soccer players. *Am J Sports med*, **36**(80), 1476–83.

Chapter 6

Statistics used in observational studies

Will G. Hopkins

Many outcomes in research are quantified with continuous dependent variables, which take on a wide and finely graded range of values: blood pressure measured in mmHg, body mass index in kg/m^2, performance time in seconds, and so on. The outcome is usually a difference, change, or difference in the change in the mean value of the variable between groups or treatments, and the outcome can be expressed in the original units of the variable: e.g. a change in mean blood pressure of 10 mmHg. The analysis often includes log transformation of the variable to improve estimation of the outcome as a percent or factor difference or change, and standardization is also an option to interpret the magnitude of the outcome. One makes inferences about the outcome using a t-test to derive some measure of uncertainty in the true value (p-value, confidence interval, and chances of benefit and harm), or one uses a general linear model to estimate and adjust for other factors affecting the dependent variable. Analyses with variables of this kind are straightforward and can often be performed with a spreadsheet. On the other hand, the variables used to quantify injury outcomes – risk, odds, count, rate, hazard, time to injury, severity of injury, and burden of injury – usually require approaches that are more challenging.

The variables used in injury research and the statistics summarizing outcomes depend partly on study design (also see Chapter 2). Most studies are concerned with factors affecting injury incidence, the development of injuries analysed either by comparing injury outcomes in subgroups of a cohort of initially uninjured individuals or by comparing characteristics of individuals who are cases of injury with those of uninjured controls. Prevalence studies – which characterize currently injured and uninjured individuals in a cross-section of a population – can also be analysed to produce estimates of incidence. This chapter will, therefore, focus on incidence and its related measures of injury.

Risk, risk difference, and risk ratio

An individual's injury status can be represented by a binary variable, with the values of 0 (uninjured) or 1 (injured). The mean of this variable in a group of individuals is the proportion of the group injured and is known as the risk of injury. The risk can also be interpreted as the probability that any given individual in the group will get injured. A proportion or probability is a number between 0 and 1, but is often multiplied by 100 and referred to as (percent) chances of injury.

A value of exposure to something causing an injury, such as participation in sport, always underlies the value of the risk. Exposure can be calendar time (in days, weeks, months, etc.), time spent active in training or competition (hours), the number of practices or games, the number of inciting events (e.g. tackles), or even simply part or all of a season. Example: a risk of 0.21 for injury in the first month of a season for players in a particular sport means that a proportion of the players (0.21, 21%, or about one-fifth) was injured. A longer exposure leads to a greater proportion of injuries. Eventually the proportion approaches 1, or 100%, as can be seen in Fig. 6.1. Risk is calculated for a group, but it applies equally to the average person in the group: thus, if you

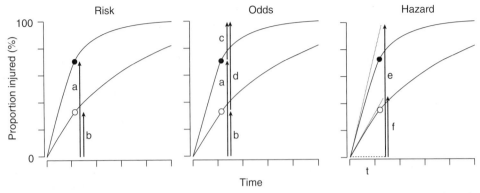

Fig. 6.1 Accumulation of injuries in two populations (or very large samples) that are initially free of injury and that differ in their developing incidence of injury. The three panels illustrate the calculation of risks and odds at a time when injuries are counted, and calculation of hazards at the beginning of the monitoring period (Time = 0).

Risks: a and b. Risk difference: a − b. Risk ratio: a/b.
Odds: a/c and b/d. Odds ratio: (a/c)/(b/d).
Hazards: e/t and f/t, where t is arbitrary. Hazard ratio: e/f.

The hazard is the instantaneous risk per unit of time, or the rate of appearance of new injuries expressed as a proportion of uninjured individuals. At Time = 0 the hazard is therefore the slope (as shown), and at later times the hazard is the slope divided by the proportion still uninjured. In these figures the two groups have different but constant hazards.

are a player in this sport and you are similar to the average player in the study that provided the estimate of risk, your chances of getting injured are 21% in the first month of the season. The risk for specific individual players varies from 21%, depending on how factors such as subject and game characteristics alter the risk. Much research on sports injury is devoted to identifying characteristics that alter risk – hence the term risk factors.

The effect of a risk factor should be presented initially by showing the risks in the different groups represented by the factor. Example: the risk for male players over a certain period is 30%, while the risk for female players over the same period is 20%. These two numbers automatically tell the reader that males appear to be at greater risk of injury and that gender is, therefore, a risk factor for injury. What is not clear from the two numbers is the uncertainty in the extent to which gender really is a risk factor. The main source of uncertainty is sampling variation, which one accounts for by showing a confidence interval (or lower and upper confidence limits) for the population or true value. The usual levels of confidence for a confidence interval are 90, 95, and 99%, depending on the design and aim of the study. It is possible to show confidence intervals for the risk of injury in females and males separately, but this approach does not address directly the uncertainty in the effect of gender. For that, the two estimates of risk have to be combined into a single effect statistic that summarizes the effect of the risk factor, then its confidence interval has to be derived.

The most obvious effect statistic for injury risk is the risk difference. In the example above, the risk difference is 10%, and with a small sample its 99% confidence interval might be −3% to 23%. A more common effect statistic is the risk ratio: the risk of injury in one group divided by that of the other. In the example, the ratio is 1.50 and the confidence interval might be 0.88 to 2.60. A ratio of 1.50 is usually interpreted as 50% higher risk, and a ratio of 2 is 100% higher risk or twice the risk. Risk ratios less than 1 indicate reduced risk: 0.90 is 10% less risk or 90% of the risk, and so on. Fig. 6.1 illustrates risk and the legend illustrates the calculation of risk difference and risk ratio for two groups.

With a binary variable scored as 0 or 1 to represent the injury status of each individual, the risk difference is simply the difference in the means. Calculation of the confidence interval for the risk difference is not so simple: it can be derived accurately via the unequal-variances t-statistic applied to the binary variable, but only when there are more than a few injured and uninjured individuals in each group. The assumption of normality of the sampling distribution that underlies the use of the t statistic is otherwise no longer valid and the resulting confidence limits are therefore untrustworthy and sometimes unrealistic (less than 0 and/or greater than 1, which are obviously impossible). The problem is even more serious when using a linear model to estimate and adjust for other factors affecting injury risk. In linear models, predicted values of the dependent variable can range from minus infinity to plus infinity, so with a binary variable as a dependent, the estimates of risk as well as the confidence limits can be outside the permissible range of 0–1.

Odds, odds ratio, and generalized linear modelling

Statisticians have attempted to overcome the problem of impossible risks in their analyses by using a dependent variable related to risk of injury, but in a form that can have a range of minus infinity to plus infinity. The variable in question is the log of the odds of being injured. As already noted, the probability of injury itself is not suitable to model, because its range is only 0–1. The odds of injury is the probability of injury (p) divided by the probability of non-injury ($1-p$), as illustrated in Fig. 6.1. The odds has the desired upper limit of infinity as p tends to 1 but an unsuitable lower limit of zero as p tends to 0. The log of the odds keeps the upper limit at infinity and pushes the lower limit out to minus infinity ($= \log(0)$). The transformation of p into the log of the odds, $\log(p/(1-p))$, is called a logit transformation or link function, and using the log of the odds as the dependent variable in a linear model is called logistic regression. This procedure also takes into account the fact that the frequencies of 0s and 1s in a sample have a binomial distribution. Logistic regression is not available with the standard functions in a spreadsheet, but it is available in all statistical packages, usually as part of a suite of procedures known as generalised linear modelling.

The generalized linear model allows inclusion of a variable representing time or other measure of exposure as an 'offset', to adjust for any differences in the amounts of exposure between individuals or groups. With an advanced stats package it is also possible to analyse re-injury using a repeated-measures version of the generalized linear model known as generalized estimation equations.

In logistic regression, the difference in injury risk between two groups is estimated as the difference in the log of the odds. This number then has to be converted by back-transformation into something that makes sense in the real world. A difference in logs corresponds to a ratio of the original numbers: $\log(A/B) = \log(A) - \log(B)$. Hence, the effect of a risk factor derived by logistic regression is an odds ratio. To perform the back-transformation exponential e is raised to the power of the effect provided by the linear model. Back-transformation of the confidence limits expressed in '±' form produces limits for the odds ratio as a '×/÷' factor. Back-transformation of the upper and lower limit produces the equivalent upper and lower limit for the odds ratio.

Researchers and readers often misinterpret the odds ratio as a ratio of risks; e.g. an odds ratio of 2.0 becomes 'twice as likely to be injured' or 'twice the risk of injury'. These interpretations are accurate only when the actual risks in both groups are low (<10%), which can be demonstrated with the formula for odds. If either risk is higher, an odds ratio >1 is larger than the corresponding risk ratio; e.g. risks of 60% and 30% make an odds ratio of 3.5 (= (60/40)/(30/70)) but a risk ratio of 2.0 (= 60/30). With very high risks, a risk ratio can only ever be slightly greater (or less) than 1.0, but the odds ratio can tend to infinity (or zero). When risks are substantial, it is therefore important to convert the odds ratio and its confidence limits into actual risks in one group, using known or estimated risk in the other group as a reference. One thereby ends up with the effect of the risk factor as a risk ratio or risk difference, which are easier outcomes to interpret. If the risk or proportion injured in the reference group is p and the odds ratio is OR, the risk in the comparison group can be derived by simple algebra as $p.OR/(1 + p(OR - 1))$, and the relative risk and risk difference follow therefrom. This formula should not be used to convert confidence limits for the odds ratio into confidence limits for the risk ratio or risk difference, and it is only approximate when the odds ratio has been adjusted for other risk factors[1].

Linear models often include continuous predictor variables, and the effects of these variables are expressed as slopes: differences in the dependent variable per unit of the predictor. When the model is logistic regression, a slope back-transforms to an effect that has units of odds ratio per unit of the predictor. For example, if age is included in the model as a simple linear effect, the effect of age adjusted for other predictors in the model would be expressed as an injury odds ratio per year. The units of such predictors can make a huge difference to the interpretation of the magnitude of the effect. For example, an odds ratio of 1.05 per year may seem tiny, yet age may actually have a substantial effect. How so? Because the differences in age between subjects in the study might be typically ±10 years, the effect of at least this many years should be estimated. In the logistic model the slope is multiplied by 10, then back-transformed. The same results can be achieved by raising the odds ratio per year to the power of the number of years. Here, $1.05^{10} = 1.63$. It has been argued elsewhere that the most appropriate difference in the predictor to assess the magnitude of its effect is actually two standard deviations[2], so the effect of age on injury in this example is 1.05^{20} or $1.63^2 = 2.7$! These remarks about the effect of continuous predictors apply also to the other injury models that produce ratios as outcomes.

Logistic regression is based on the assumption that factors affecting injury affect the odds of injury in a multiplicative manner. Alas, real risk factors almost certainly do not work in this manner, so the widespread use of logistic regression in injury research is inappropriate and sometimes provides wrong answers. A more reasonable assumption is that risk factors affect the short-term risk of injury throughout the period of exposure to risk. For example, in any brief instant of time, risks of injury for males and females are both miniscule, but the risk for males might always be 1.50 times the risk for females. When the short term is infinitesimal, risk expressed per unit of time or its equivalent in games, practices, or other measures of exposure is a measure of incidence known as the hazard. This measure and its associated effect statistic – the hazard ratio – is discussed in more detail later. When the proportions of injuries in a study end up at less than 10%, the effects will be practically identical whether estimated and expressed as odds or hazard ratios. However, when injuries accumulate to substantial proportions, the odds diverge from the risk, so if it is right to model the hazard, it must be wrong to model the odds.

The odds ratio nevertheless has to be used when data come from a case-control study in which controls are selected at the end of monitoring: so-called cumulative sampling. In the analysis the cases of injury are subdivided into subgroups differing in the potential risk factor, and the controls are subdivided similarly. The log of the counts becomes the dependent variable, the Poisson distribution (not the binomial distribution) is invoked to account for the sampling variation in the counts, and the effect of the risk factor is estimated as a ratio of counts of injured to uninjured individuals in exposed and unexposed subgroups. As explained in Box 6.1, this effect is formally an odds ratio with a value the same as can be expected in a cohort study, so the outcome can be interpreted as if it came from a cohort study. In the majority of case-control studies, injuries are

Box 6.1 Odds and hazard ratios in case-control studies

In an analysis of injury incidence the aim is to develop a model in which one or more measures of exposure predict some measure of incidence. The outcome statistic in a case-control study is analysed with a generalized linear model by coding injury status as 1 (cases) or 0 (controls) and by using a logit link function and a binomial distribution. The outcome is then a ratio of ratios of counts: cases/controls in the exposed individuals divided by cases/controls in unexposed.

With cumulative sampling (controls sampled at the end of the period of monitoring), the cases represent some fraction α of injured individuals in the population, and the controls represent some fraction β of the uninjured individuals. The ratio cases/controls in exposed individuals therefore equals $(\alpha \times$ injured$)/(\beta \times$ uninjured$)$ in the population, and there is a similar expression for the unexposed individuals. The ratio of the ratios of cases/controls therefore equals the ratio of the ratios of injured/uninjured in the population, because the α and β all cancel out. This expression is the odds ratio in a cohort study.

With incidence-density sampling (controls sampled as cases appear), the above ratio of counts becomes a hazard ratio for the effect of exposure, provided the hazard ratio is constant. The proof is not trivial. In any small increment of time, the sampled number of cases with exposure is proportional to the hazard for exposure, and the sampled number of cases without exposure is proportional (with a different constant of proportionality) to the hazard for non-exposure. Because of the way controls are sampled in fixed proportion to the cases (e.g., four times as many), the numbers of controls sampled with and without exposure are also each proportional to some linear sum of the hazards. Now, in the next increment of time, a substantial factor change in one hazard (a doubling, say) must be accompanied by the same change in the other hazard, because the hazard ratio is constant. Hence, the numbers of cases and controls with and without exposure change by the same factor, a doubling. Therefore, the sum of the cases with exposure over the two increments is equal to three times the cases in the first increment, as are the sums of cases without exposure and of controls with and without exposure. The ratio of the counts over the two increments is therefore the same as the ratio over the first increment, which is the hazard ratio, because the increment of time is infinitesimal. By induction, the ratio of the sum of the counts over any number of increments of time is the hazard ratio.

uncommon (incidences <10%) in unexposed and exposed groups. Therefore, in these cases the odds ratio can be treated as a risk or hazard ratio. With more common injuries, one cannot use the usual formula for converting an odds ratio into a relative risk, because the proportion of injured in unexposed individuals is unknown. This problem may arise when performing a meta-analysis of some risk factor. It is better to perform case-control studies by sampling controls as cases appear: so-called incidence-density sampling. It is also better to analyse these studies via proportional-hazards regression, as explained later, but when opting for generalized linear modelling of the accumulated counts, the outcome statistic is now automatically a hazard ratio, and it is an unbiased estimate when the hazard ratio is constant.

A common analysis in injury studies is a comparison of the proportions of different kinds of injury in a group of injured athletes, e.g. arm (23%), body (31%) and leg (46%). The data consist of individual cases of injury, each with different values of predictor variables. One way to understand such data is to regard them as coming from an injury study in which there are not simply two values of the outcome variable (injured or uninjured) but three or more (injured arm, injured body, injured leg, etc.). If data for uninjured individuals are available, they can be included as another value of the outcome variable (uninjured). The generalized linear model appropriate for such data uses not the binomial distribution but the multinomial distribution, reflecting the fact that there are more than two values for the dependent. If only injured individuals are analysed, the appropriate link function is the cumulative logit, but if uninjured individuals are included and there is a defined period of monitoring, the appropriate link is the cumulative complementary log–log. Corresponding effects of predictors are expressed as odds ratios and hazard ratios. Be sure to use back-transformation to get values of risk for important levels of predictors (e.g. affected body part) adjusted for other predictors (e.g. gender, level of competition, etc.).

Count and count ratios

If the research question concerns the number of injuries each individual has experienced, the variable characterizing each individual's injuries is an integer: 0, 1, 2, 3, etc. This variable has problems similar to those of a binary variable, and as with a binary variable, the only kind of analysis that can be done with the raw numbers is an unequal-variances t-test. The rescue package statisticians have devised for modelling an injury count is the form of generalized linear modelling known as Poisson regression: the dependent variable is the injury count over the monitoring period, the link function (transformation) is the log, and the analytical procedure takes into account the fact that the counts in a sample have a Poisson distribution – hence the name of the procedure. The use of log transformation is based on the reasonable assumption that the effects on risk are manifested as factors, which, after back-transformation, are expressed as ratios. These count ratios are sometimes referred to as rate ratios, because counts of injury over the period of monitoring are indeed rates. These ratios are not usually converted into rate differences.

Two assumptions underlying Poisson regression are that injury events are independent and that they occur with the same probability in individuals who have the same values of risk factors in the linear model. If these assumptions are violated, the dispersion of the counts in the sample may be different from that expected for a Poisson distribution. Some stats packages take this scenario into account by allowing specification and estimation of an additional parameter describing the dispersion of the counts, and the resulting distribution is known as negative-binomial. The parameter is the amount by which the variance of the counts is greater or less than the expected value, the mean of the counts. (The sampling standard deviation of a count of independent events is the square root of the count.) This parameter does not have a practical interpretation, but the estimates of effects and confidence limits are more trustworthy when it is included in the model.

Rate and rate ratios

The period or other value of exposure that provided the data for the estimate of injury risk or injury count can be included overtly in the risk or count in various ways. For example, if 20% of athletes in a team of 25 sustained an injury in a 4-week period consisting of 20 exposures to practices and games per athlete, there were five injured athletes per 500 athlete-exposures, which can be expressed as 10 injured per 1 000 athlete-exposures. Injuries can also be expressed as a number per 1 000 athlete-hours or per 10 000 athlete-minutes of participation in practices and/or games. Such measures of injury are called rates, and they are useful when comparing risks of injury between groups or sports derived from different exposures.

Be aware that direct comparison of rates that are derived from proportions are inaccurate when the proportions are different and one of them is >10%. For example, a sport with an injury rate of 10 injured athletes per 1 000 athlete-exposures derived from a study in which 60% of the athletes were injured is actually more risky than a sport with the same rate derived from a study in which only 10% of the athletes was injured. For appropriate comparison, rates should be either derived from the same period of monitoring, or estimated from the hazard, or (especially when re-injury is an issue) estimated from counts of injuries for each athlete. In the latter case, Poisson regression is the appropriate form of the generalized linear model. Poisson regression should also be used to compare summary statistics from different sports or other groups, but it is important to do the analysis with the actual counts of injury and to use an offset variable if the exposure differs between the sports or groups.

In calculating injury rates, some researchers simply add up all the injuries in a given period without regards to whether the injuries come from the same individual or whether reduction in exposure to risk during the individual's period of injury should be taken into account in the denominator used to calculate the rate. The resulting statistic nevertheless represents a practical rate for comparing sports or groups, but estimation of its confidence limits and estimation of confidence limits of factors affecting the rate become problematic when incidence is high enough (e.g. >10%) for re-injury to be an issue. If there is concern about violating the assumptions underlying Poisson regression even with the negative binomial distribution, bootstrapping should be used to estimate confidence limits (see also Chapter 10). For bootstrapping, the study sample needs to have at least 30 observations. A new sample of the same size is generated by drawing observations at random from the original sample. This bootstrapped sample will have repeats of some observations while others are not represented, but no matter. One can then calculate the outcome statistic for this sample, repeat the process at least 1 000 times, and rank-order the values of the outcome statistic. The percentiles corresponding to a chosen level of confidence are the confidence limits (e.g. the 50th and 950th percentiles for 90% confidence from 1000 bootstrapped samples). When the outcome statistic comes from a general or generalized linear model, the linear model is applied to each bootstrapped sample and the confidence limits are derived from the adjusted estimates, ignoring the confidence limits derived from the model for the original and bootstrapped samples. This approach can be used for any analysis where one is confident the model itself is appropriate but where violation of assumptions underlying the model could make confidence limits derived from the model untrustworthy.

Hazard, time to injury, and their ratios

In the section on odds and odds ratios the notion of the hazard was introduced: the risk evaluated over a very short period of time. For example, an injury hazard of 0.08 per week for a particular group implies that a proportion of 0.08 (or 8%) of the group will become injured in 1 week. The time interval here is arbitrary: the hazard is estimated in principle for an infinitesimally small time interval but expressed for a time interval that makes the hazard something important but small enough (~1–10%) to be interpreted reasonably accurately as a risk. A hazard of 8% per week is the same as a hazard of 1.1% per day, 0.05% per hour, 32% per month and even 400% per year, but for a hazard referring to sports injuries, the 8% per week would probably be the most informative and least likely to be misinterpreted. The hazard can also be interpreted as a mean injury count per athlete per unit of time: a hazard of 0.08 per week means 0.08 injuries per individual per week, but to express it as 4.0 injuries per individual per year is justifiable only if injuries continue to occur independently in the same individuals at the same hazard rate over the entire year.

The hazard is a useful concept for understanding how injuries gradually accumulate over time. Thus, if the hazard is 0.01 or 1% per day, one can assume that 2% of the group will be injured in 2 days, 3% in 3 days, and so on. However, this process can not continue indefinitely, because after

100 days more than 100% of the group will be injured! In fact, when working out the proportion of athletes who are injured over some period of time, the hazard of 1% per day applies only to those individuals who have not yet become injured. As injuries accumulate, there are less people without an injury, so the 1% refers to an ever diminishing number of people; after 100 days the proportion injured would have reached only 63%. This estimate is based on the assumption that the hazard stays constant, but it will increase with time if increasing fatigue during the season increases the risk of injury, and it will decrease with time as the more injury-prone individuals get injured and removed from the remaining pool of uninjured individuals.

Another useful concept is the inverse of the hazard, which has units of time per injury. Thus, a hazard of 0.08 per week when inverted is $1/0.08 = 12.5$ weeks per injury. If the hazard is constant, 12.5 weeks represents the time to injury for the average individual. Even if the hazard changes with time, the inverse of the hazard at any given time can be interpreted as the time that would elapse typically before an injury occurred, if the hazard stayed constant. This injury statistic is possibly the easiest for non-specialists to understand, but researchers seldom report it.

The outcome statistic based on hazards is the hazard ratio. For example, an analysis might provide an estimate of the injury hazard ratio of 1.50 for maleness, which would mean that males are 1.5 times more likely than females to get injured in any small interval of time at any time during the study. An alternative practical interpretation is that on average females will take 1.50 times longer than males to get injured, if the hazards do not change from that point forwards. (If the hazards do change, the hazard ratio no longer estimates the ratio of the actual mean times to injury, even if the hazard ratio stays constant.) It is not usual to express outcomes as differences in hazard or differences in mean time to injury, although the latter is a candidate for the single most informative statistic in injury research.

There are two approaches to modelling hazards and estimating their ratio. When the data consist of counts of injured and uninjured individuals in a cohort study, the dependent variable in a generalized linear model with a complementary log–log link function and a binomial sampling distribution is effectively an estimate of the log of the hazard (apart from an additive constant), and the outcomes are hazard ratios[2]. See Box 6.2 for an explanation. Surprisingly, the hazards can change during the monitoring period, but provided the hazard ratio stays constant, this model provides an unbiased estimate of it. A constant hazard ratio is a reasonable default assumption in injury research, and the fact that the estimated hazard ratio is independent of the monitoring period gives it a great advantage over the odds and risk ratios. The complementary log–log link can also be used with prevalence studies, in which a population is surveyed to identify individuals currently injured and uninjured. In these studies the duration of the injury affects the prevalence, but assuming the mean duration of injury is the same in groups defined by the potential risk factor (e.g. females and males), effects derived from the model are independent of duration of injury and are hazard ratios for injury incidence, as explained in Box 6.2.

The second approach to modelling hazards is proportional-hazards or Cox regression – the method of choice when the time of occurrence of each injury is known. The log of the time to injury is effectively the dependent variable, so after back-transformation and inversion the effects are hazard ratios – which are assumed not to change as time progresses and more people get injured. Time to injury cannot be analysed with general or generalized linear modelling, because these do not allow proper inclusion of times for subjects who withdraw from a study or who have still not become injured at the close of the study. In proportional-hazards regression such times are included, but the procedure is instructed that they are right-censored; i.e. an injury would have occurred for these subjects eventually, but we do not know when that would have been. Other advantages of proportional-hazards regression include: the capacity to model time-dependent changes in a risk factor's hazard ratio; the capacity to model times between repeated

Box 6.2 Use of the complementary log–log transformation

In a population in which N individuals are still uninjured and the probability of injury per unit time (the hazard) is a constant h, the reduction in N through injury in an infinitesimal of time δt is given by $\delta N = - N.h.\delta t$. Integration yields $N = N_0.(1 - e^{-h.t})$, where N is the number of uninjured individuals at time t, and N_0 is the number of uninjured individuals at time zero. But $N/N_0 = p$, the proportion injured or the probability or risk of injury, so $p = 1 - e^{-h.t}$. The curves shown in Fig. 6.1 are derived from this equation.

Rearranging, $1 - p = e^{-h.t}$. Taking natural logs, $\log(1 - p) = -h.t$, or $-\log(1 - p) = h.t$.

Taking logs again, $\log(-\log(1 - p)) = \log(h) + \log(t)$.

Thus, at a given time t, the complementary log-log transformation of the proportion injured represents an estimate of the log of the hazard plus a constant $(\log(t))$. For two groups in a cohort study, the difference in the complementary log–log of their proportions is an estimate of the difference of the log of their hazards. Back-transformation yields the hazard ratio. Equivalently, if the proportion of injuries is p_1 and p_2 after the same time t, the hazard ratio is $\log(1 - p_1)/\log(1 - p_2)$. For simplicity it is assumed that the hazards are constant, but it is easy to show that this approach provides an unbiased estimate of a constant hazard ratio, no matter how the hazards change during the monitoring period.

In a survey of injury prevalence in a population, a sampled individual will be uninjured only if the injury has not occurred in a time prior to the survey equal to the mean duration of injury, T. For a constant hazard h, this probability is $e^{-h.t}$. The probability of being injured is therefore $1 - e^{-h.T}$. As above, the complementary log–log of this probability is an estimate of the injury hazard, and back-transformed differences between groups are estimates of injury hazard ratios.

injuries when estimating risk of re-injury; and the capacity to produce estimates even when every individual in a group gets injured. One might think that use of injury time rather than a binary injury variable would also lead to greater precision in the estimate of the hazard ratio, but it is not so: when data can be analysed with the same linear model, proportional-hazards regression and generalized linear modelling provide similar unbiased estimates and confidence intervals.

When times of occurrence of injury are available, the time-course of the gradual increase in injuries can be shown in graphical form by plotting the proportion injured (p) in each group against the injury time. The curves are similar to those in Fig. 6.1, but the occurrence of each event is shown as a small-step change in the observed proportion rather than as a smooth change in the predicted proportion. The same information is conveyed in a so-called survival or Kaplan-Meier plot, which displays the gradual fall in survival or proportion uninjured $(1 - p)$ against time. With a log scale on the Y-axis of a survival plot, the negative slopes of the curves are the hazards, so a time-dependent change in the slope indicates a change in the injury process that may be important. Any asynchrony between groups in the change represents a violation of the assumption of a constant hazard ratio. Such plots have yet to appear in the sports-injury journals.

Severity and burden of injury

Severity of injury is a measure representing the cost of an injury to an individual, calculated either in monetary terms or in time off work, practice or competition. The best statistics to summarize severity are the mean and standard deviation. The distributions of dollar cost and time lost are usually skewed by infrequent severe injuries, so analysis after log transformation provides a better comparison of group means (as percent or factor differences) and better adjustment when other factors impacting severity are included in a linear model. Back-transform the standard deviation into a coefficient of variation or a factor variation. Be aware that the back-transformed means are not the same as the arithmetic means: they should be considered as similar to (but better than) medians. For administrative costing, always use the arithmetic means.

The total cost of injury to a sport or other group in money or time lost can be termed the burden of injury, and it is derived by combining severity of injury with injury incidence. When the cost of each individual's injury is known, the variable used to calculate the burden is the same as that characterizing severity, but it now includes values of zero for the uninjured individuals. As such, this variable is likely to be grossly non-normal, which is not a problem for simple comparisons of means using the unpaired t-statistic, but which can make outcomes from more complex linear models untrustworthy. See Box 6.3 for approaches to this problem. When the mean cost of injury and the incidence of injury have been estimated separately, derive the burden from their product and express differences between groups (gender, types of injury, athletes, sports, etc.) as percents or factors. The method for deriving confidence limits is explained in Box 6.3.

Box 6.3 Modelling injury burden

When the cost of each individual's injury is known, there are several approaches to increase confidence in the analysis of injury burden. First, use the linear model to derive the outcomes with the raw variable, but get confidence limits for the outcomes using the same model applied to several thousand bootstrapped samples. The outcomes are probably best expressed as percents: e.g. 'injuries in this sport carry a 35% greater burden (99% confidence limits . . .) than in that sport'. This approach keeps outcomes closest to the original data, but the effects and adjustments in the model will be biased towards individuals with high costs. Log transformation is the usual solution to this problem, but log transformation produces missing values for the individuals with no injuries. To keep these observations in the analysis, replace the values of zero cost with half the smallest non-zero cost in the data-set, then log-transform and derive effects and confidence limits as percents or factors from the model. This approach is acceptable if the zeros are in the minority and if the scatter of residuals is reasonably uniform (but not necessarily normal) in plots against the predicted and the predictors in the model. It also avoids the challenge of bootstrapping. If the residuals are still grossly non-uniform after log transformation, as a last resort try rank-transformation of the costs before using the linear model and bootstrapping. Back-transform the rank effects and confidence limits into real costs at some chosen value of cost, such as the median.

When the mean cost of injury and the risk of injury have been estimated separately, derive the approximate confidence limits for the injury burden by combining confidence intervals of log-transformed values, as follows: express the confidence intervals of injury cost and injury risk as factors, square the logs of these factors and add together, take the square root, back-transform to a factor, then convert the factor to lower and upper confidence limits. For the confidence limits of the percent or factor difference in burdens, repeat the process of transforming, combining, and back-transforming the confidence intervals of the two burdens. (See reference 7 for examples of this approach.)

Magnitude thresholds for injury outcomes

The value of an effect statistic helps make a decision about clinical or practical importance of an effect only when the uncertainty in the statistic is considered in relation to smallest beneficial and harmful values of the statistic. If the uncertainty represented by the confidence interval indicates that the effect could be beneficial and harmful, one is obliged to conclude that the outcome is unclear and that more subjects need to be studied. Otherwise, the outcome is clear and one may decide that the effect is beneficial, harmful, or trivial, depending on the possible true value of the effect represented by the confidence interval. Actual chances that the true value is beneficial and harmful can be calculated to refine the decision. This magnitude-based approach to inferences about clinical utility should be used instead of the traditional null-hypothesis test, which can result in clinically unethical decisions[3–5].

The magnitude-based approach to inferences requires overt use of the least clinically important value of an effect. For the continuous measures that were mentioned in the opening paragraph of this chapter, a widely accepted default is 0.20 of the between-subject standard deviation (averaged over the groups being compared). Values of 0.60, 1.2, 2.0, and 4.0 can also be used as thresholds of moderate, large, very large, and extremely large effects[5] (see also the section on magnitudes at www.newstats.org). These thresholds for magnitude are appropriate to assess differences in the cost of injury. If the cost is log-transformed, then the assessment of magnitude has to be performed with the log-transformed values.

Little or no published or informal consensus on the least clinically important values for any of the other measures of injury is available, let alone the other magnitude thresholds. Therefore, one needs to develop reasonable default estimates. The thresholds depend on whether the injury is common (most individuals can expect to get injured during the period of exposure) or uncommon (only a small proportion is injured, however long the period of exposure).

With sports injuries that become common during a season, athletes are aware that they are likely to become injured, and they will want to remain uninjured for as long as possible. In Box 6.4 thresholds have been developed by considering two groups with different but constant hazards. Risk difference increases to maximum and then declines as the proportion injured approaches 1.0 in both groups. The thresholds for small, moderate, large, very large, and extremely large maximum risk differences are 0.1, 0.3, 0.5, 0.7, and 0.9, or differences in chances of injury of 10%, 30%, 50%, 70%, and 90%. The corresponding thresholds for the hazard ratio are 1.3, 2.0, 4.0, 10, and 100. Thresholds for a decrease in injury are negative values of risk difference (−0.1, −0.3, ...) and the inverse of the ratios (1/1.3, 1/2.0, ...). Hazard ratios are not translated into odds ratios, because odds ratios should not be interpreted directly. For rare injuries, hazard-ratio thresholds of 1.1, 1.4, 2.0, 3.3, and 10 are justifiable on the grounds that the corresponding proportions of cases attributable to the exposure or effect under investigation would be 10%, 30%, 50%, 70%, and 90%.

An estimate of the smallest important effect is required for estimation of sample size, which can be investigated using a spreadsheet that provides estimates based on clinical error rates and statistical error rates[6]. When exposures to risk and injury incidences are ~50%, a risk difference of 0.1 and a hazard ratio of 1.3 give sample sizes similar to those for continuous dependent variables in other observational designs: ~300 for clinically based and ~800 for statistically based estimates. A hazard ratio of 1.1 requires sample sizes 10 times as large, and if only a small proportion of the population is exposed to risk, sample sizes can range from thousands for case-control studies to tens of thousands or more for cohort studies.

Box 6.4 Magnitude thresholds for risk difference and hazard ratio with common injuries

When injury hazards are constant but differ between two groups, the risk difference builds to a maximum sometime during the season, then declines to zero as the proportion injured approaches 1 in both groups, as can be seen in any of the three panels in Fig. 6.1. It is suggested that a maximum risk difference of 10% represents the smallest important difference, because at this stage in the season it is equivalent to becoming injured in only one season in 10 as a result of the risk factor. Similarly, maximum risk differences of 30%, 50%, 70%, and 90% seem reasonable as thresholds for moderate, large, very large, and extremely large. These thresholds for risk difference can also be derived from a scale of magnitudes for correlation coefficients, first suggested by Jacob Cohen (0.1, 0.3, and 0.5 for small, moderate, and large) and augmented (0.7 and 0.9 for very large and practically perfect), as explained in the section on magnitudes at www.newstats.org.

Now, the time at which the maximum risk difference occurs can be derived by elementary calculus, as follows. The risk difference between two groups with hazards h and k is $(1 - e^{-h.t}) - (1 - e^{-k.t}) = e^{-k.t} - e^{-h.t}$. The maximum occurs where the first derivative of this difference is zero, i.e., where $h.e^{-ht} - k.e^{-k.t} = 0$. Therefore the maximum occurs where $t = (\log(k) - \log(h))/(k - h)$. A spreadsheet was used to calculate t and the resulting risk difference for $h = 1$ and various values of k. The values of k corresponding to risk differences of 10%, 30%, 50%, 70%, and 90% are 1.3, 2.3, 4.4, 10, and 50. These are therefore the hazard-ratio thresholds for small, moderate, large, very large, and extremely large.

Similar thresholds for common injuries were derived by focussing on the time to injury. First, simulation with a spreadsheet was used to generate samples of time to injury in two groups with different constant hazards. The log-transformed times in each group turned out to have the same standard deviation, regardless of the hazard. When this standard deviation was used to standardize the difference in the means of the log-transformed times, the hazard ratios corresponding to the standardized magnitude thresholds of 0.2, 0.6, 1.2, 2.0, and 4.0 were found. The hazard ratios are 1.3, 2.2, 4.5, 13, and 180.

Combining the remarkably similar results of these two disparate approaches, the suggested simplified thresholds for the hazard ratio are 1.3, 2.0, 4.0, 10, and 100.

Box 6.5 Magnitude thresholds for hazard ratio with rare injuries

With rare injuries, most individuals do not end up injured, and most would therefore be unconcerned about changes in risk of a factor of 2 or even more. (We all engage in risky behaviours without much concern when we perceive the risks to be low.) However, if the focus is on the group of individuals who end up injured, hazard ratios as low as 1.1 become important. A hazard ratio of 1.1 represents a 10% increase in the incidence of an injury and therefore a 10% increase in the workload and expenses for clinical services dealing with the injury. I think such an increase would be regarded as substantial, whereas anything less might go unnoticed or be accommodated without fuss. A similar argument applies when someone is accountable for an increase in incidence of an uncommon injury: amongst the injured individuals, one in every 11 represents an extra case that could have been avoided and that could therefore qualify for compensation; to this group and to the person accountable, a hazard ratio of 1.1 is also substantial.

> **Box 6.5 Magnitude thresholds for hazard ratio with rare injuries** *(continued)*
>
> The other magnitude thresholds for rare injuries can be generated by a consideration of the proportion of cases that would be attributable to the exposure or effect under consideration: in the population or group giving rise to the cases that normally arise without exposure, hazard-ratio thresholds of 1.1, 1.4, 2.0, 3.3, and 10 would result in proportions of cases attributable to the exposure of 10%, 30%, 50%, 70%, and 90%. For example, if 65 cases of a rare injury occurred normally in a population in a given period, and exposure of the population to something produced 35 extra cases in the same period, 35% of the cases would be due to the exposure, the hazard ratio would be 1.54, and the magnitude would therefore be moderate. These thresholds apply also to risk and odds ratios, because these have practically the same values as hazard ratios for rare outcomes. As with common injuries, the threshold for a decrease in hazard, odds, or risk ratio is the inverse of the corresponding threshold for an increase. These thresholds should all be suitable for injury burden.

Acknowledgements

Ian Shrier, Ken Quarrie, and Steve Marshall provided valuable suggestions for improvement that were incorporated into the final version.

Suggested reading

Hopkins WG, Marshall SW, Quarrie KL, Hume PA (2007). Risk factors and risk statistics for sports injuries. *Clin J Sport Med*, **17**, 208–10.

Greenland S (2004). Model-based estimation of relative risks and other epidemiologic measures in studies of common outcomes and in case-control studies. *Am J Epidemiol*, **160**, 301–5.

References

1. Shrier I (2006). Understanding the relationship between risks and odds ratios. *Clin J Sport Med*, **16**, 107–10.
2. Perneger TV (2008). Estimating the relative hazard by the ratio of logarithms of event-free proportions. *Contemp Clin Trials*, **29**, 762–6.
3. Batterham AM, Hopkins WG (2006). Making meaningful inferences about magnitudes. *Int J Sports Physiol Perform*, **1**, 50–7.
4. Hopkins WG (2007). A spreadsheet for deriving a confidence interval, mechanistic inference and clinical inference from a p value. *Sportscience*, **11**, 16–20.
5. Hopkins WG, Marshall SW, Batterham AM, Hanin J (2009). Progressive statistics for studies in sports medicine and exercise science. *Med Sci Sports Exerc*, **41**, 3–12.
6. Hopkins WG (2006). Estimating sample size for magnitude-based inferences. *Sportscience*, **10**, 63–7.
7. Quarrie KL, Hopkins WG (2008). Tackle injuries in professional rugby union. *Am J Sports Med*, **36**, 1705–16.

Chapter 7

Reviews – using the literature to your advantage

Quinette Louw and Karen Grimmer-Somers

Staying on top of current evidence is essential for researchers, teachers, and clinicians to ensure that clinical decisions and treatments are well founded and defensible. However, it is generally frustrating for any health professional in the sports-health industry to stay on top of current literature. One reason for this is that it takes time to read sufficiently, across the breadth of relevant journals, to be familiar with what is being written. Literature is also often of variable quality and value to clinical practice. Health professionals consequently need to be critical about what they are reading so that they can prioritize evidence into what is believable and what is useful to their needs. This chapter outlines different types of literature reviews and identifies important elements.

Definitions and classifications

There is a range of ways in which sports-injury research has been undertaken and reported across the globe, resulting in a significant volume of published research. Traditionally, however, sports-related researchers have taken individual routes to classifying conditions and defining exposures and outcomes. This has resulted in major differences in the definitions and classifications of diagnoses, in playing and injury exposures, in risks related to the sustaining of injuries, and in obtaining good health outcomes. Consequently, sports-injury studies cannot be readily compared to obtain a global picture of injury incidence and prevalence. These differences have also lead to conflicting research findings, which have confused clinicians, coaches, and sports participants alike.

For example, consider the identification of the risks of sustaining an injury from sports participation. The prevention of sports injuries requires a sound understanding of injury-risk factors. In sports-injury preventive research, however, there are significant gaps in understanding, which are a direct result of the use of the variable definitions and classifications of study factors. Consequently, although a wide range of both extrinsic and intrinsic risk factors has been defined for sports injuries, their impact is often differently reported across studies. This makes it difficult for clinicians and researchers to obtain a clear picture of relevant risk factors for a specific injury or sport, which thus constrains effective planning for preventative strategies.

Coming to grips with literature

We live in an era of scientific-information overload, where more than 2 million research articles are published annually[1]. Thus, finding answers to clinical questions by synthesizing research studies is no longer a trivial task[2]. To conduct a rigorous synthesis of literature, reviewers need knowledge about research methodology, skills to search for information, time, resources, and access to databases. Many researchers, teachers, and clinicians, however, may not be in a position to undertake their own reviews and they may therefore seek access to the published syntheses of literature for the research questions of interest to them. They may look in published literature or even on the Internet for reviews on their topic of interest. Even when reading reviews written by others, however, they should be critical and understand the limitation of published literature reviews. Thus, when they read a review, they should ask critical questions about the methodology of the review, which will assist them to put findings into context.

Function of literature reviews

A new body of research – secondary evidence production – has emerged over the past two decades, which summarizes primary research evidence. Primary research reflects studies undertaken on humans. Evidence syntheses – or secondary evidence – collate the findings of individual primary studies that have been conducted in the same research area. These are often called literature reviews. Reviews offer a way of synthesizing current research evidence and making sense of the findings of separate primary studies. Reading secondary evidence has a number of benefits. One major benefit is time efficiency, as health-care professionals do not have to read through individual research papers themselves in order to produce a synthesis of the evidence. Reading secondary evidence also assists health professionals with keeping on top of current research findings readily and it assists them in identifying gaps in knowledge. This is particularly important in preventing the unnecessary duplication of research efforts when undertaking primary research. Being aware of literature gaps supports researchers in planning research efforts that are focused on the research areas, which, if addressed appropriately, will add to the body of knowledge.

Types of literature reviews

There are two main types of reviews: general (traditional) literature reviews and systematic reviews. The type of review depends on its aim, methodology, and intended audience.

General or traditional reviews (or narrative) are usually a qualitative summary of evidence, which is based on the authors' views and preferences, for a given topic[3]. Traditional reviews usually present a broad overview of what has been written on a range of issues related to a topic (e.g. studies that report on the prevalence, risk factors, and management of knee-overuse injuries). Papers included in traditional reviews are often selected according to the authors' personal preference, which often supports their opinion, philosophy, and viewpoint. Because authors of traditional reviews rarely state how they selected and analysed their primary studies, readers cannot assess whether the review process was comprehensive or the extent to which the authors' prejudice influenced the choice of literature cited in the reviews. Furthermore, because the methodological quality of included research is often not considered, conclusions from traditional reviews may be biased, leading to inaccurate and inappropriate recommendations[4]. However, traditional reviews are often considered to be useful to sports clinicians, as they provide an overview of the range of important issues related to the topic of interest. Traditional reviews may also be useful in the early stages of a research project, since they present a broad overview of the topic, which can assist researchers with setting the background for a research project proposal or thesis.

Systematic reviews, on the other hand, are a synthesis of all relevant primary studies related to a carefully constructed research question (e.g. 'What is the effectiveness of pre-season proprioceptive training in reducing lateral ankle-sprain injuries in adolescent soccer players?'). They contain explicit statements about research objectives and are conducted with the use of a systematic and reproducible methodology[5]. Additional requirements of systematic reviews are that they should include a comprehensive and exhaustive search of all literature pertaining to the research topic, clear study-selection criteria, the systematic identification of studies, the critical appraisal of the methodology of studies, and the synthesis of results[3]. The explicit methodology applied in systematic reviews aims to reduce potential bias in literature selection and provides conclusions that are more reliable than those provided by traditional reviews. Reasons for conflicting study findings can also be examined in order for the generalizability of review findings to be established and for new areas of research to be identified. The process of conducting a systematic review is time consuming and may be overwhelming to many researchers. However, it provides a wealth of useful information about the extant literature on a given topic. Information yielded from systematic reviews can assist in the design of new primary research questions and, if possible, should be conducted prior to any new research study.

Systematic reviews are nowadays accepted to be superior in quality compared with traditional/narrative reviews. This chapter thus focuses on the methodology of systematic reviews in order to clarify the synthesis of evidence for a specific question.

Writing the systematic review protocol and conducting the review

Conceptualizing a secondary research project or secondary research question is similar to conducting a primary research question. The research question should be justified by existing knowledge or theories. The rationale of the review requires reasonable thought and the review should address a pertinent clinical or scientific issue that will produce useful information for clinicians, researchers, or policy-makers. Conducting a good systematic review is a time-consuming process and it is therefore important to prevent duplication by ascertaining if a similar review has already been published or is in progress. Databases, such as the Cochrane Library, can be searched for the protocols of systematic reviews that are in progress. Because very few sports-related systematic reviews are published in the Cochrane Library or PubMed (limiting searches to systematic reviews), it may be useful to network with experts or authors in the field to ascertain if a similar review to the one that is being planned is being undertaken by other research groups.

It is impossible for a single researcher to conduct a systematic review and thus it is common (and advisable) for systematic reviews to be conducted by teams of researchers. Well-conducted reviews usually involve a review team of three to four individuals. Review-team members should have knowledge of research methodology and skills in searching for information and at least one of the team members should be a content expert. The principal reviewer should manage the project and ensure that the role of each team member is clearly defined early in the review process. The review process can span several months, depending on the extensiveness of the research question and the resources available. To keep track of the review methodology and decisions, a review protocol should be developed by the review team. This should include:

1. background information;
2. setting an explicit review question;
3. review objectives linked to the review question;
4. setting inclusion and exclusion criteria;
5. search strategies for databases;
6. a method of selecting eligible papers;
7. hierarchy for assigning levels of evidence, critical appraisal of study quality and the process of dealing with inconsistencies between raters;

   8. data extraction and analysis

   9. statistical synthesis; and

  10. references.

Background information

The background sets the scene for what is currently known in the area – provides the rationale for why the review needs to be undertaken, the clinical implications of the review, and issues associated with the review findings. It can include information from a traditional review and should provide an overview of the area and the clinical problem.

Setting an explicit review question

The next step in conducting a systematic review is to define a specific review question. A well-designed focused research question is a crucial element of a good systematic review (also see Chapter 1). A broad and poorly defined question wastes time and resources and may fail to produce a definitive answer. A poorly defined question also constrains the conduct of focused searches in library databases and may require the screening of a large amount of potentially eligible studies to assess their eligibility for the review. Designing a review question requires up-to-date knowledge of the field of interest to ensure that the review makes a contribution to the body of knowledge. Sports researchers interested in conducting systematic reviews should not feel limited to reviews addressing the effectiveness of interventions, as a range of systematic review questions can be addressed. The type of question dictates the type of research designs that will provide the most appropriate data with which to answer the systematic review question (Table 7.1).

    The review team, in designing the research question, can use methods such as PICO or PECOT (Population, Exposure/Intervention, Comparator, Outcomes and Time) to ensure that the question is well structured. PICO refers to defining Population, Intervention, Comparison and Outcomes. This method requires that at least three PICO components be included in the question[6]. Although this method can be applied to questions relating to aetiology, it is most useful for effectiveness reviews. Newer methods, such as PECOT, are useful for questions addressing aetiology[7, 8].

Review objectives linked to the review question

The primary objective of the systematic review is to synthesize available and relevant scientific evidence for a specific question. Secondary objectives may be to assess study heterogeneity and identify gaps in literature. In the aforementioned study by Abernethy and Bleakly (Box 7.1)[9],

Table 7.1 Examples of systematic review questions and the primary research designs that they may be relevant for inclusion

Examples of systematic review questions	Appropriate study designs to answer the questions
What is the effectiveness of proprioceptive training in the prevention of ankle injuries in soccer players?	Experimental studies and case studies
What are the prevalence and risk factors of knee injuries in youth soccer?	Epidemiological (descriptive, cause–effect) studies
Are females more at risk of sustaining an anterior cruciate ligament injury?	Epidemiological (case-control, cohort) studies
What is the validity of test X in diagnosing ACL injury?	Diagnostic accuracy studies

---

Box 7.1 Examples of the key components of a systematic review question described with the use of the PICO and PECOT methods

Question: What is the effectiveness of strategies to prevent injury in adolescent school sport compared to no or any other intervention on injury rate and injury severity?[9]

Examples of operationalized review questions:

PICO		PECOT	
Population	Adolescents	*Population*	Adolescents
Intervention	Any preventive intervention	*Exposure/ Intervention*	Any preventive intervention
Comparison	No intervention or any other interventions	*Comparison*	No intervention or any other interventions
Outcomes	Injury rate and injury severity	*Outcomes*	Injury rate and injury severity
		Time	Long term

---

the objectives were to review randomized controlled trials to evaluate the effectiveness of preventive strategies in adolescent sport and to make injury-prevention recommendations based on the strength of evidence.

Setting inclusion and exclusion criteria

Due to the wide availability of published scientific information for many review questions, it is essential to define unambiguous inclusion and exclusion criteria to identify studies that address the review question appropriately. Inclusion and exclusion criteria usually relate to the preferred type of study design for the review, a clear definition of study participants, intervention, exposure, comparison, and outcomes, the time frames of research to be included in the review (e.g. the last 10 years of publications) and the language of articles. Setting eligibility criteria requires that reviewers clearly and carefully define the key elements. Once again, the PICO or PECOT method can be used to identify the key elements of the review question.

   For example, Abernethy and Bleakly[9] defined the population (*P*) as 12- to 18-year-old adolescents involved in supervised physical education and sport (including school sport but excluding sport that only a minority has the opportunity to experience, such as motorized sport, unsupervised skate and extreme sport). The Intervention element (I) involved any type of preventative intervention. The comparison (C) was defined as no intervention or an intervention that did not involve prevention. The outcomes (O) were injury severity (defined as 'time missed from sports participation, training practice or match because of injury') and injury rate (defined as injury per participant, injury per 1000 exposures, and injury per 1000 exposure hours).

   Each clinical area usually involves specific inclusion/exclusion criteria. Additional important outcomes that could be considered for sports-injury preventive-effectiveness reviews therefore could include complications, adverse effects, measures of service utilization, and subjective symptoms, such as instability[10].

Search strategies for databases

Data to answer the review question can be obtained from peer-reviewed scientific literature published in scientific journals and from unpublished information (grey literature), such as

Table 7.2 List of useful sources of information for finding information on sports-related review questions

Free databases	Subscription databases
GoogleScholar	SportDiscus
PubMed	EMBASE
OTSeeker	Cochrane Databases
PEDro	Medline
TRIP – www.tripdatabase.com/	AMED
SUMSearch (http://sumsearch.uthscsa.edu/)	CINAHL
Scirus (http://www.scirus.com/)	

policy reports and student theses. There is a range of freely available databases and subscription library databases that can be used in the search for information. Examples of useful databases for sports-related research are provided in Table 7.2.

The functions of information databases vary and, for the most appropriate information to be found efficiently, it is often necessary to develop specific search strategies according to the way in which the databases operate. Librarians and information specialists are particularly useful in assisting reviewers to develop effective search strategies that yield the greatest number of potentially eligible papers for review in the most efficient manner.

A search strategy usually comprises the key subject terms related to the review question. All major information databases can be searched by specifying more than one word and by using Boolean operators, such as 'AND' and 'OR'. In general, 'AND' is used to combine (mandate) more than one subject term and 'OR' is used to search for variants or synonyms of the search term[11]. Most databases have the facility to use wild cards or truncations. These are useful in identifying word variants of the same word stem. For instance, in PubMed, an asterisk symbol (*) is used to indicate a wild card, in other words 'injur*' searches for words 'injury', 'injured', and 'injuries'.

Because databases comprise thousands of electronic records, records are indexed according to index terms or subject headings called MeSH (Medical subject headings) in PubMed, for example. By applying MeSH terms, key subjects are translated by terms recognized by the database. For example, using the MeSH 'athletic injuries' optimizes the chances of retrieving all studies dealing with sports-related injuries. Box 7.2 illustrates the steps involved in designing a search strategy.

The most appropriate search strategy requires practice and is usually defined by trial and error. A balance should be obtained between the number of hits (potentially relevant articles) produced by the strategy and the relevance of the hits (are they useful?). For instance, if the search strategy provides too many hits, the strategy may be too broad and should be redefined. The number of hits yielded by the search strategy is usually in the hundreds, and keeping track of the search history and hits requires a practical organisational plan that can be stated in the proposal. Some reviewers prefer to print all the hits from each database to provide a permanent record, while others save the hits in clearly marked electronic files. Whichever method is followed, the process should be transparent and retrievable.

A method of selecting eligible papers

Screening hits is a time-consuming process and, to avoid bias, hits are usually screened by two reviewers independently. A third member may be consulted to resolve disagreements. The first

Box 7.2 Key steps in developing a search strategy

Consider searching PubMed for literature to answer the research question: *What is the occurrence and risk factors of knee injuries in adolescents who participate in sport or recreational activities?*

Step 1	Identify the main concepts of the review question, but it is not necessary to incorporate all four aspects of the PICO research question. The key components selected for this example are "knee injuries", "adolescents", and "sport/recreational activities".
Step 2	Check if subject headings (MeSH in PubMed) for the key components are available by searching the MeSH database e.g. "Recreation" [MeSH] is the subject heading for recreational and sporting activities.
Step 3	Identify synonyms or variants of key terms and combine terms using "OR", consider different spellings.
Step 4	Set search "Limits" e.g. The "Age" limit can be set for adolescents, aged 13–18 years.
Step 5	Review the inclusion and exclusion criteria to set additional limits e.g. publication dates, study design, and language.
Step 6	Use wildcards or truncation where appropriate e.g. kne* will search knee and knees.
Step 7	Search each of the key components; "Athletic Injuries" [MeSH],"Recreation" [MeSH] and kne*.
Step 8	Use the History function to combine the different searches (# is used before the search number).
	Example of search strategy
	#1 Search "Recreation"[MeSH] #2 Search "Athletic Injuries"[MeSH] #3 Search #1 AND #2 Field: All fields, Limits: Adolescents: 13–18 years, Publication Date from 1980/01/01 to 2005/10/10, English, Humans #4 Search #3 AND kne*
Step 9	Review the number and relevance of the hits

round of screening aims to identify potentially eligible papers by reviewing titles and abstracts. The second round of screening aims to screen the full texts of eligible papers to decide which studies should be included in the review. Reasons for the exclusion of studies should also be documented, as peer reviewers of systematic reviews to be published may request reasons why some studies are not included in the review. For this reason, the screening process should be retrievable and it is useful to use a flow-chart or consort-diagram (Fig. 7.1) to illustrate the study-selection process.

Levels of evidence and a critical appraisal of study quality

Assigning levels of evidence

Identifying primary research designs required to answer the review question is an intrinsic step in a systematic review. There are many examples of evidence hierarchies developed by different organizations around the world and review teams can choose whichever hierarchy best suits their

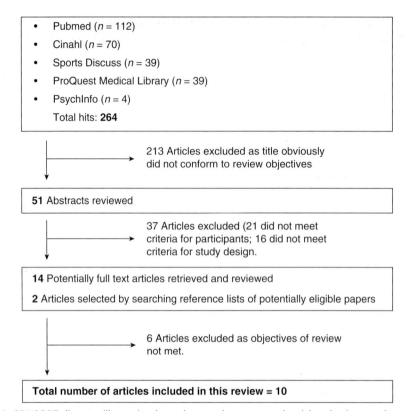

Fig. 7.1 CONSORT diagram illustrating how the search output and article selection can be summarized.

purpose. The example chosen for this chapter is the hierarchy developed by the National Health & Medical Research Council (NH&MRC) in Australia (Table 7.3)[12]. It is important to apply a hierarchy of evidence to each article once it is included in the review.

Some review teams limit the type of research designs to be included in the review (e.g. only randomised controlled trials to answer effectiveness questions), while other review teams take a

Table 7.3 NH&MRC Quantitative evidence hierarchy

Level I	*Systematic review of level II studies*
Level II	*Randomized controlled trial*
Level III-1	*Pseudo randomized controlled trial (e.g. alternate allocation)*
Level III-2	*Comparative study with concurrent controls*
	Controlled trials (non-randomized)
	Cohort study
	Case-control study
Level III-3	*Comparative study without concurrent controls*
	Historical control study
Level IV	*Case series with pre- and post-test outcomes*

broader approach and include any other relevant study design. It is usually recommended that researchers use the data generated by the 'gold standard' study design for a specific question. For instance, randomized controlled trials are viewed to be the 'gold standard' design for answering effectiveness questions. The advantage is that the review findings will be least biased. However, often there is an absence or very few randomized controlled trials available to answer the specific effectiveness question. The reviewers may then select to include controlled trials in addition to randomized controlled trials. When this approach is followed, the strength of the evidence will need to be interpreted with caution, due to the increased risk of bias inherent to designs not considered to be the gold standard.

Critical appraisal of study quality

Appraising the methodological quality of included articles is an important step in determining the strength of evidence available for the review question. However, appraising quality sports-related papers using appropriate critical appraisal tools may pose a challenge to review teams, as reviewers should decide on the appraisal process and tools. Critical appraisal tools are structured checklists that assist reviewers with grading the methodological quality of studies included in the review. There are currently more than 100 critical appraisal tools from which sports researchers can choose[13]. These tools are broadly classified as generic tools, which can be used to appraise any design, and each specific tool is designed for a specific type of study design. Critical appraisal tools are very accessible to researchers nowadays. One source for critical appraisal tools has been developed by the Centre for Allied Health Evidence (CAHE) Critical Appraisal Tools (CATs) (www.unisa.edu.au/cahe/cats). However, selecting the most appropriate tool is more complex, as there is no gold-standard tool and sports researchers should consider the critical appraisal elements relevant to their review. This may require the team deciding on the standard critical appraisal instrument to be used or adapting or developing a tool that is specific to the review. When adapting or developing a tool, the review team should reach consensus on the most relevant aspects of the critical appraisal tool for the specific review.

The critical appraisal process should also be conducted independently by two members of the review team. Similar to the study-selection process, disagreements should be resolved by a third reviewer. The kappa statistic (Box 7.3) is commonly used to measure agreement between reviewers. Kappa values between 0.4 and 0.59 may be considered fair agreement, between 0.6 and 0.74 good agreement and a value more than 0.75 is viewed as excellent agreement.

Data extraction and analysis

Data extraction tables or forms can be used to retrieve relevant data from eligible papers. Standard data-extraction tables have been developed by organisations such as the Joanna Briggs Institute[14]. Reviewers may also choose to develop a study-specific data-extraction instrument. This should comprise at least basic descriptive information, such as demographics, study variables, study-design specifics (such as sample size), data to answer the review question, main study findings, and clinical recommendations. If a new data-extraction table is designed, it is useful to validate it with all members of the review team and with experienced systematic reviewers who are not involved with the review in order to assess whether the data to be extracted are adequate in addressing all review objectives.

Data extracted from studies included in the review assist reviewers in assessing study heterogeneity. This refers to the diversity among studies with respect to participants, interventions, and outcome studies[15]. Examining the heterogeneity of studies assists reviewers in deciding how to analyse and report study findings in a meaningful manner. When all studies (or a subgroup)

Box 7.3 Cohen's Kappa

The Cohen's Kappa coefficient (κ) is a general statistical measure for inter-rater agreement. It measures the agreement between two *raters* who each classify N items into C unique categories. In the case of this chapter κ measures agreement between two reviewers who independently score N papers on C unique quality criteria.

As κ takes into account that some agreement occurs by chance, it is generally considered to be a more robust measure than the percent of agreement amongst raters.

The equation for κ is $\Pr(a) - \Pr(e)/1 - \Pr(e)$, where $\Pr(a)$ is the relative observed agreement between raters, and $\Pr(e)$ is the agreement expected to occur by chance.

Example

Suppose one is analysing knee X-rays of professional soccer players in order to determine the prevalence of sustained Osgood–Schlatter episodes. Each X-ray was examined by two radiologists, and either said 'Yes' or 'No' to the presence of residual symptoms. Suppose the data are as follows:

		Assessor B	
		Yes	No
Assessor A	Yes	10	9
	No	6	45

The observed percentage of agreement is $\Pr(a)$ is then equal to $(10 + 45)/70 = 0.79$. To calculate the probability of random agreement $\Pr(e)$ note that:

- Assessor A said 'Yes' to 19 X-rays and 'No' to 51. Thus assessor A registered 'Yes' 37% of the time.

- Assessor B said 'Yes' to 16 X-rays and 'No' to 54. Thus assessor B registered 'Yes' 30% of the time.

Then the probability that both assessors would say 'Yes' randomly is $0.37 * 0.30 = 0.11$ and the probability that both would say 'No' is $0.63 * 0.70 = 0.44$. This makes the overall probability of random agreement $\Pr(e) = 0.11 + 0.44 = 0.55$.

Applying these numbers to the formula for Cohen's Kappa one gets:

$$\kappa = \Pr(a) - \Pr(e)/1 - \Pr(e) = 0.79 - 0.55/1 - 0.55 = 0.24/0.45 = 0.53$$

included in the review are homogeneous, a meta-analysis can be conducted as the findings of only clinically similar studies can be combined. A meta-analysis is a statistical approach used to combine the results of two or more homogeneous studies to produce a summary statistic (or measure of effect). The summary statistic is not simple the 'average', but is a weighted value as the relatively larger trials contribute more than smaller studies to the calculation of the summary statistic. Meta-analyses increase the power and precision of the effect of the intervention as well as the generalizability of the findings[3]. When a meta-analysis is possible, software such as Review Manager developed by the Cochrane Collaboration can be used to conduct the analysis. The latest version, Review Manager Version 5, is user-friendly and freely available from the Cochrane Collaboration's website (www.cochrane.org). However, often insufficient data are provided in the published paper and reviewers have to contact the authors to obtain the data required to

Box 7.4 Example forest plot and explanation

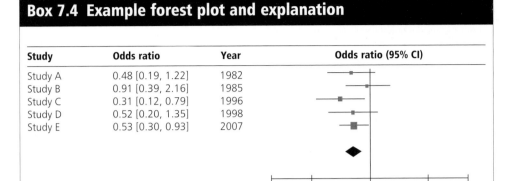

Study	Odds ratio	Year	Odds ratio (95% CI)
Study A	0.48 [0.19, 1.22]	1982	
Study B	0.91 [0.39, 2.16]	1985	
Study C	0.31 [0.12, 0.79]	1996	
Study D	0.52 [0.20, 1.35]	1998	
Study E	0.53 [0.30, 0.93]	2007	

0.02   0.1   1   10   50
Favours stretching   Favours not stretching

The first column represents the included randomized controlled trials that were clinically homogeneous and investigated whether stretching regimes (intervention) reduced the onset of patellofemoral pain (outcome) compared to not performing stretching (comparison) in adolescent basketball players (population). The year the study was published is indicated in the third column. In this example, the odds ratio is the measure of effect. The odds ratio of each trial is indicated by the corresponding dark rectangle and the horizontal line crossing each rectangle indicates the width of the confidence interval. Each study's odds ratio and 95% confidence interval values are indicated in the second column. The size (sample size) of each study is illustrated by the size of the rectangles. The summary statistic (combined, weighted odds ratio) is indicated by the vertical midline of the black diamond and the odds ratio value is 0.53. The confidence interval for all trials combined is indicated by the width of the black diamond (0.37–0.75). The central, solid black vertical line is the line of no effect (odds ratio = 1). The summary statistic indicates a protective effect (0.53), therefore there is less likelihood that a player will develop patellofemoral pain if a stretching regime is performed. The confidence interval of the summary statistic does not cross the line of no effect (solid black vertical line) and therefore the results indicate that the benefit of performing a stretching regime is statistically significant.

conduct the meta-analysis. When a meta-analysis is conducted, a forest plot is used to present the review findings. An example of a forest plot is illustrated in Box 7.4.

Meta-analyses present an opportunity to sports researchers, as they lack the resources to conduct large-scale studies that produce credible results. More meta-analyses will be possible in sports related research if the variability in injury-definitions, injury-classifications, and exposures can be eradicated by the researchers.

Sensitivity analysis may also be required to answer all the 'what if' questions. For instance, when conducting a meta-analysis, reviewers may want to assess the impact of lower-quality studies on the summary statistic. The researchers can then formulate two forest plots to illustrate the difference in the findings if all studies are pooled compared to only high-quality studies.

When studies are heterogeneous, the synthesis of primary research generally cannot produce a meta-analysis and findings should be reported qualitatively (or descriptively) (this is often called a meta-synthesis). Sports-related studies are often heterogeneous and a qualitative/descriptive synthesis of included studies should present an unbiased summary of the evidence for a specific question by including all studies identified in the search. However, a disadvantage of a descriptive synthesis is that it cannot provide a statistical estimate or the size of the effect. Researchers should therefore guard against over-stressing the findings of such studies.

Statistical synthesis

One of the most difficult tasks in undertaking a review is to present review findings in a sensible manner, to ensure that all objectives are met and to provide a useful summary of literature to assist clinicians in making clinical decisions. Therefore, it is important to review objectives and the primary research question when results are presented. Flow-charts, tables, and graphs are often used when systematic reviews are reported in order to present findings in a reader-friendly, synthesized format.

Often reviewers follow all the steps in the review process carefully but may not present the interpretation of findings and clinical recommendations clearly. When interpreting findings, reviewers should consider the following factors:

- The body of evidence (the number of studies reviewed).
- The homogeneity of the studies, the quality of the studies and the impact of the methodological shortcomings on the study findings.
- The appropriateness and descriptions of the interventions.
- The costs and risks associated with the interventions.
- The validity and reliability of the methods used to measure the outcomes.
- The relevance of the outcomes of the studies reviewed with respect to important stake-holders including patients, health-care providers, health-care funders, etc.
- The appropriateness of the key study-variable definitions.
- Countries where studies have been conducted.
- Whether all studies have been conducted by the same research group.
- Possible reasons if the study findings are equivocal between studies.
- The relevance of the clinical recommendation emanating from the review findings to different contexts.
- The potential impact of the clinical recommendation based on the review findings.

Referring to studies

All the references considered for the review should be reported in the reference list. It is common for the references to be separated into those relevant to the background section, those that were considered but excluded (and for what reason) and those that were included in the review process. A standard referencing style is also required. Because of the number of words involved in many literature reviews, a numerical referencing system is suggested, as this removes a large number of words from the body of the text. The Vancouver referencing style is therefore the most common numeric referencing style used for academic work and is generally the preferred style by journals. When an in-text citation is referenced, a number is placed beside the text either in superscript (i.e. 1) or in brackets (i.e. (1) or [1]), which corresponds to the number in the reference list. Each reference is given a number and this number is used each time that the reference is cited, whether once only or whether multiple times. The full reference (the author and publication details) is then provided in numerical order in the reference list. Other numeric referencing styles, such as endnotes and footnotes, which number the in-text citation, provide a footnote (at the bottom of the page) or an endnote (at the end of the chapter) with the reference. Full references are then included in the reference list. Each reference has a new number each time that it is cited. One reference may therefore have multiple numbers linked to it.

Publishing the review

While narrative reviews are published less often these days, the number of systematic review publications is increasing exponentially. In sports medicine, relatively fewer systematic reviews have been published compared with other related fields, such as general orthopaedics. It is thus crucial for sports scientists to consider doing systematic reviews and publishing them, as the outcomes of secondary research can inspire new and innovative primary research projects to enhance the sports-medicine knowledge base. It is important to publish reviews in journals that are widely read by sports clinicians, so that the full value of the review findings are realized in clinical practice. Many sports journals now accept one review per issue and, if review teams therefore have a review in progress, it is a good idea for them to make contact with the editors of the journals in which they would like to have their reviews published well ahead of completing their reviews to gauge the potential for having the reviews published in a timely manner. The questions that review teams could ask are whether the journals will consider a review on their specific review questions, the turn-around times of the review processes, the manner of publication (whether it is paper-based and/or electronic), the number of words and references allowed for reviews, and the impact factor of the journals. Once a review team has selected the journal in which it has decided to have its review published, it is also important for the team to consider the journal's specific author instructions/requirements when writing the review. For example, the journal may have slight variations on the punctuation and formatting for the reference list. Following the author instructions/requirements assists the review team in minimizing the potential for outright rejection (for not meeting the journal requirements). Being prepared can also reduce the review and revision time.

References

1. Ball R, Tunger D (2006). Science indicators revisited: Science Citation Index versus SCOPUS: A bibliometric comparison of both citation databases. *Information Services and Use*, **26**, 293–301.
2. Volmink J (2007). Literature review, in Joubert G, Ehrlich R (eds) *Epidemiology: A research manual for South Africa*, pp. 66–74. Oxford University Press.
3. Pai M, McCulloch M, Gorman JD, Pai N, Enanoria W, Kennedy G, Tharyan P, Colford JM (2004). Systematic reviews and meta-analysis: An illustrated, step-by-step guide. *Natl Med J India*, **17**(2), 86–95.
4. Akobeng AK (2005). Understanding systematic reviews and meta-analysis. *Arch Dis Child*, **90**, 845–8.
5. Greenhalgh T (1997). Papers that summarise other papers (systematic reviews and meta-analyses). *BMJ*, **315**(7109), 672–5.
6. Sackett DL, Straus SE, Richardson WS, Rosenberg W, Haynes RB (2000). *Evidence-based medicine: How to practice and teach EBM*. Churchill Livingstone, Edinburgh.
7. Toouli J (2007). Editorial. *HPB: Official journal of the International Hepato Pancreato Biliary Association*, **9**(4), 249–50.
8. Van der Wees PJ, Hendriks EJM, Custers JWH, Burgers JS, Dekker J, De Bie RA (2007). Comparison of international guideline programs to evaluate and update the Dutch program for clinical guideline development in physical therapy. *BMC Health Services Research*, **7**(191), DOI:10.1186/1472–6963–7–191.
9. Abernethy L, Bleakly C (2007). Strategies to prevent injury in adolescent sport: A systematic review. *Br J Sports Med*, **41**, 627–38.

10. Handoll HHG, Rowe BH, Quinn KM, De Bie R (2001). Interventions for preventing ankle ligament injuries (review). *Cochrane Database Syst Rev*, **3**, DOI:10.1002/14651858.CD000018.

11. Jansen BJ, Spink A, Saracevic T (2000). Real life, real users, and real needs: A study and analysis of user queries on the web. *Inform Process Manag*, **36**(2), 207–27.

12. NHMRC hierarchy of evidence. [cited 2009 Jan 27]. Available from: http://www.nhmrc.gov.au/ guidelines/_files/Stage%202%20Consultation%20Levels%20and%20Grades.pdf.

13. Katrak P, Bialocerkowski A, Massy-Westropp N, Kumar VS, Grimmer K (2004). The content of critical appraisal tools. *BMC Research Methodology*, **4**(22), DOI:10.1186/1471–2288–4–22.

14. Joanna Briggs Institute Reviewer's Manual: Data extraction sheets. 2008 [cited 2009 Jan 27]: 155–8 Available from: http://www.joannabriggs.edu.au/pdf/JBIReviewManual_CiP11449.pdf.

15. Cochrane handbook. [cited 2009 Jan 27]. Available from: http://www.cochrane-handbook.org.

Part 3

Establishing injury aetiology

Chapter 8

The multi-causality of injury – current concepts

Willem Meeuwisse and Brent Hagel

Whether in life, or in conducting research, we are often trying to ascertain truth. This is also the case when applied to the area of injury prevention. We want to be able to understand what can be done to reduce injury and then implement programmes to lessen the burden in society. In seeking solutions to complex problems such as this, how we think is often more important than what we think. As such, our goal in this chapter is to outline methods of evaluating or understanding injury prevention.

Models of injury prevention

Haddon (1972) developed a matrix, modelled on motor-vehicle collisions, that examined different phases (pre-event, event, and post-event) across a number of parameters including host, vehicle, physical environment, and social environment[1]. The pre-event phase is where we would like to focus most of our attention, since our aim is to prevent injuries from occurring in the first place. Traditional epidemiological separation of injury prevention employs categories of primary (where the injury does not occur), secondary (rapid diagnosis and treatment and prevention of associated morbidity), and tertiary (return to full function and prevention of re-injury). Using this terminology, we will focus on primary prevention.

Willem van Mechelen (1992) outlined steps in injury prevention where (i) the extent of the problem is outlined, (ii) the risk factors or causes are identified, (ii) preventive measures are introduced, and (iv) the effectiveness of prevention is measured by going back to the first phase (the extent of the injury problem)[2]. In this next section we would like to focus on the second stage, that being identifying the risk factors or cause.

Understanding risk factors and cause

Origins of causal thinking in epidemiology

This chapter is concerned with addressing the issue of sports-injury aetiology. In essence, aetiology may be defined as causal origin[3]. Rothman, Greenland, and Lash discuss in detail the notion of causality[4]. Any such discussion would be incomplete without considering Hill's criteria for attempting to evaluate causal vs. non-causal relationships[5]:

1. strength
2. consistency
3. specificity
4. temporality

5. biological gradient

6. plausibility

7. coherence

8. experimental evidence

9. analogy

Many acknowledge that the only absolute criteria that is necessary, but not sufficient, is temporality. Rothman, Greenland, and Lash ultimately have this to say about 'causal criteria':

> Causal criteria appear to function less like standards or principles and more like values…which vary across individual scientists and even vary within the work of a single scientist, depending on the context and time. Thus, universal and objective causal criteria, if they exist, have yet to be identified.

In 1976 Rothman wrote an elegant paper outlining the difference between necessary and sufficient cause[6]. A necessary cause exists when a factor must always precede an effect and, furthermore, the outcome or disease cannot occur without the presence of this necessary factor. This differs from a sufficient cause which is, in fact, a collection or constellation of factors. It is, essentially, a set of minimal conditions and events that inevitably can produce the outcome. In Fig. 8.2 adapted from Rothman (1976), factor A is a necessary component to complete a sufficient cause[6]. However, factors B, C, and F are not necessary causes as there are sufficient causes that occur without them.

Central to any discussion of causation is the notion of a causal contrast. To say that artificial turf causes lower-extremity injuries is a vacuous statement. Would it be a risk factor for lower-extremity injury if the athletes played on artificial turf or asphalt? With a contrast of these two surfaces, we might find that artificial turf is actually protective for lower-extremity injury. A more meaningful causal contrast would be to compare artificial turf with natural grass surfacing. The point is that inherent in any statement of causation is an appropriate causal contrast of an index with a referent category of the determinant of injury.

Following from this point, is the notion that aetiology is inherently retrospective[3]. That is, atiological time zero is the time of outcome occurrence (e.g. head injury when evaluating snowboarding helmet effectiveness; wrist injury when evaluating wrist-guard effectiveness). The key is that one should look back from the time of case occurrence to an aetiologically relevant period of time. Here we mean the time period over which the determinant is expected to act to increase

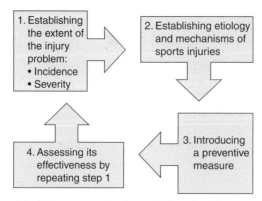

Fig. 8.1 A four stage model of injury prevention by van Mechelen[2].

Reproduced from van Mechelen W, Hlobil H, Kemper H (1992). Incidence, Severtiy, Etiology and Prevention of Sports Injuries – A review of concepts. *Sports Med*, **14**(2), 82–99 with permission from Wolters Kluwer Health | Adis (© Adis Data Information BV 1992. All rights reserved.)

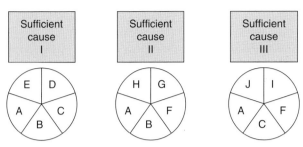

Fig. 8.2 Rothman's sufficient cause model.
Adapted from Rothman[6].

or decrease the risk of injury. For example, one might evaluate the effect of ski and snowboard helmets just prior to an injury-producing event or a non-injury-producing crash. It is easy to see that this is a more aetiologically relevant time period than, say, asking a group of skiers and snowboarders at the start of the season whether they plan to wear helmets in the upcoming season over which time evaluation of injury status will take place.

To summarize, when examining aetiology, we need to understand that we are always looking back to a relevant time period for the determinant of interest. In addition, a contrast of an index and referent category for the determinant (e.g. helmet users compared with non-users) is an essential element for evaluating causation.

Sport and recreational injuries

In 1994 Meeuwisse developed a multi-factorial model of injury where intrinsic risk factors that predispose the athlete are first identified[7]. Exposure to extrinsic risk factors then occurs, which may make the athlete more susceptible to injury. All of these factors are considered to be distant from the outcome. Then, there is an inciting event producing an injury with, usually, an identifiable mechanism of injury that is proximal to the outcome. One of the issues raised repeatedly questions which risk factors, of all those possible, are actually important in causing injury? Intrinsic factors can include player characteristics such as past history, flexibility, and strength, to name a few. Extrinsic risk factors include items such as equipment, footwear, and the playing surface. The important questions are as follows:

1. Which factors are associated with an increased rate of injury (risk factors)?

2. Are those factors the 'cause' of injury?

3. Are those factors modifiable?

If it is possible to establish a correlation between an injury and a (risk) factor, one must ascertain whether or not that correlation represents a causal relationship. Sometimes there is an undetermined variable that the risk factor and the injury have in common. This is often referred to as a confounder[7]. For example, are irregular menses in female runners a causal factor for running injuries? While there may be an association, a relationship with a third factor may prove to be the more important element. In this case, running mileage may be the true causative factor. Running mileage is both associated with amenorrhea and also associated with higher rates of injury. If we control for running mileage, the first apparent relationship (irregular menses and injury) may disappear.

The reason this is important is because, irrespective of the causal relationship, the risk factor is usually a valid predictor of injury. However, removing the risk factor may not necessarily prevent injury if a causal relationship does not exist.

There are some limitations to the model proposed by Meeuwisse in 1994 that were addressed in a manuscript by Bahr and Krosshaug[8]. They identified that the inciting event can be a complex group of key components that include the playing situation, player and opponent behaviour, gross biomechanical description, and detailed biomechanical description (Fig. 8.3).

This model describes the mechanism of injury in more detail and allows assessment in the context of intrinsic and extrinsic risk factors. However, since exposure in the context of sport injury is both possessing a risk factor and participating with it, athletes may be exposed to the same or different risks repeatedly. Furthermore, injuries may or may not result in the removal from sport (and therefore further exposure). As such, a linear approach, with a start and endpoint, does not reflect the true situation.

Connor Gissame wrote a paper in 2001 that described an operational model to investigate contact-sport injuries. His model represents a more cyclic picture beginning with a healthy, fit player who is exposed to various factors that may or may not produce injury (Fig. 8.4).

The model allowed for the possibility of no injury occurring and going back to a healthy, fit status. The model also allows that injury might occur, contributing to injury incidence and prevalence, and resulting in certain outcomes. From there, Gissane outlined the possibility of injury recurrence, a return to the healthy and fit status, or removal from sport. This model factors in the repetitive nature of athletic participation and allows multiple outcomes from injury. At the same time, it does not account for the fact that athletes may return to participation in an unhealthy state or have further recurrence after return. It is important to recognize that adaptation occurs after injury and also after non-injury.

Taking these notions into consideration, a modification of the model by Meeuwisse was developed and published in 2007[10]. Building from the original base, it was recognized that while sometimes an inciting event occurs to produce injury, more often events occur that result in no injury (Fig. 8.5). However, adaptations in the athlete may occur due to participation itself.

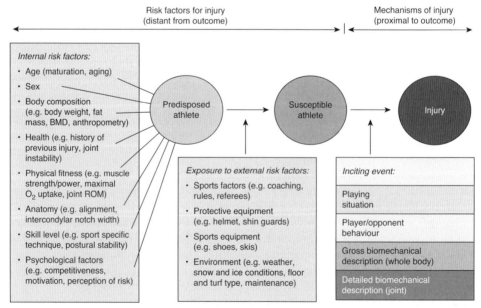

Fig. 8.3 Bahr and Krosshaug's multifactorial model of mechanisms of injury.
Reproduced from Bahr and Krosshaug[8] with permission from BMJ Publishing Group Ltd.

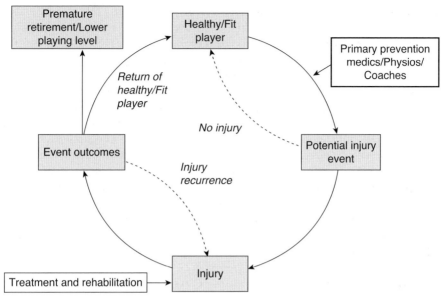

Fig. 8.4 Gissane's Operational Model to Investigate Contact Sports Injuries[9].
Adapted from Gissane et al. [9]

If an injury does occur, the athlete may be removed from participation if they do not fully recover. However, some degree of recovery may allow the athlete to return to participation and, therefore, repeat participation.

For example, it is possible that increased strength reduces risk of injury. If an athlete participates in a body-contact sport, participation itself may produce weakness or it may result in

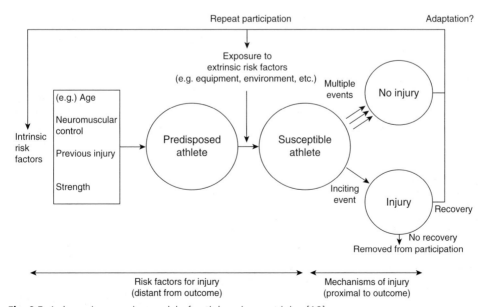

Fig. 8.5 A dynamic, recursive model of aetiology in sport injury[10].
Reproduced with permission from: Meeuwisse WH, Tyreman H, Hagel B, Emery CA (2007). Dynamic Model of Etiology in Sport Injury: The recursive nature of risk and causation. *Clin J Sport Med*, **17**(3), 215–19.

strengthening. If they adapt and get stronger, their risk decreases, but if they mal-adapt and get weaker, their injury risk increases. In this setting, exposure to other (constant or unchanging) risk factors may produce an injury. This example illustrates how intrinsic predisposition can change with repeat participation.

This model also allows different outcomes including no injury, injury removal, injury and recovery (which could be either full or partial), and adaptation versus mal-adaptation. Athletes may also enter into the cycle at any point from the beginning of the season or year or at specific events such as a heavy training period or competition.

One other question that needs to be identified is the implication of no injury. Often events occur which appear to be mechanisms of injury, but likewise very similar events can occur that produce no injury. We have to ask ourselves, why does an injury occur in some situations and not in others with similar mechanisms? This question was raised in an editorial by Meeuwisse (2009) where identifying the 'mechanism of no injury' (MONI) was identified as important[11]. It is critical when studying mechanisms of injury to first consider the mechanism of no injury and try and identify the difference between the two. If the difference can be articulated, we may be well on our way to identifying the most important aetiological elements of injury.

Implications for study design

This has implications for study design. We can do cross-sectional studies, but this does not allow us to establish a time factor that separates cause from effect. Case-control and cohort studies are superior in this regard as they allow observation over time, whether historically or prospectively and therefore allow us to establish cause. Likewise, intervention studies, which ideally should be randomized controlled trials (RCTs), produce time-dependent variables that also allow establishment of cause and effect. There are limitations with randomized controlled trials that include compliance and therefore, 'exposure to the intervention'. A critical examination of the differences between randomized controlled trials and non-experimental studies is beyond the scope of this chapter, but see Sorensen et al. for an excellent overview[12].

Within the context of sport, we need to consider the specificity of risk factors, whether at a team level or individual level. If we are going to apply this dynamic recursive model of injury cause, we need to consider whether we should be using the same variables but changing the way we measure them.

We have to ask whether it is appropriate to measure variables at a single point in time, or whether they should be measured at multiple points in time. The other possibility is that new time-dependent variables are created. Placing this in the context of non-experimental designs, cohort studies could be done with repeated measures to account for changes over time, allowing for an accounting of exposure implications, specifically, with time-dependent variables. In conducting case-control studies we have to consider what point in time to measure prior exposure and, perhaps, whether we should consider a summary measure or whether we should consider each exposure unique.

Object of study

The first step in assessing a causal relationship is careful consideration of what Miettinen defines as the object of study or 'the outcome's incidence density in causal relation to the etiologic determinant in a defined domain'([3] p. 485). Some examples include:

+ the occurrence of head injuries in relation to helmet use among skiers and snow-boarders.
+ the occurrence of lower-extremity injuries in relation to past injury in intercollegiate football players.
+ the occurrence of concussion in relation to body checking in minor ice hockey players.

This relationship must be with respect to potential effect-modifiers and conditioned on all potential confounders. Thus, it is crucial to develop appropriate conceptual and, ultimately, operational definitions of each of the outcome(s), determinant(s), and confounder(s) to be considered in a given study.

Outcome, determinant, and confounder definitions

The outcome definition must be as homogeneous as possible. Miettinen suggests that cases of an outcome be 'severe' and 'typical'[3]. This avoids the problem of outcome misclassification. Our own work in both intercollegiate football and skiing and snowboarding has shown that determinants have different effects depending on the body region injured[13,14]. Therefore, it is appropriate to be very specific in the outcome definition (wrist injury vs. upper-extremity injury or knee injury vs. lower-extremity injury).

Precision in the operational definition of the determinant of interest is important as well. One might consider age as a determinant of injury. If the categorization is old versus young, this will likely be insufficient to demonstrate an effect, unless age is a strong risk factor for injury. However, categorizing age into smaller, but still meaningful groups (<5; 6–10, 11–14, etc.) will likely lead to adequate operationalization of age as a determinant of injury. Treating age as a continuous variable provides the most efficient use of all the information, but mis-specification of the functional relationship between this variable and outcome (incidence, prevalence, odds, etc.) becomes more likely.

If aetiology is truly of interest, then of outcome, exposure, and confounders, it is most important to adequately measure confounders to guard against residual confounding. For example, any past injury versus none is a very broad operational definition. For example, if we are interested in the effect of knee bracing as a protective factor for knee injury, then past injury would be a potentially important confounder as it is associated with bracing and would be an independent risk factor for knee injury. In this case, not adjusting for past injury would potentially remove the protective effect of knee bracing, if such a protective effect truly existed. But adjusting for any past injury (arm fracture, concussion, leg injury, etc.) would be inadequate to control confounding. A better operational definition might be knee injury within the past year.

Ideally, one would design the occurrence relation down to the regression model before conducting the study. This is facilitated by adding a table to the study protocol detailing how the variable will be treated in the analysis. This conveys the thought behind the definition of each type of variable to be captured in the study.

We have recently published on the dynamic, recursive nature of sport injury. The model is meant to guide the researcher's thinking about the factors that may influence the occurrence of injury in a given athlete and environment. However, the complexity involved in considering the conditions producing the injury event, gives way to simplicity in the analysis. In designing the analysis, fundamentally, we have merely to consider the causal contrast of interest, that is, the contrast of the index and reference category of the determinant. This is true irrespective of whether the system of data collection is prospective ('cohort study') or retrospective (case-control) study[3]. In this sense, aetiological time zero is the time of case occurrence, and it is in reference to this time, that the causal contrast is made. In addition, inherent in this conceptualization is the timing of the exposure of interest. Miettinen[15] considers sub-populations of a source population for a study:

1. The index population, consisting of those from the study domain with recent exposure.

2. The reference population from the study domain that has no recent exposure and that is comparable to the index population for extraneous determinants of injury (i.e. confounders).

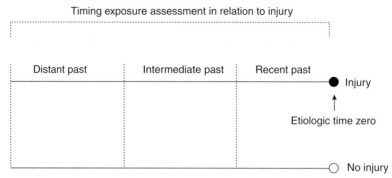

Fig. 8.6 Conceptualization of aetiological research analysis including aetiological time zero and timing of the assessment of exposure status.

The index and reference populations make up the study population. Fig. 8.6 graphically depicts the conceptual elements of aetiological research. Fig. 8.7 illustrates the elements that go into the analysis of aetiological data. As stated above, the simple depiction of the comparison in Fig. 8.7 in terms of the parameter of interest (incidence-density ratio) is to be conditioned on the relevant confounding factors either through stratification or regression modelling.

Taking action

Before developing and introducing preventive measures, we must consider the question of benefit versus harm. It is obvious that we desire to reduce injury. However, introducing preventive measures can produce 'side effects' that might include an increased risk of the same injury, increased risk of some associated injury, or a change in the nature or style of sport that makes participation more dangerous.

For example, the concept of risk compensation discussed by Hagel and Meeuwisse[14] relates to potential athlete behavioural change in response to a safer sport or recreational environment. The same concept of risk compensation applied to mechanisms of injury was outlined in a paper

	Injured	Study base sample
Index	a	b
Reference	c	d

a = injured subjects in index category of determinant
b = sampled subjects in index category of determinant
c = injured subjects in reference category of determinant
d = sampled subjects in reference category of determinant

a/b = quasi rate of injury in index category of determinant
c/d = quasi rate of injury in reference category of determinant

(a/d)/(c/d) – ad/bc – odds ratio – unbiased estimate of incidence density ratio

Fig. 8.7 Analysis of data collected from an aetiological research study.

by MacIntosh[16]. He identified on-field behaviour and skills leading to certain events which produced mechanical load, followed by a mechanical response, an injury mechanism, and finally injury. These elements can be influenced by training, tolerance levels, and even preventive methods.

The evaluation of preventive measures is particularly important. The intervention itself must be based on the dynamic nature of risk and cause. The researcher must decide where or when to intervene; that is, the number of stages, cycles, and whether on a group or individual basis.

When preventive measures are developed, an assessment of efficacy and effectiveness should be conducted. The concept of translating research into injury-preventive practice was outlined by Caroline Finch[17]. She elaborated on the mid-stage of van Mechelen's 4-stage approach[2]. A more detailed description was provided, including the development of preventive measures under ideal or scientific conditions, and then describing the intervention context to inform implementational strategies before evaluating the effectiveness in that context. Knowledge translation and engaging the sport community is a key ingredient of effective preventive programmes.

Conclusion

Our goal is to understand risk factors and to consider whether they can be modified. It appears that most risk factors are sport specific and interact with other factors to increase the chances of injury; and they do so in a dynamic recursive manner where risks change over time with repeat participation. Our approach to studying risk factors must take this into consideration. To develop effective preventive measures, we need to decide how far back to look at causal factors, addressing aetiologically relevant time and the number of cycles. Ultimately, it is hoped that novel approaches will lead to reduction in sport injuries and healthy participation.

References

1. Haddon J (1997). A logical framework for categorizing highway safety phenomena and activity. *J Trauma*, **12**, 193–207.
2. van Mechelen W, Hlobil H, Kemper H (1992). Incidence, Severtiy, Etiology and Prevention of Sports Injuries – A review of concepts. *Sports Med*, **14**(2), 82–99.
3. Miettinen O (1999). Etiologic Research: Needed revisions of concepts and principles. *Scand J Work Environ Health*, **25**(6), 484–90.
4. Rothman K, Greenland S, Lash T (2008). *Modern epidemiology, 3rd Edition*. Lippincott Williams & Wilkins, Baltimore.
5. Hill A (1965). The Environment and Disease: Association or Causation? *Proceedings of the Royal Society of Medicine* **58**, 295–300.
6. Rothman K (1976). Causes. *Am J Epidem*, **104**(6), 587–92.
7. Meeuwisse W (1994). Athletic Injury Etiology: Distinguishing between interaction and confounding. *Clin J Sport Med*, **4**(3), 171–5.
8. Bahr R, Krosshaug T (2005). Understanding Injury Mechanisms: a key component of preventing injuries in sport. *Br J Sports Med*, **39**, 324–9.
9. Gissane C, White J, Kerr K, Jennings D (2001). An Operational Model to Investigate Contact Sports Injuries. *Med Sci Sports Exerc*, **33**(12), 1999–2003.
10. Meeuwisse WH, Tyreman H, Hagel B, Emery CA (2007). Dynamic Model of Etiology in Sport Injury: The recursive nature of risk and causation. *Clin J Sport Med*, **17**(3), 215–19.
11. Meeuwisse W (2009). What is the Mechanism of No Injury (MONI)? *Clin J Sport Med*, **19**(1), 1–2.
12. Sorensen H, Lash T, Rothman K (2006). Beyond randomized controlled trials: a critical comparison of trials with non-randomized studies. *Hepatology*, **44**(5), 1075–82.

13. Hagel B, Fick G, Meeuwisse W (2003). Multivariate Analysis of Injury-Related Risk Factors in Intercollegiate Football. *Am J Epidem*, **157**(9), 825–33.

14. Hagel B, MeeuwisseW (2004). Risk Compensation: A "side effect" of sport injury prevention? *Clin J Sport Med*, **14**(4), 193–6.

15. Miettinen O, Caro J (1989). Principles of Nonexperimental Assessment of Excess Risk, With Specific Reference to Adverse Drug Reactions. *J Clin Epidemiol*, **42**(4), 325–31.

16. McIntosh A (2005). Risk Compensation, Motivation, Injuries and Biomechanics in Competitive Sport. *Br J Sports Med*, **39**, 2–3.

17. Finch C (2006). A New Framework for Research Leading to Sports Injury Prevention. *J Sci Med Sport*, **9**, 3–9.

Chapter 9

Investigating injury risk factors and mechanisms

Tron Krosshaug and Evert Verhagen

The previous chapter described the intricate relationship between risk factors, mechanisms of injury, and injury. In an attempt to prevent an injury from occurring, insight into the components that form (part of) a causal link in the events that lead to injury is required. Straightforwardly stated, minimizing the role of a causal component or completely removing this component from the equation will in theory reduce the likelihood of an injury occurring. Thereby, effective injury prevention requires thorough knowledge on risk factors and mechanisms of injury that are a vital part in the injury-causing pathway.

Such a causal relationship between a causal component and injury occurrence is commonly referred to as injury aetiology. In general the term 'aetiology' refers to the causes of diseases or pathologies. Thereby, by definition, an aetiological component may sometimes only be part of a chain of causation. In addition, one must distinguish 'causation' from 'statistical correlation' or 'association'. Instead of an injury being caused by a certain risk factor or mechanism, events may simply be present together due to chance, bias, or confounding. Specific statistical techniques that are able to provide evidence of a causal relationship are discussed in Chapter 10. However, in order to determine causation, careful sampling and measurement of potential risk factors and thorough investigation of the mechanism of injury is equally important to sophisticated statistical analysis. This chapter will focus specifically on the techniques that may be used to investigate potential injury risk factors and mechanisms of injury.

Epidemiological criteria for causation

In 1965 Sir Austin Bradford Hill laid out nine criteria for evaluating statistical associations[1]. This list of 'criteria' continues to be used today, and outlines the minimal conditions required to establish a causal relationship between two events. While it is effortless to claim that factor A (e.g. previous injury) causes injury B (ankle sprain), it is another matter to establish a meaningful and statistically valid connection between these two circumstances (Fig. 9.1).

Temporality

Exposure to a causal factor always precedes the outcome. If factor A (previous injury) is believed to cause injury (ankle sprain), then it is clear that factor A must necessarily always precede injury onset. Of all nine criteria this is the only absolutely essential criterion that must be met in order to speak of a causal relationship.

Strength

This is defined by the size of the association as measured by appropriate statistical tests. The stronger the relationship between the risk factor and injury risk, the less likely it is that the detected

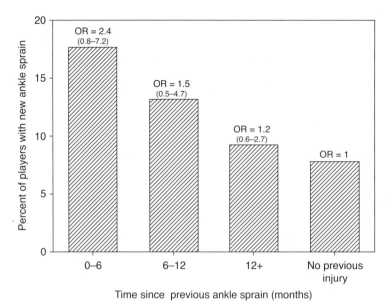

Fig. 9.1 The relationship between previous injury and risk of recurrent injury.
Reproduced from Verhagen et al.[2] with permission from BMJ Publishing Group Ltd.

relationship is due to an extraneous variable. As can be seen in Fig. 9.1, the risk of sustaining an ankle sprain is about twofold when one has experienced an ankle sprain within the preceding 12 months[2]. This can be considered a strong association, especially keeping the multi-causality that underlies onset of injury in the mind.

Dose–response relationship

The presence of a dose–response relationship is a strong evidence for a causal relationship. Fig. 9.1 shows that risk of an ankle-sprain recurrence declines over time. This is evidence of a dose (impaired proprioception)–response (ankle-sprain recurrence) relationship. It should be noted that the absence of a dose–response relationship does not rule out a causal relationship. A threshold may exist above which a relationship may develop. The presence of a dose–response relationship, in fact, is the underlying premise of injury prevention. Usually one tends to visualize a dose–response relationship in the upwards sense; the stronger the presence of a specific factor, the stronger the risk of injury. However, at the same time, if a specific factor is the cause of an injury, the incidence of the injury should also decline when exposure to the factor is reduced or eliminated.

Consistency

An association needs to be consistent when results are replicated in studies in different settings using different methods. If a relationship is truly causal, one would expect to find it consistently in throughout a variety of studies in a variety of populations. The data presented in Fig. 9.1 stem from a single descriptive study on ankle sprains in volleyball players[2]. Similar conclusions can be drawn from other descriptive studies in volleyball[3]. Moreover, studies in other sports have also indicated that previous injury is a factor associated with recurrence risk[4]. Having said so, there are also injury risk factors that are, for instance, sports, region, or situation specific. This limits the extent to which one may consistently find a certain factor to be causally related to injury.

Plausibility

Perhaps the most logical of all criteria for causality, there needs to be a rational basis for positing an association between a risk factor and injury. Especially when studying a multitude of risk factors in a single trial it is likely to find an association simply by chance. For instance, in a prospective trial one may find a relationship between ankle-sprain risk and a preference for Italian cuisine. Although such a relationship may be statistically sound, it is not plausible. The causal relationship depicted in Fig. 9.1 can be pragmatically described. After an index ankle sprain, damage to the mechanoreceptors of the ankle ligaments can produce a proprioceptive impairment in the ankle[5]. This might explain the increased risk of re-injury within 1 year after an ankle sprain[6–8].

Coherence

This criterion elaborates on 'plausibility', and states that a causal association should be compatible with existing theory and knowledge. In other words, it is necessary to evaluate claims of causality within the context of the current state of knowledge. However, as with the 'plausibility' criterion, evidence that contradicts established theory and knowledge is not automatically false. This, in fact, may force a reconsideration of accepted beliefs and principles.

Consideration of alternate explanations

When judging whether a reported association is causal, it is always necessary to consider multiple hypotheses before making conclusions about the causal relationship between a risk factor and an injury. In case of the relationship illustrated in Fig. 9.1, it could well be that player position is an injury-causing factor. In volleyball the majority of ankle sprains occur at the net-zone due to landing on another player's foot after a block or spike[2, 3]. While players tend to have specific tasks on the field, it will consistently be the same players that perform a block or spike. Ankle sprains will repeatedly occur in these players, linking a previous injury to a recurrence, while in fact it could be the player's position that is the causing factor. For that reason the data presented in Fig. 9.1 has been corrected for player position and only shows the relationship between previous injury and injury-recurrence risk.

Experiment

The injury can be prevented or the severity can be minimized by an appropriate experimental regimen.

Specificity

This is the weakest of all the criteria and is observed rarely in the causality of sports injury. Specificity is established when a single alleged risk factor produces a specific injury. However, sports-injury causality is usually, as described in Chapter 8, an intricate pathway of multiple risk factors and mechanisms of injury acting together. This makes it is necessary to examine causal relationships within a larger systemic perspective.

Risk factors

Risk factors are in concept different than injury mechanisms. As stated in Chapter 8, risk factors occur distant from the injury outcome, whereas mechanisms of injury occur proximal to the outcome and mark the onset of injury. The position that risk factors and injury mechanisms have on the timeline that precedes injury defines to a certain extent the methods by which they can be assessed or measured. Risk factors need to be assessed in all athletes that are part of the population at risk. In contrast, injury mechanisms are ascertained only when an injury occurs. Nevertheless, it may also be necessary to describe situations where no injury occurs in order to identify the causative mechanism. However, as explained further on in this chapter, assessing mechanisms of injury poses challenges as well.

The strongest design for an aetiological study is a prospective cohort study One takes a population at risk, measures potential risk factors, and follows the population over time while mapping injuries. In the end one can analyse whether differences exist between the injured and non-injured participants. As injury causation is multi-factorial (also see Chapter 8), it may be clear that large study samples are required in order to register enough injuries and to define something useful about injury causation. This severely limits the methods that can be practically used to asses potential risk factors. Whereas it may be possible to objectify biomechanical or physiological in a laboratory setting in about 100 athletes, this would prove an impossible feat in larger samples. For this reason, when studying risk factors one is usually confined to questionnaires and assessment methods that can be applied practically in the field.

A multitude of practical measures that assess muscle strength, physical fitness, co-ordination, etc., can be found throughout the literature, and it is beyond the scope of this chapter to deal with such assessment methods in full detail. However, when looking for a suitable assessment technique (or when developing one) one needs to be aware of two key issues – validity and reliability.

Validity

Validity is an important term in epidemiology, referring to the degree to which a study supports the intended conclusion drawn from the results. Validity is a broad term that can be applied in every aspect of a study. In short, validity answers three questions: (i) does an instrument measure what it is intended to measure; (ii) do study results correspond to real life; and (iii) the absence of systematic error. Different types of validity exist, and with increasing level of evidence these are:

Face validity

Face validity is an estimate of whether a test appears to measure a certain criterion. The judgement whether the test is valid is made on the 'face' of the test. Usually, demographic questions in a questionnaire (e.g. age, weight, height, etc.) are considered to be face valid.

Content validity

Closely related to face validity, content validity is also a non-statistical type of validity. In contrast to face validity, content validity is built into a test by careful selection of which items to include, preferably by a team of experts on the topic at hand.

Construct validity

Construct validity is the correspondence between empirical findings and theoretical expectations of a given test or instrument. This type of validity is used when there is no 'golden standard', and thus no 'truth' to compare the test outcome to.

Criterion validity

Considered the highest level of validity, criterion validity determines the correspondence of a test or instrument with a 'golden standard'. This type of validity is most often used in diagnostic studies (does a test predict the outcome) and thus is also of interest when determining risk factors for injury.

Two types of criterion validity exist, concurrent validity and predictive validity. The term concurrent validity is used when the test and criterion are measured at more or less the same time, e.g. a physical examination of the ankle and X-rays in case of a suspected ankle fracture. Concurrent validity says something about the diagnostic value of a given test, but also on the correspondence between e.g. an elaborate biomechanical test on ankle proprioception and an easy-to-use field test like the single-leg balance test. Predictive validity refers to the type of validity where the criterion (injury) is being determined after the test or measurement. Although different in concept, both types of validity can be determined using the same statistical techniques. Most often validity is expressed as the correlation between the values derived from a gold-standard as opposed to the values derived from a specific test. Nevertheless, the literature is unclear on which methods should be used and where the cut-off points for validity lie.

Box 9.1 gives an example of different measures of validity between a field-test and a 'gold-standard'. It should be noted that the positive predictive value (PPV) and negative predictive value (NPV) are proportional to the prevalence of the condition tested for. If in the example presented in Box 9.1 the proportion of subjects with ankle instability would be higher, the PPV would probably be greater and the NPV lower. In this case, the low prevalence of instability increases the value of the NPV. This can be explained by the simple fact that, with a low prevalence of a specific condition, the chance of a negative test result being truly negative increases. To overcome this problem, likelihood ratios may be reported, as these do not depend on prevalence.

Reliability

Reliability describes the uniformity of a set of measurements, measuring instruments, or assessors. This can either be whether repeated measures using a single instrument will give similar outcomes (test–re-test), whether multiple measures by a single assessor gives similar results (intra-rater reliability), or whether two independent assessors give similar scores (inter-rater reliability). A reliable method or measure is measuring something consistently. Thereby, reliability does not imply validity (Fig. 9.2).

Various methods to determine reliability exist, each with a specific use and with well-described cut-off scores for reliability. It goes beyond the scope of this chapter to discuss these methods in detail. Any book or website on statistics can provide a full explanation on the use of any of these methods.

Joint probability of agreement

This is the most simple and weakest measure of reliability. It assumes that data are distributed nominally, and does not take into account that agreement also occurs by chance. It is the number of times each outcome (e.g. 1, 2,..., 5) is assigned by each measurement or assessor. This number is then divided by the total number of outcomes.

Kappa statistics

Kappa statistics are usually used when quantifying agreement between independent assessors. Cohen's kappa works for two assessors. Fleiss' kappa works for any fixed number of assessors. Kappa statistics do take into account that a certain amount of agreement is based on chance and is, therefore, an improvement upon the joint probability of agreement. However, kappa

Box 9.1 Validity assessment of a field test determining ankle stability in comparison to a biomechanical test in a controlled laboratory setting (gold-standard).

Laboratory test

		+	−	
Field test	+	8	7	15
	−	2	83	85
		10	90	100

Sensitivity $= P(T^+ \mid D^+) = a/a + c = 8/10 = 0.80 = 80\%$
Sensitivity is the number of field test positives divided (T^+)by the 'true' number of positives as determined by the gold standard (D^+), in this case the lab test. A sensitivity of 100% means that the test recognizes all unstable ankles as such. Thus in a high sensitivity test, a negative result is used to rule out ankle instability.

Specificity $= P(T^- \mid D^-) = d/b + d = 83/90 = 0.92 = 92\%$
Specificity is the number of field test negatives (T^-) divided by the 'true' number of negatives as determined by the lab test (Z^-). A specificity of 100% means that the test recognizes all healthy ankles people as stable. Thus a positive result in a high-specificity test is used to confirm ankle instability.

Positive predictive value $= P(D^+ \mid T^+) = a/a + b = 8/15 = 0.53 = 53\%$
The positive predictive value (PPV) is the proportion of field-test positives who are correctly diagnosed as having ankle instability, showing the probability whether a positive test result reflects the underlying condition being tested for.

Negative predictive value $= P(D^- \mid T^-) = d/c + d = 83/85 = 0.98 = 98\%$
In contrast to the PPV, the negative predictive value (NPV) is the proportion of field test negatives who are correctly diagnosed as not having ankle instability. The NPV shows the proportion of subjects with negative test results who are correctly diagnosed.

Positive likelihood ratio $= P(T^+ \mid D^+)/P(T^+ \mid D^-) = \text{Sensitivity}/1 - \text{Specificity} = 0.80/0.08 = 10$
The positive likelihood ratio gives insight into the proportion field test positives who are correctly diagnosed as having ankle instability as opposed to the proportion field-test positives who do not have ankle instability.

Negative likelihood ratio $= P(T^- \mid D^+)/P(T^- \mid D^-) = 1 - \text{Sensitivity}/\text{Specificity} = 0.20/0.92 = 0.22$
The negative likelihood ratio gives insight into the proportion field-test negatives who are correctly diagnosed as not having ankle instability as opposed to the proportion field-test negatives who do have ankle instability.

statistics also treat the data as a nominal distribution and assume that ratings have no natural ordering.

Correlation coefficients

Correlation coefficients can be used to measure pair-wise correlation among measurements or assessors using an ordered scale. Spearman correlations can be used for ordinal data, Pearson

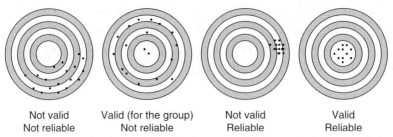

Not valid   Valid (for the group)   Not valid   Valid
Not reliable   Not reliable   Reliable   Reliable

Fig. 9.2 A schematic example of the relationship between reliability and validity. The circles depict a shooting target, the dots are the shots taken at the target. The centre of the target is the true value of the criterion that is measured.

correlation in case of a continuous scale. However, neither coefficient takes into account the magnitude of the differences between measurements or assessors.

Intra-class correlation coefficient

The intra-class correlation coefficient (ICC) is the proportion of variance of an observation due to between-subject variability in the true scores. The ICC takes the differences in ratings for individual segments and the correlation between assessors into account, and is thereby an improvement over correlation coefficients. The ICC ranges from 0 to 1 and will be high when there is little variation between the scores produced by measurements or assessors.

Limits of agreement

Another approach to reliability is to determine the mean of the differences between the two measurements or assessors. Confidence limits around this mean provide insight into how much outcomes are influenced by random variation. If the measurements or assessors tend to agree, the mean will be near zero. If one measurement or assessor is consistently different than the other (systematic error), the mean have a narrow confidence interval, but will be far from zero. If the measurements or assessors disagree without a consistent pattern (random error), the mean of the differences will be near zero with a wide confidence interval.

Mechanisms of injury

As stated earlier, injury mechanisms directly precede or occur at injury onset. Therefore, although the concepts of validity and reliability are of use here as well, different methodologies apply. A number of different methodological approaches have been used to describe the inciting event (Fig. 9.3). These include interviews of injured athletes, analysis of video recordings of actual injuries, clinical studies (where the clinical joint damage findings are studied to understand the injury mechanism, mainly through plain radiography, MRI, arthroscopy, or CT scans), *in vivo* studies (measuring ligament strain or forces to understand ligament-loading patterns), cadaveric studies, mathematical modelling, and simulation of injury situations, or measurements/estimation from 'close to injury' situations. In rare cases, injuries have even occurred during biomechanical experiments.

Interviews

One of the most commonly used approaches in studying mechanisms of injury is the description of the injury as reported either by the athlete, the coach, medical personnel, or others who

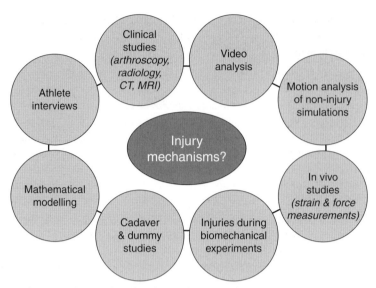

Fig. 9.3 Research approaches to describe the mechanisms of injuries in sports.
Reproduced from krosslaug et al. [9] with permission from *BMJ* Publishing Group Ltd.

witnessed the accident[9–19]. The advantage of using this approach is that it is relatively easy to obtain data, e.g. through a personal interview or a questionnaire. Information on mechanisms of injury is therefore often collected as part of routine injury-surveillance systems, where it is possible to gather data on a large number of injured athletes[20, 21].

There are, however, several challenges associated with athlete interviews. Categorization of mechanisms of injury into predefined descriptions may result in incomplete or even erroneous interpretation, e.g. if the categories are created to fit with a specific theory on the mechanism of injury. Interestingly, in one study[22] on anterior cruciate ligament (ACL) injuries where the description of the injury mechanism was written down as stated by the patients, 17 different mechanisms of injury were reported, whereas normally the number of categories is much fewer. Unfortunately, mechanism-of-injury descriptions based on the athlete-interview approach commonly use widely different terminology and categories, and definitions are rarely provided and sometimes it seems somewhat arbitrary which variables are reported[23, 24]. Detailed descriptions of the mechanism of injury should therefore be interpreted with caution, if based on athlete interviews alone.

Another important limitation with the athlete-interview approach is the ability of injured players to comprehend and recall what actually took place when they were injured. Injuries usually happen quickly and often involve several players, opponents, and team-mates. It is therefore difficult to determine to what extent the injured athlete or the witnesses are able to assess the playing situation and, perhaps even more difficult, the biomechanical aspects of the mechanism of injury.

However, for some types of injury and sports where playing actions and mechanisms of injury are easily categorized and the mechanisms of injury are consistent, questionnaire data may provide an accurate description of the mechanisms, at least for the playing (sports) situation and athlete/opponent behaviour. For example, questionnaire studies from volleyball have clearly documented the mechanisms for ankle sprains. These mainly occur at the net when landing on the foot of an opponent or a team-mate after blocking or attacking[25]. This information on mechanisms of injury was then successfully used as the basis for an intervention study focussing on exercises to teach correct approach, take-off, and landing technique when blocking or attacking[26]. This example shows that data from athlete interviews can be important for developing preventive methods.

Clinical studies

Another approach to understand the mechanism of injury is to analyse the pathology of the injury and associated damage. For instance, magnetic resonance imaging (MRI) or computed tomographic (CT) scans of the head can diagnose the location of brain and skull damage accurately, and thereby form the basis for an estimate of the location and direction of the forces causing the observed damage.

Studies investigating the associated joint damage after ACL injury may indeed be helpful in generating new hypotheses, and possibly rejecting others. However, it is not possible to determine the sequence of events leading to the observed findings reliably based on such studies alone. The essential question – and main limitation of clinical studies in general – is whether the damage occurs before, during, or as a result of the ACL rupture.

Although exact descriptions of joint pathology can be obtained from arthroscopy, MRI, and other imaging studies, an accurate prediction of the detailed joint biomechanics leading to injury is therefore difficult. Information on joint biomechanics alone may not be sufficient to develop ideas for prevention. Therefore, it may be that the most important role of data from clinical examinations is that the information can be used to support or contradict observations from other methods, such as interviews of the injured athlete or analysis of videotapes of the incident. This requires a prospective approach where data from all the three methods are collected in a standardized manner.

Video analysis

Systematic video analysis of injuries can potentially contribute information on the sports situation and athlete-movement patterns, which can be used directly to prevent injuries. As an example, several research groups have used video analysis to study the mechanisms of football injuries in a series of studies[27–32]. These studies have mainly focussed on describing the playing situation, athlete–opponent interaction, and refereeing, confirming results from questionnaire studies pointing to tackling duels and heading duels as high-risk situations. Until now, whole-body or joint biomechanics have been studied to a lesser degree in football injuries, but two studies by Andersen et al. have recently examined the mechanisms of ankle[14] and head[33] injuries. For ankle injuries, the joint kinematics showed mostly supination trauma as expected (Fig. 9.4). However, several of the incidents were triggered by an external medial force of the ankle (late tackle from the side) that brought the player out of balance, causing unanticipated foot motion just prior to landing. This illustrates the importance of describing not only the joint-specific biomechanics, but also the playing situation leading up to the injury.

Although video analysis has the potential to be a more detailed and reliable way of analysing mechanism of injury than athlete interviews, current methods for estimating kinematics from uncalibrated video sequences are inadequate[34]. It has been shown that simple visual inspection, i.e. trying to estimate joint angles by just looking at video sequences, has an unacceptable error[35]. Therefore, the video-analysis approach has been more useful to describe the playing situation and athlete/opponent movements than detailed joint biomechanics. However, recently a new model-based image-matching technique has recently been described and applied to get detailed joint kinematics in ACL injuries[36] and ankle sprains[37].

An obvious limitation of the video-analysis approach is the quality of the video recording, e.g. the image quality, the resolution of the athlete of interest, and the number of views available

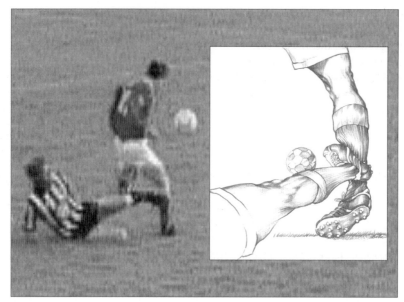

Fig. 9.4 Typical mechanism for lateral ligament injury in football as observed from systematic video analysis: opponent contact to the medial side of the leg, causing the player to put weight on an inverted ankle.
Illustration reproduced with permission from ©Oslo Sports Trauma Research Center/T. Bolic.

indicates that additional camera views increases the accuracy of a model-based image-matching technique to extract human motion from uncalibrated video images[34]. In addition, the viewing angle relative to the athlete will determine what variables are more reliable[34]. A significant challenge is to determine the exact point of injury. In studies of ACL injuries, one report claims that they could determine the 'precise point of injury'[38], while another stated that finding the exact moment of ACL disruption was impossible[39].

Another limitation, which must be kept in mind when interpreting the results, is that not all of the injuries reported by team medical personnel can be identified on the game tapes. In fact, about half of all injuries in football can be found on video[40, 41]. This also means that studies based on video analysis alone[28, 42], without reliable medical information from the same matches, must be interpreted with caution. The completeness and diagnostic accuracy of the medical information is an important factor to consider when planning a video study.

A range of potential selection biases can result from the availability of video tapes. The video approach is more likely to be used for matches played by elite professional athletes, where TV coverage is regular, and less likely in amateur, female, or youth sports. Moreover, training videos are often not available, and the mechanisms of injury may differ from training to match play, since we would expect there to be less aggression and foul play in training. Finally, most video-analysis studies only describe events and situations leading to injury. Unless there is a representative control sample of non-injury situations, it cannot be determined if the characteristics of the injury situations are different from what normally takes place without resulting in injury.

Laboratory motion analysis

The strength of laboratory motion analysis is that kinetics and kinematics can be estimated with much greater precision than what is possible from analysing video recordings. However, injuries cannot be replicated in the laboratory for obvious reasons, and studies using motion analysis are therefore generally designed to mimic typical injury situations. For example, several laboratory studies have recently investigated side-step cutting or jump landings in relation to non-contact ACL injuries[43, 47]. However, although it is possible to quantify the motion patterns for movements that are assumed to be similar to the situations where the injuries mainly occur[10, 48], it is difficult to predict to what extent the joint dynamics are in fact comparable. Unfortunately, comparisons of laboratory and game biomechanics have not been studied so far. However, in order to create more 'match-like' situations, different research groups have tried to simulate the game setting, e.g. by introducing unanticipated cutting[47, 49], a static defender[43], or catching a ball while landing[50]. All of these factors proved to increase joint loading, indicating that there are indeed significant differences between controlled laboratory trials and match situations that may lead to injury.

There are also other problems to traditional motion-analysis techniques which introduce errors in the estimates, e.g. skin movement artefacts[51, 52], identification of bony landmarks[53], and signal noise[54, 55]. Key variables like knee internal/external rotation and rotation moments have proved to be unreliable in a high-impact sporting motion[51].

In vivo strain/force measurements

In vivo studies of strain or forces represent another approach that can provide useful information on the tissue loading in situations with similar characteristics as injury situations, and thus perhaps also relevant for injury. Some of the most utilized methods are strain gauges (e.g. the Differential Variable Reluctance Transducer[56]) and buckle transducers[57] or fiberoptic sensors[58] for measuring force. Lately, additional non-invasive methods, e.g. ultrasonography[59] and magnetic resonance imaging[60], have shown their potential.

However, due to the technical challenges[56], the ability to perform sport-specific movements using invasive techniques is presently limited. In addition, the non-invasive studies are limited in that they cannot be applied in a sports-relevant situation. *In vivo* studies have therefore generally focussed on e.g. muscle-tendon biomechanics and rehabilitation, rather than mechanism-of-injury research.

Injuries during biomechanical experiments

For obvious ethical reasons one cannot replicate injury situations in a experimental study on live subjects. In a few rare cases[61, 62] accidental sports injuries have occurred during research experiments. Of course, studies in this category are both rare and undesired. We must therefore consider other approaches for gaining insight in the mechanisms of injury.

Cadaveric and dummy studies

Cadaveric studies looking into the anatomy and function of joints and ligaments are numerous [62, 65]. A common approach has been to measure the kinematics before and after cutting one or more ligaments of, e.g. the knee[66, 67]. Based on such studies, gross estimates of ligament function can be obtained, classifying the ligaments into 'primary restraints' and 'secondary restraints', depending on their effect on joint angular or translational motion. It is also possible to mimic the assumed mechanism of injury and load an intact cadaver joint to failure to see if the mechanism produces the intended pathology. A technically more sophisticated approach is using strain gauges or force transducers to assess ligament function under different loading conditions.

Although these studies are important in understanding ligament function, their value in mechanism-of-injury research is limited, since lower loads can not be extrapolated to failure-level with confidence[68]. Unfortunately, the validity of cadaveric studies is also often hampered by the fact that specimens are old and/or not representative of an athletic population[69]. In addition, the freezing and thawing process reduces the ultimate load of the tissue[70].

In most studies muscular support is lacking, although some cadaveric studies have also simulated muscle forces in, e.g. the quadriceps and/or hamstrings[71–73]. However, the actual muscle force patterns that contribute to the joint dynamics in a real-injury situation are unknown, and would probably be difficult to reproduce in such a set-up even if they were known.

Another approach used within sports-injury research is using dummies or physical models, which are well known from car crash testing. Such dummies, e.g. the Hybrid III family of dummies, have excellent biofidelity, and can be instrumented with, e.g. load sensors and accelerometers[74]. Since dummies are passive (i.e. lack muscles), the types of injuries that can be investigated using this approach are obviously limited. Nevertheless, in those situations where the assumptions are met, dummy studies have proven to be helpful.

Mathematical modelling

Lately, sophisticated mathematical modelling and estimation of 'close to injury situations' or simulation of injurious situations has become increasingly popular. The advantage with the simulation approach is that one can study different mechanisms of injury in a virtual environment, thus avoiding any hazard to athletes. Depending on the models, one can study cause–effect relationships, e.g. between neuromuscular control and knee loading[75], or intercondylar geometry and ACL impingement[76].

Due to the complexity in anatomy and neuromuscular control, a sophisticated mathematical simulation model will necessarily have to rely on assumptions and simplifications to deal with the inherent indeterministic nature of the equations describing the dynamics. Because of this, a more complex model may be able to reproduce the measured kinematics more precisely, but the ability to predict new (e.g. injury-producing) situations may possibly suffer[75].

The fact that an injury model nearly always needs to be validated, either in a non-injury situation or *in vitro*, clearly adds a degree of uncertainty to its use. However, the biggest challenge is probably how to verify that the simulated injury pattern actually resembles what is experienced in real life.

Conclusion

Risk factors and mechanisms of injury are both causally related to injury. Although both form part of the multi-causal pathway leading to injury, by concept risk factors and mechanisms require different measurement techniques. Within this variety of techniques the terms validity and reliability play a crucial role in deciding which measure or method to use when quantifying a specific factor or mechanism.

As seen from the description of the various research approaches, evidence relevant to understand the mechanisms for sports injury can be obtained from widely different methods and study designs. Therefore, the traditional evidence hierarchy[77] cannot be applied in this setting. Important insight can be gained from studying the events preceding (e.g. the velocity at impact, the playing situation), at (e.g. the loads), or following (e.g. the associated joint damage to the knee) the point of injury.

For most types of injury, a single research approach alone will not be sufficient to describe all aspects of the injurious situation, and it is therefore necessary to combine a number of different research approaches to describe the mechanisms fully. For example, relevant combinations of research approaches which could provide a broader and more precise understanding could be combining athlete interviews, video analysis, and clinical studies, or combining video analysis and cadaveric/dummy/mathematical simulation studies.

References

1. Hill AB (1965). The environment and disease: association or causation. *P Roy Soc MEd*, **58**, 295–300.

2. Verhagen EALM, van der Beek AJ, Bouter LM, Bahr RM, van Mechelen W (2004). A one season prospective cohort study of volleyball injuries. *Br J Sports Med*, **38**(4), 477–81.

3. Reeser JC, Verhagen E, Briner WW, Askeland TI, Bahr R (2006). Strategies for the prevention of volleyball related injuries. *Br J Sports Med*, **40**(7), 594–600.

4. Murphy DF, Connolly DAJ, Beynnon BD (2003). Risk factors for lower extremity injury: a review of the literature. *Br J Sports Med*, **37**, 13–29.

5. Freeman MA (1965). Instability to the foot after injuries to the lateral ligament of the ankle. *J Bone Joint Surg Br* **47**, 669–77.

6. Brand RL, Black HM, Cox JS (1977). The natural history of inadequately treated ankle sprain. *AmJ Sports Med*, **5**(6), 248–53.

7. Ekstrand J, Gillquist J (1983). Soccer injuries and their mechanisms: a prospective study. *Med Sci Sports Exerc*, **15**(3), 267–70.

8. Tropp H, Odenrick P (1988). Postural control in single limb stance. *J Orthop Res*, **6**, 833–9.

9. Krosshaug T, Andersen T E, Olsen O-E O, Myklebust G, Bahr R (2005). Research approaches to describe the mechanisms of injuries in sport: limitations and possibilities. Br J *Sports Med*, **39**, 330–9.

10. Arendt E, Dick R (1995). Knee injury patterns among men and women in collegiate basketball and soccer. NCAA data and review of literature. *Am J Sports Med*, **23**(6), 694–701.

11. Orchard J, Seward H (2002). Epidemiology of injuries in the Australian Football League, seasons 1997-2000. *Br J Sports Med*, **36**(1), 39–44.

12. Junge A, Dvorak J, Graf-Baumann T, Peterson L (2004). Football injuries during FIFA tournaments and the Olympic Games, 1998–2001: development and implementation of an injury-reporting system. *Am J Sports Med*, **32**(1 Suppl), 80S–9S.

13. Ekstrand J, Walden M, Hagglund M (2004). A congested football calendar and the wellbeing of players: correlation between match exposure of European footballers before the World Cup 2002 and their injuries and performances during that World Cup. *Br J Sports Med*, **38**(4), 493–7.

14. Andersen TE, Floerenes TW, Arnason A, Bahr R (2004). Video analysis of the mechanisms for ankle injuries in football. *Am J Sports Med*, **32**(1 Suppl), 69S–79S.

15. Natri A, Beynnon BD, Ettlinger CF, Johnson RJ, Shealy JE (1999). Alpine ski bindings and injuries. Current findings. *Sports Med*, **28**(1), 35–48.

16. Gray J, Taunton JE, McKenzie DC, Clement DB, McConkey JP, Davidson RG (1985). A survey of injuries to the anterior cruciate ligament of the knee in female basketball players. *Int J Sports Med*, **6**(6), 314–16.

17. Fetto JF, Marshall JL (1980). The natural history and diagnosis of anterior cruciate ligament insufficiency. *Clin Orthop*, **147**, 29–38.

18. Myklebust G, Maehlum S, Engebretsen L, Strand T, Solheim E (1997). Registration of cruciate ligament injuries in Norwegian top level team handball. A prospective study covering two seasons. *Scand J Med Sci Sports*, **7**(5), 289–92.

19. Myklebust G, Maehlum S, Holm I, Bahr R (1998). A prospective cohort study of anterior cruciate ligament injuries in elite Norwegian team handball. *Scand J Med Sci Sports*, **8**(3), 149–53.

20. Ronning R, Gerner T, Engebretsen L (2000). Risk of injury during alpine and telemark skiing and snowboarding. The equipment-specific distance-correlated injury index. *Am J Sports Med*, **28**(4), 506–8.

21. Langran M, Selvaraj S (2004). Increased injury risk among first-day skiers, snowboarders, and skiboarders. *Am J Sports Med*, **32**(1), 96–103.

22. Nakajima H, Kondo M, Kurosawa H, Fukubayashi T (1979). Insufficiency of the anterior cruciate ligament. Review of our 118 cases. *Arch Orthop Trauma Surg*, **95**(4), 233–40.

23. Feagin JA, Jr., Curl WW (1976). Isolated tear of the anterior cruciate ligament: 5-year follow-up study. *Am J Sports Med*, **4**(3), 95–100.

24. Harner CD, Paulos LE, Greenwald AE, Rosenberg TD, Cooley VC (1994). Detailed analysis of patients with bilateral anterior cruciate ligament injuries. *Am J Sports Med*, **22**(1), 37–43.

25. Bahr R, Bahr IA (1997). Incidence of acute volleyball injuries: a prospective cohort study of injury mechanisms and risk factors. *Scand J Med Sci Sports*, **7**(3), 166–71.

26. Bahr R, Lian O, Bahr IA (1997). A twofold reduction in the incidence of acute ankle sprains in volleyball after the introduction of an injury prevention program: a prospective cohort study. *Scand J Med Sci Sports*, **7**(3), 172–7.

27. Fuller CW, Junge A, Dvorak J (2004). An assessment of football referees' decisions in incidents leading to player injuries. *Am J Sports Med*, **32**(1 Suppl), 17S–22S.

28. Hawkins RD, Fuller CW (1998). An examination of the frequency and severity of injuries and incidents at three levels of professional football. *Br J Sports Med*, **32**(4), 326–32.

29. Fuller CW, Smith GL, Junge A, Dvorak J (2004). An assessment of player error as an injury causation factor in international football. *Am J Sports Med*, **32**(1 Suppl), 28S–35S.

30. Giza E, Fuller C, Junge A, Dvorak J (2003). Mechanisms of foot and ankle injuries in soccer. *Am J Sports Med*, **31**(4), 550–4.

31. Andersen TE, Larsen O, Tenga A, Engebretsen L, Bahr R (2003). Football incident analysis: a new video based method to describe injury mechanisms in professional football. *Br J Sports Med*, **37**(3), 226–32.

32. Fuller CW, Smith GL, Junge A, Dvorak J (2004). The influence of tackle parameters on the propensity for injury in international football. *Am J Sports Med*, **32**(1 Suppl), 43S–53S.

33. Andersen TE, Arnason A, Engebretsen L, Bahr R (2004). Mechanisms of head injuries in elite football. *Br J Sports Med*, **38**(6), 690–6.

34. Krosshaug T, Bahr R (2005). A model-based image-matching technique for three-dimensional reconstruction of human motion from uncalibrated video sequences. *J Biomech*, **38**(4), 919–29.

35. Krosshaug T, Nakamae A, Boden B, Engebretsen L, Smith G, Slauterbeck J, Hewett TE, Bahr R (2007). Estimating 3D joint kinematics from video sequences of running and cutting maneuvers – assessing the accuracy of simple visual inspection. *Gait Posture*, **26**(3), 378–85.

36. Krosshaug T, Slauterbeck J, Engebretsen L, Bahr R (2007). Biomechanical analysis of ACL injury mechanisms: three-dimensional motion reconstruction from video sequences. *Scand J Med Sci Sports*, **17**(5), 508–19.

37. Fong DT, Hong Y, Shima Y, Krosshaug T, Yung PS, Chan KM (2009). Biomechanics of supination ankle sprain: a case report of an accidental injury event in the laboratory. *Am J Sports Med*, **37**(4), 822–7.

38. Teitz CC (2001). Video analysis of ACL injuries, in Griffin LY (ed) *Prevention of noncontact ACL injuries*. pp. 87–92. American Association of Orthopaedic Surgeons, Rosemont, IL.

39. Boden BP, Dean GS, Feagin JA, Jr., Garrett WE, Jr (2000). Mechanisms of anterior cruciate ligament injury. *Orthopedics*, **23**(6), 573–8.

40. Andersen TE, Tenga A, Engebretsen L, Bahr R (2004). Video analysis of injuries and incidents in Norwegian professional football. *Br J Sports Med*, **38**(5), 626–31.

41. Arnason A, Tenga A, Engebretsen L, Bahr R (2004). A prospective video-based analysis of injury situations in elite male football: football incident analysis. *Am J Sports Med*, **32**(6), 1459–65.

42. Rahnama N, Reilly T, Lees A (2002). Injury risk associated with playing actions during competitive soccer. *Br J Sports Med*, **36**(5), 354–9.

43. McLean SG, Lipfert SW, Van Den Bogert AJ (2004). Effect of gender and defensive opponent on the biomechanics of sidestep cutting. *Med Sci Sports Exerc*, **36**(6), 1008–16.

44. Salci Y, Kentel BB, Heycan C, Akin S, Korkusuz F. (2004). Comparison of landing maneuvers between male and female college volleyball players. *Clin Biomech (Bristol, Avon),* **19**(6), 622–8.

45. Pollard CD, Davis IM, Hamill J (2004). Influence of gender on hip and knee mechanics during a randomly cued cutting maneuver. *Clin Biomech (Bristol, Avon),* **19**(10), 1022–31.

46. Hewett TE, Myer GD, Ford KR, Heidt RS, Jr., Colosimo AJ, McLean SG, van den Bogert AJ, Paterno MV, Succop P (2005). Biomechanical measures of neuromuscular control and valgus loading of the knee predict anterior cruciate ligament injury risk in female athletes. A prospective study. *Am J Sports Med,* **33**(4), 492–501.

47. Ford KR, Myer GD, Toms HE, Hewett TE (2005). Gender differences in the kinematics of unanticipated cutting in young athletes. *Med Sci Sports Exerc,* **37**(1), 124–9.

48. Olsen OE, Myklebust G, Engebretsen L, Bahr R (2004). Injury mechanisms for anterior cruciate ligament injuries in team handball: a systematic video analysis. *Am J Sports Med,* **32**(4), 1002–12.

49. Besier TF, Lloyd DG, Ackland TR, Cochrane JL (2001). Anticipatory effects on knee joint loading during running and cutting maneuvers. *Med Sci Sports Exerc,* **33**(7), 1176–81.

50. Cowling EJ, Steele JR (2001). The effect of upper-limb motion on lower-limb muscle synchrony. Implications for anterior cruciate ligament injury. *J Bone Joint Surg Am,* **83-A**(1), 35–41.

51. Reinschmidt C, Van Den Bogert AJ, Nigg BM, Lundberg A, Murphy N (1997). Effect of skin movement on the analysis of skeletal knee joint motion during running. *J Biomech,* **30**(7), 729–32.

52. Cappozzo A, Catani F, Leardini A, Benedetti MG, DellaCroce U (1996). Position and orientation in space of bones during movement: Experimental artefacts. *Clinical Biomechanics,* **11**(2), 90–100.

53. Della Croce U, Cappozzo A, Kerrigan DC (1999). Pelvis and lower limb anatomical landmark calibration precision and its propagation to bone geometry and joint angles. *Med Biol Eng Comput,* **37**(2), 155–61.

54. Cappello A, LaPalombara PF, Leardini B (1996). Optimization and smoothing techniques in movement analysis. *Int J Biomed Comput,* **41**(3), 137–51.

55. Woltring HJ (1985). On optimal smoothing and derivate estimation from noisy displacement data in biomechanics. *Hum Mov Sci,* **4**, 229–45.

56. Beynnon BD, Fleming BC (1998). Anterior cruciate ligament strain in-vivo: a review of previous work. *J Biomech,* **31**(6), 519–25.

57. Fukashiro S, Komi PV, Järvinen M, Miyashita M (1995). *In vivo* Achilles tendon loading during jumping in humans. *Eur J Appl Physiol,* **71**, 453–8.

58. Finni T, Komi PV, Lepola V (2000). *In vivo* human triceps surae and quadriceps femoris muscle function in a squat jump and counter movement jump. *Eur J Appl Physiol,* **83**(4–5), 416–26.

59. Maganaris CN, Paul JP (2002). Tensile properties of the in vivo human gastrocnemius tendon. *J Biomech,* **35**(12), 1639–46.

60. Bey MJ, Song HK, Wehrli FW, Soslowsky LJ (2002). A noncontact, nondestructive method for quantifying intratissue deformations and strains. *J Biomech Eng,* **124**(2), 253–8.

61. Zernicke RF, Garhammer J, Jobe FW (1977). Human patellar-tendon rupture. *J Bone Joint Surg Am,* **59**(2), 179–3.

62. Barone M, Senner V, Schaff P (1999). ACL injury mechanism in alpine skiing: Analysis of an accidental ACL rupture, in Johnson RJ (ed) *Skiing trauma and safety, 12th edition,* pp. 63–81. American Society for Testing and Materials, West Conshohocken, PA.

63. Girgis FG, Marshall JL, Monajem A (1975). The cruciate ligaments of the knee joint. Anatomical, functional and experimental analysis. *Clin Orthop,* **106**, 216–31.

64. Furman W, Marshall JL, Girgis FG (1976). The anterior cruciate ligament. A functional analysis based on postmortem studies. *J Bone Joint Surg Am,* **58**(2), 179–85.

65. Rong GW, Wang YC (1987). The role of cruciate ligaments in maintaining knee joint stability. *Clin Orthop,* **215**, 65–71.

66. Veltri DM, Deng XH, Torzilli PA, Warren RF, Maynard MJ (1995). The role of the cruciate and posterolateral ligaments in stability of the knee. A biomechanical study. *Am J Sports Med*, **23**(4), 436–43.

67. Matsumoto H, Suda Y, Otani T, Niki Y, Seedhom BB, Fujikawa K (2001). Roles of the anterior cruciate ligament and the medial collateral ligament in preventing valgus instability. *J Orthop Sci*, **6**(1), 28–32.

68. Berns GS, Hull ML, Patterson HA (1992). Strain in the anteromedial bundle of the anterior cruciate ligament under combination loading. *J Orthop Res*, **10**(2), 167–76.

69. Woo SL, Hollis JM, Adams DJ, Lyon RM, Takai S (1991). Tensile properties of the human femur-anterior cruciate ligament-tibia complex. The effects of specimen age and orientation. *Am J Sports Med*, **19**(3), 217–25.

70. Clavert P, Kempf JF, Bonnomet F, Boutemy P, Marcelin L, Kahn JL (2001). Effects of freezing/thawing on the biomechanical properties of human tendons. *Surg Radiol Anat*, **23**(4), 259–62.

71. Markolf KL, O'Neill G, Jackson SR, McAllister DR (2004). Effects of applied quadriceps and hamstrings muscle loads on forces in the anterior and posterior cruciate ligaments. *Am J Sports Med*, **32**(5), 1144–9.

72. DeMorat G, Weinhold P, Blackburn T, Chudik S, Garrett W (2004). Aggressive quadriceps loading can induce noncontact anterior cruciate ligament injury. *Am J Sports Med*, **32**(2), 477–83.

73. Renstrom P, Arms SW, Stanwyck TS, Johnson RJ, Pope MH (1986). Strain within the anterior cruciate ligament during hamstring and quadriceps activity. *Am J Sports Med*, **14**(1), 83–7.

74. Mertz HJ (2002). Anthropometric test devices, in Nahum AM, Melvin JW (eds) *Accidental injury. Biomechanics and prevention. 2nd edition*, pp. 89–102. Springer-Verlag, New York.

75. McLean SG, Huang X, Su A, Van Den Bogert AJ (2004). Sagittal plane biomechanics cannot injure the ACL during sidestep cutting. *Clin Biomech (Bristol, Avon)*, **19**(8), 828–38.

76. Fung DT, Zhang LQ (2003). Modeling of ACL impingement against the intercondylar notch. *Clin Biomech (Bristol, Avon)*, **18**(10), 933–41.

77. Brighton B, Bhandari M, Tornetta P, III, Felson DT (2003). Hierarchy of evidence: from case reports to randomized controlled trials. *Clin Orthop*, **413**, 19–24.

Chapter 10

Statistics in aetiological studies

Ian Shrier and Russell J. Steele

The objective of aetiological research is to determine the causes of disease. In sports-injury research, this often begins with examining the frequency of different types of injuries in a group of subjects, or comparing patterns across groups of subjects. Because one expects to see more outcomes as the frequency of exposure increases, injury rates provide more interesting causal comparisons than counting the number of injuries. However, data to calculate injury rates are not always available (e.g. emergency room data) and investigators and clinicians need to make the best inferences possible given the data available. Even when data come from randomized controlled trials (RCTs), simple statistical analyses may sometimes lead to biased estimates and inappropriate causal inferences. It is important that investigators and clinicians understand the limitations of the general approaches used so that the results are interpreted with appropriate caution. The purpose of this chapter is to highlight some common errors in the more advanced analyses that are often conducted in sports-injury (and other types) research. Data analysis is similar to other aspects of research and needs to be conducted with the appropriate rigour, and based on sound reasoning for the choices made. This chapter only touches on a few of the more common errors, and investigators are strongly encouraged to seek out the help of a qualified statistician whenever possible.

Do some injuries occur more often than others?

Most articles in sports-injury research will describe the pattern of injuries that were observed, and this is often stratified by some other factor such as gender (Fig. 10.1). The investigator is interested in knowing if some injuries are more common than others, and if the injury patterns differ across groups. In this example, the investigator does not know the amount of exposures (i.e. how many games) and, therefore, there is no denominator to calculate injury rate (number of injuries/number of exposures). Because there is no denominator, these types of data are sometimes referred to as numerator-only data. Looking at the left panel in Fig. 10.1, are the differences likely to have occurred by chance? To determine this, some measure of uncertainty is needed and this is provided by confidence intervals in the right panel.

All inferences from statistical analyses require that one estimates:

1. The point estimate for the true population value (e.g. 20% of injuries occur to the head and neck)

2. An uncertainty for the point estimate, which is often given as the 90% or 95% confidence intervals as shown by 'error bars' (e.g. if a study is repeated 100 times, the true value for the population would fall within the various studies' confidence intervals in 90% (or 95%) of the studies).

In sports-injury research, the usual practice is to present the data as per the left panel in Fig. 10.1. There are usually no confidence intervals, and there is often no statistical comparison to see if the

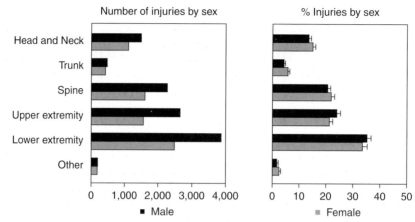

Fig. 10.1 The left graph is a plot of the number of injuries in each category for male and female Cirque du Soleil artists between 2002–06. The right-hand-side graph is a plot of the percentage of injuries for males within each category, and for females within each category. The bars represent the upper 95%CI boundary calculated using bootstrap methods that account for the lack of data-independence.

differences within a group or between groups are likely to have occurred by chance. In the worst case, authors will ignore the uncertainty surrounding their measure and inappropriately state that one type of injury is more common than another, or that the two groups have different patterns of injury.

Because the above analyses are so common, it might seem surprising that such practices occur. However, calculating the measure of uncertainty requires a certain measure of expertise because the statistical procedures are often not available within the user-friendly interfaces of the well-known statistical packages (e.g. SPSS, Statview); therefore, they are not done.

The difficulty with calculating the uncertainty is that the regular measures, require that the probability of an event occurring (e.g. injury) is independent of the probability of other events occurring. In most other areas of research, each person contributes only one data-point in the entire figure (e.g. a person only dies once) and the appropriate analysis would be the simple chi-square test. However, in sports-injury research, each person is contributing many data-points and this violates the assumptions underlying the chi-square analysis. For example, a subject can have multiple lower-extremity injuries, and can have injuries to both the upper and lower extremities. In addition, some athletes are considered more injury prone than others, and a previous injury is believed to be a strong risk factor for a subsequent injury. Therefore, to make appropriate inferences, one must account for the lack of data independence.

In the context of the data shown in Fig. 10.1, an appropriate and straightforward statistical method to construct uncertainty intervals is the bootstrap[1]. In brief, imagine there were 500 subjects with a total of 4000 injuries. The bootstrap approach samples and re-samples the data in order to obtain a reliable estimate of uncertainty. For example, one first randomly chooses one of the 500 subjects and records the subject's types of injuries. Then, one repeats this process as many times as there are subjects (i.e. 500 times in this example) and each time, the random choice is one of the full list of 500 subjects (i.e. the same subject can be chosen several times). This list of 500 'subjects' (in which some subjects are duplicated) represents one sample of the bootstrap method. The process is then repeated in order to obtain many samples (typically $n = 1\,000$)[1]. Because subjects can be duplicated in each sample, and the choice of subjects is random, the duplicated subjects within each of these samples will be different, and the proportion of injuries in each category (and across each stratification group) will be different for each sample. It may be surprising to non-statisticians, but there are indeed statistical proofs showing that these differences in proportions can be used to obtain accurate 95% confidence intervals which can be interpreted in the traditional sense[1].

In the above example, we were comparing men and women. In sports-injury research, one is often interested in comparing the injury patterns during training to the injury patterns during games. In this case, each subject contributes to both each outcome category and each exposure category, so the problem of data-dependence is even greater. However, the principles of the boot-strap method are the same and the method is appropriate to obtain estimates of uncertainty.

There are limitations to the bootstrap method. First, there are several ways to obtain estimates of confidence intervals and although the details are beyond the scope of this chapter, the advantages/disadvantages of each depend partly on whether the data is skewed (e.g. some individuals have many more injuries than most individuals)[1]. Second, the fewer number of individuals, the less likely the bootstrap method is to provide an appropriate estimate. There is no definitive number below which it cannot be used, but the rule-of-thumb is that less than 50 subjects is problematic. Lastly, care must be taken when looking at complicated population-summary measures, but these are unlikely to be used in most standard injury-research problems.

Data-dependence does not only occur with numerator-only data but is a more general problem for all of sports-injury research. In population-based epidemiological research, the problem is often known as 'clustering'. For example, subjects within a study of hockey injuries are naturally grouped by teams. Players on a more aggressive team may be more likely to become injured com-pared to subjects on a less aggressive team, i.e. it is more likely for two players of the same team to have the same injury rate compared to two players of different teams. Therefore, the data from different subjects is not independent: if this is not taken into account, measures of uncertainty will be too narrow and the risk of inappropriate inferences increases. The same problem can exist at many levels: subjects on teams, teams within leagues, leagues within sports, etc. In all of these cases, the bootstrap method can be used to obtain appropriate estimates of uncertainty but other methods are also sometimes appropriate depending on the research question and the data. These can be grouped into two general groups: (i) 'fixed-effects modelling' (include the clustering vari-able as a covariate in the model), and (ii) 'random effects modelling', which is also known in various disciplines as 'cluster-analysis', 'mixed-modelling', 'multi-level modelling', or 'hierarchi-cal modelling'. The method of including the clustering covariate in the model assumes that each level of the covariate (e.g. team A, team B, team C) has one true mean that remains fixed over time (hence, known as the fixed-effects model), and that these are the only clusters of interest (i.e. the investigator does not intend to make inferences on teams not in the study). However, there are theoretical reasons to think that each group of the cluster represents only a sample of a variety of sub-populations with variability between these sub-populations. The fixed-effects covariate approach does not take this form of variability into account. In random-effects modelling, the grouping factor is not usually considered of interest – the investigator is only trying to account for the lack of independence but is not trying to measure the actual difference between the clusters. For example, in a randomized trial of sport injuries in soccer with and without warm-up exer-cises, one might randomize 20 teams to the intervention and 20 teams to control. In this study, athletes from one team are more likely to have similar injury rates compared to athletes of another team and this lack of data-independence needs to be accounted for. In addition, one is not inter-ested in estimating the injury rate for each team because the teams are only samples of a larger population of teams. Therefore, including team as a random effect in the model would be the most appropriate method of analysis in this situation.

Injury rates

When exposure data are available, injury rates provide for more definitive causal inferences. An injury rate is simply the number of injuries divided by the number of exposures. If one has data for each individual, then one can calculate an injury rate for each individual, and then describe the distribution of injury rates for the entire group (e.g. mean ± 95%CI). However, data in sports-injury research are often collected at the team level (population-level data) and individual-level data are not available. This is typically partly for feasibility reasons and partly for confidentiality reasons.

When analysing population-level data, the point estimate for the injury rate in the population is the sum of injuries across all individuals divided by the sum of exposures across all individuals. The formula for the uncertainty surrounding this estimate is based on the fact that the number of injuries for an individual is 'expected' to follow the Poisson distribution. If this assumption is true, the standard error (a measure of uncertainty) is equal to the (sum of injuries across all individuals)$^{1/2}$/(sum of exposures across all individuals). The standard error is then used to calculate confidence intervals. This is the method used in most sports-injury research[2].

Although this is a very common method, problems will arise if the data violate the underlying assumptions. First, the Poisson distribution is a very specific distribution (e.g. the mean of the distribution is assumed equal to the variance of the distribution) and the above standard formula will not provide accurate measures of uncertainty if the data follows a different distribution. Second, the formula assumes that there is one fixed overall injury rate that is the same for every individual. In reality, one expects some groups of individuals to have higher injury rates than other groups (e.g. strikers in soccer/football are expected to have different injury rates compared to mid-fielders). This is another example of non-independence of data (or clustering) and the standard formulae cannot account for it. For example, the variance in the injury rates among Cirque du Soleil artists was greater than the mean injury rate (called over-dispersion), and the standard formulae suggested the overall injury rate was 9.7 (95%CI: 9.4–10.0)[3, 4]. However, bootstrap methods that accounted for the over-dispersion and the lack of data independence suggested a 95%CI of 9.1–10.3[3, 4]. This may seem like a small difference but there were thousands of injuries in this analysis and data with less injuries will show greater differences.

In aetiological research, we are interested in knowing if a particular factor is associated with an increased injury rate. The standard method is to compare the injury rates as either a rate ratio, or a rate difference[2]. Again, these estimates are based on an expectation that the frequency of injuries follows a Poisson distribution. Both the standard formula and a univariate Poisson regression (i.e. the main exposure is the only covariate) will yield identical answers because they are based on the Poisson distribution. However, these answers will be incorrect if the underlying assumptions are not valid. In the data from Cirque du Soleil[3], the standard-formula injury-rate ratio and univariate Poisson regression for males to females was 0.93 (95%CI: 0.87 to 0.97, $p = 0.014$). However, the injury-rate ratio using a regression model that incorporated the over-dispersion in the data suggested the rate ratio was 0.93 (95%CI: 0.83–1.04, $p = 0.21$). This latter calculation was almost identical to the rate ratio calculated based on the injury rates from the individuals and bootstrap methods[3], i.e. methods that did not assume a specific underlying data distribution. This example illustrates that a violation of the underlying assumption can have dramatic effects for readers who focus on p-values (0.014 vs. 0.21) and some effect for those who focus on confidence intervals. Most statistical software provide an option to show indicators of data dispersion when using Poisson regression methods, and this is the recommended procedure if data for both injuries and exposures are available for each individual. Where data per individual are not available, the standard formulae can be used but should be interpreted with caution.

Choosing covariates in multiple regression

The previous sections of this chapter were concerned with associations as a first step, whereas etiological research is concerned with causes. There are many nuances to the definition of cause. In counterfactual theory, cause is deterministic at the individual level and can be defined as 'Had the exposure not been present at that time, the outcome would have differed'[5]. Because we can never know what would have happened had something not been present (known as 'counterfactual' because it contradicts the factual circumstances of what occurred), our causal inferences are limited to comparative risks at the population level[7]. In essence, the underlying assumption is that the comparison group is equivalent to what the exposure group would have been like had the exposure not occurred.

Causal inferences can be made from both observational and experimental studies. In experimental studies, there is an expectation that the two groups will be balanced with respect to prognostic factors, but differences may occur by chance (the probability of such differences is actually quite high for small studies)[7]. In observational studies, there is the additional problem that differences may occur specifically because a particular treatment or exposure is strongly associated with some other factor (e.g. a subject stretches frequently because they have had many previous injuries). In both RCTs and observational studies, causal inferences about the intervention programme may be biased due to differences in baseline prognosis and investigators often try to 'adjust' for these potential bias factors.

One common practice used to decide which covariates need to be 'adjusted' for is to include a covariate if it is associated with the exposure, associated with outcome, and changes the effect estimate when included in the model. Standard textbooks also emphasize that the covariate should not be affected by exposure and needs to be an independent cause of the outcome[8]. In fact, following the methods described above may still result in the investigator introducing bias where none existed without adjustment[6, 9, 10], which is especially problematic if the objective is to test for causal relationships. Some published examples where this has occurred include the effectiveness of HIV treatment[11], and why birth weight should not be included as a covariate when examining the causal effects of exposure during pregnancy on perinatal outcomes[12].

Is there an alternative to the current common practice noted above? One method that may help decide which statistical models are more likely to lead to unbiased causal estimates is the directed acyclic graph (DAG) approach. There are several papers explaining different nuances to this approach and the steps necessary to carry out the individual procedures, each with strengths and weaknesses[5, 10, 13, 14]. Investigators are encouraged to read these references to learn how to apply the methods; this chapter is limited to an explanation of the general concepts on how the DAG method can be used to determine which statistical models are likely to reduce bias, and which are likely to increase bias.

In the following example, which has been previously published[6], one is interested in establishing whether warm-up exercise (or lack thereof) is an aetiological factor of sports injury. Fig. 10.2 represents one possible DAG showing the relationships between different variables.

In the DAG approach, arrows are drawn between two factors that are believed to be causally related to each other, with the arrow directed from the cause to the effect. In the DAG in Fig. 10.2, the coach has a causal effect on team motivation and aggression, which may affect whether warm-up exercises are performed; team motivation/aggression may also be a cause of previous injury. Contact sports are believed to increase the probability of previous injury, and the contact occurring during a game may affect proprioception after the warm-up has occurred. The coach may cause changes in fitness levels (through training practices, not shown on the diagram), which causes changes in pre-game proprioception, which causes changes in warm-up exercises.

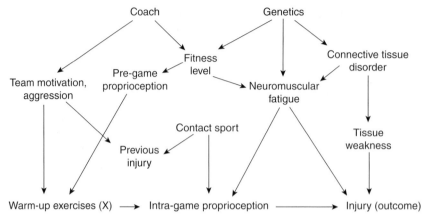

Fig. 10.2 A directed acyclic graph (DAG) noting potential causal relationships from the causal variable (blunt end of line) to the effect variable (arrow head).

If this diagram is correct, it can be shown that including previous injury in an observational study may lead to an increase in bias[5]. This occurs because inclusion of previous injury in the model creates an association between team motivation and contact sport (called 'conditional association' because it only occurs if previous injury is included in the model)[5]. This is extremely important because previous injury is considered a risk factor for subsequent injury, and almost all researchers would automatically include it as a covariate, or would stratify their analysis on it (i.e. calculate independent injury rates for those with and without previous injury). However, both of these methods would lead to a more biased estimate compared to other more appropriate analyses. Two possible examples that would minimize the bias in the estimate are to include (i) Team Motivation as a covariate in addition to previous injury, and (ii) the only covariates included are measures of neuromuscular fatigue and tissue weakness.

From the DAG approach, it is clear that an appropriate statistical model depends on identifying the actual causal relationships that exist. Some readers may disagree with the DAG as drawn and might prefer the DAG in Fig. 10.3.

In this example, investigators believe there are additional causal relationships between previous injury and pre-game proprioception, and between pre-game proprioception and intra-game proprioception. If this were the correct DAG, the situation is more complicated because bias is introduced whether one includes previous injury, or omits previous injury without including specific other variables. Rather, to minimize bias, one option would be to include only pre-game proprioception and team motivation (previous injury is not required).

Finally, Meeuwisse has recently proposed that investigators adopt a recursive model approach to sports-injury research[15] (also see Chapter 8). This model reflects the reality of what occurs in sport as subjects get injured and progress through the healing process. However, some of the questions that naturally arise from using such a model require very specialized analyses. This is because a regression analysis that includes a variable that is caused by the exposure of interest will almost always produce a biased effect for the total causal effect of that exposure, and this problem is not solved by using time-dependent covariates (because they are also affected by exposure)[11]. Therefore, the ability to use Meeuwisse's model will almost always require alternatives to traditional multiple regression techniques such as marginal structural models[11, 16, 17] and g-estimation[18, 19] to obtain unbiased estimates. Readers are encouraged to find statisticians in their area who understand these techniques and are available for collaboration.

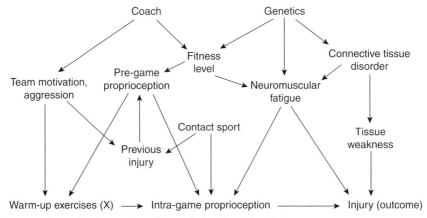

Fig. 10.3 An alternative directed acyclic graph (DAG) to Fig. 10.2.

Determining mediating effects through multiple regression

Investigators are often interested in 'decomposing' total causal effects into different mechanistic causal effects. The overall idea is that by identifying the magnitude of the total effect that acts through each mechanism, one can increase the impact of the prevention programmes. One method often suggested is to calculate the causal effect (i) without the mediating covariate in the model (total causal effect), and (ii) including the mediating covariate in the model (direct effect; i.e. independent of this covariate). The effect due to the mediating variable is then taken to be the difference between the two[20]. The purpose of this section is to review some of the limitations to this method that often go unrecognized[20–22].

Most importantly, there is no statistical test to determine with great certainty which variables are the mediating variables because all tests require specifying the correct DAG[23]; the fact that an effect estimate is changed after inclusion of a covariate could also be due to reducing confounding bias or increasing selection bias (which are unrelated to the question of mediating effects), changes due to effect modification, or because something is a marker of a mediator. Assuming we are confident that the chosen variable is a mediating variable, there remain statistical and philosophical challenges to decomposing total causal effects into partial causal effects[20, 21].

First, interventions are not always more effective if they target a mediating variable. For example, interventions that penalize players in sport for dangerous play address a direct cause of injury and may have some effect. On the other hand, interventions aimed at changing the culture of the sport (e.g. Fair Play rules[15] or teaching parents what is appropriate and inappropriate behaviour) address an indirect cause and could have a more generalized effect for many sports.

Second, decomposing causal effects requires that there is no confounding between the effect of the mediating variable and the outcome[21]. If there is confounding here, the effect estimate for the mediating variable may be biased (this is true in both observational and randomized studies). For example, let us assume the DAG in Fig. 10.4 is correct.

In this situation, an effect estimate of intra-game proprioception on Injury would be biased because 'fitness' causes both the intra-game proprioception and the outcome, even though the total causal effect estimate for warm-up is unbiased[20]. If we assume direct and indirect effects sum to the total effect, and the estimate for indirect effect acting through the mediator is biased, then it follows that the 'direct causal effect' of Warm-up Exercise on Injury is biased. Therefore, any inferences based on these decomposed analyses may lead to inappropriate conclusions.

Finally, what does the difference between the total causal effect and the calculated direct/indirect causal effects really mean even when there is no confounding of the mediating variable

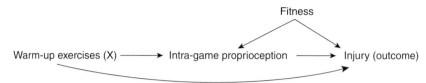

Fig. 10.4 A directed acyclic graph showing hypothetical causal relationships between warm-up exercises, fitness, intra-game proprioception, and injury. The arrow from warm-up exercises to injury represents the direct effect, and the arrows from warm-up exercises to intra-game proprioception to injury represent the indirect effect. The total casual effect is the sum of the direct and indirect effects.

on the outcome? We will use the example of a study investigating the effect of implementing a Fair Play intervention (rule changes that promote mutual respect and provide advantages if no penalties occur) to decrease overly aggressive behaviour into amateur sport, which is expected to lead to a decreased injury rate. Let us say that the injury-rate ratio for Fair Play rules versus no Fair Play rules calculated without the mediating variable (aggression in this case) is 4.0. Further, the injury rate ratio with 'aggression' as a covariate in the model is 2.0 (i.e. a 50% decrease in the total causal effect). In this case, most people would assume that if a second study were conducted with Fair Play rules, and we fixed aggression to the same value in every individual, the observed injury rate ratio would be 2.0. However, this is only true if the effect of Fair Play rules is the same in those with and without aggression (i.e. no unit-level interaction); if this is not the case, then the calculated direct effect is always biased[20] and the observed effect in the second experiment would not be equal to the expected value based on regression decomposition analysis. In addition, if the calculated direct effect is biased, and the total causal effect is unbiased, then the calculated indirect effect is also likely to be biased[20].

When one uses regression techniques for decomposition analysis as above, it yields what is known as the 'controlled' direct effect. There is another approach to effect decomposition called the 'natural' (or 'pure') direct effect, and unlike the controlled direct effect, the result is not affected by unit-level interaction[20, 22, 24]. In this analysis, the investigator fixes the level of aggression (i.e. the intermediate variable) to the level the subject would have had, had the subject never been exposed (in this case, no exposure to Fair Play rules). In this analysis, a subject who would 'naturally' be aggressive without Fair Play rules is fixed at aggressive, and a subject who is naturally non-aggressive without Fair Play rules would be fixed at non-aggressive. Although unit-level interaction is not a problem, the analysis cannot be done with ordinary regression analysis and one must use other statistical techniques such as marginal structural modelling[24, 25].

The controlled direct effect and natural direct effect decomposition analyses address different research questions and each has advantages and disadvantages. The controlled direct effect decomposition analysis answers the question of what would happen if we implemented our principle intervention, and at the same time added a second intervention that fixed the mediating variable to the same value in every subject. For example, what is the effect of Fair Play rules if every person was non-aggressive? The natural direct effect decomposition analysis answers the question about the programme's effectiveness if we implement our principle intervention, and at the same time a) break the causal link from the main exposure to the mediating variable and b) still allow the mediating to vary depending on other factors[22]. This would not make sense in the example above for Fair Play rules, but may be valuable for biological or biomechanical links between variables, or complex interventions.

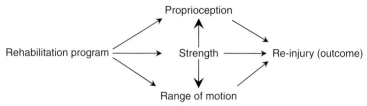

Fig. 10.5 A rehabilitation program is a complex intervention including proprioception exercises, strengthening exercises and range of motion exercises. All three types of exercises may have direct effects to reduce injuries. Strengthening exercises have been shown to improve range of motion in chronic groin pain (presumably because the underlying weakness was a cause of reduced range of motion due to joint irritation and reflex increased muscle tone) and they also improve proprioception in subjects with extreme weakness (not as relevant for sport medicine).

The following is an example where the natural direct effect can be used, and abused, in sports medicine. Rehabilitation programmes normally include strengthening, range of motion, and proprioception exercises (the causal links are likely to be those illustrated in Fig. 10.5). In a natural direct-effect-decomposition analysis, including strength as the only mediating covariate means the 'direct effect' of rehabilitation on injury is the combined effect through range of motion and proprioception. Similarly, if range of motion is the only mediating variable, then the natural direct-effect-decomposition analysis would assess the 'direct effect' that is mediated by strengthening and proprioception. Although using strength as a mediating variable leads to an appropriate analysis if the DAG in Fig. 10.5 is correct, using range of motion as the mediating variable will lead to biased estimates for two reasons. First, strength is a cause of both range of motion and injury, and therefore the effect of range of motion (the mediating variable for this analysis) on injury is confounded by strength (similar to the situation discussed in Fig. 10.4). Second, even if one includes both strength and range of motion in the analysis as mediating variables, we have no method to distinguish how much of the change in range of motion is due to the range of motion exercises and how much is due to the strengthening exercises. To accomplish this, we would need a measure of the reduced joint irritation/reflex muscle tone that is the mechanism by which strengthening exercises may improve range of motion (there are additional assumptions that must be met as well). Without this, any effect-decomposition analysis using range of motion as a mediating variable will lead to inappropriate inferences. Therefore, even though unit-level interactions are not an issue in this non-regression type of analysis, one still needs to be cautious about the other assumptions.

Conclusion

The common lack of data-independence in aetiological sports medicine research requires a more complicated analysis than is routinely observed in most other types of epidemiological research. Further, because the objective is to make causal inferences, the choice of covariates in multiple regression models is much more complicated compared to a search of risk factors. The use of DAGs can be helpful, but researchers will at times need to replace their traditional use of regression techniques with newer and more powerful statistical approaches such as marginal structural modelling. Decomposing total causal effects into direct and indirect effects may seem appealing at first, but poses its own unique challenges. User-friendly statistical software has allowed investigators to conduct many different types of analyses without a sophisticated mathematical and statistical background. However, if investigators do not conceptually understand the underlying assumptions of the different possible analyses and cannot determine if they are likely to be valid, then inappropriate causal inferences will be made that will hinder rather than advance the science of sport medicine.

References

1. De Angelis D, Young GA (2005). Bootstrap method, in Armitage P, Colton T (eds) *Encyclopedia of biostatistics. 2nd edition*. John Wiley & Sons, Chisester.

2. Knowles SB, Marshall SW, Guskiewicz KM (2006). Issues in estimating risks and rates in sports injury research. *J Athl Train*, **41**, 207–15.

3. Shrier I, Steele RJ, Rich B (2009). Analyses of count data: some do's and some don'ts. *Am J Epidemiol*, **In press.**

4. Shrier I, Meeuwisse WH, Matheson GO, Wingfield K, Steele R, Prince F, Hanley J, Montanaro M (2009). Injury patterns and injury rates in the circus arts: an analysis of 5 years of data from Cirque du Soleil. *Am J Sports Med*, **37**(6), 1143–9.

5. Shrier I, Platt RW (2008). Eliminating bias through directed acyclic graphs. *BMC Med Res Methodol*, **8**, 70.

6. Hernan MA (2004). A definition of causal effect for epidemiological research. *J Epidemiol Community Health*, **58**, 265–71.

7. Shrier I, Boivin JF, Steele RJ, Platt RW, Furlan A, Kakuma R, Brophy J, Rossignol M (2007). Should meta-analyses of interventions include observational studies in addition to randomized controlled trials? A critical examination of the underlying principles. *Am J Epidemiol*, **166**, 1203–9.

8. Rothman KJ, Greenland S (1998). Precision and validity in epidemiologic studies, in Rothman KJ, Greenland S (eds) *Modern Epidemiology*, pp. 115–134. Lippincott-Raven Publishers, Philadelphia.

9. Weinberg CR (1993). Toward a clearer definition of confounding. *Am J Epidemiol*, **137**, 1–8.

10. Greenland S, Pearl J, Robins JM (1999). Causal diagrams for epidemiologic research. *Epidemiology*, **10**, 37–48.

11. Hernan MA, Brumback B, Robins JM (2000). Marginal structural models to estimate the causal effect of zidovudine on the survival of HIV-positive men. *Epidemiology*, **11**, 561–70.

12. Hernández-Díaz S, Schisterman EF, Hernán MA (2006). The birth weight "paradox" uncovered? *Am J Epidemiol*, **164**, 1115–20.

13. Hernan MA, Hernandez-Diaz S, Robins JM (2004). A structural approach to selection bias. *Epidemiology*, **15**, 615–25.

14. Hernan MA, Hernandez-Diaz S, Werler MM, Mitchell AA (2002). Causal knowledge as a prerequisite for confounding evaluation: an application to birth defects epidemiology. *Am J Epidemiol*, **155**, 176–84.

15. Meeuwisse WH, Tyreman H, Hagel B, Carolyn E (2007). A dynamic model of etiology in sport injury: the recursive nature of risk and causation. *Clin J Sport Med*, **17**, 215–19.

16. Robins JM (1999). Association, causation, and marginal structural models. *Synthese*, **121**, 151–79.

17. Robins JM, Hernan MA, Brumback B (2000). Marginal structural models and causal inference in epidemiology. *Epidemiology*, **11**, 550–60.

18. Witteman JC, D'Agostino RB, Stijnen T, Kannel WB, Cobb JC, de Ridder MA, Hofman A, Robins JM (1998). G-estimation of causal effects: isolated systolic hypertension and cardiovascular death in the Framingham Heart Study. *Am J Epidemiol*, **148**, 390–401.

19. Hernan MA, Cole SR, Margolick J, Cohen M, Robins JM (2005). Structural accelerated failure time models for survival analysis in studies with time-varying treatments. *Pharmacoepidemiol Drug Saf*, **14**, 477–91.

20. Kaufman JS, Maclehose RF, Kaufman S (2004). A further critique of the analytic strategy of adjusting for covariates to identify biologic mediation. *Epidemiol Perspect Innov*, **1**, 4.

21. Cole SR, Hernan MA (2002). Fallibility in estimating direct effects. *Int J Epidemiol*, **31**, 163–5.

22. Petersen ML, Sinisi SE, van der Laan M (2006). Estimation of direct causal effects. *Epidemiology*, **17**, 276–84.

23. Robins JM, Wasserman L (1999). On the impossibility of inferring causation from association without background knowledge, in Glymour C, Cooper C (eds) *Computation, Causation, and Discovery*, pp. 305–21. The MIT Press, Cambridge, Mass.

24. VanderWeele TJ (2009). Marginal structural models for the estimation of direct and indirect effects. *Epidemiology*, **20**, 18–26.

25. Rosenblum M, Jewell NP, van der Laan M, Shiboski S, van der Straten A, Padian N (2009). Analysing direct effects in randomized trials with secondary interventions: an application to human immunodeficiency virus prevention trials. *J R Stat Soc Ser A*, **172**(2), 443–65.

Part 4

Developing preventive measures

Chapter 11

The pragmatic approach

Alex Donaldson

In an ideal world the development of effective, implementable, and sustainable sports-injury preventive measures would be straightforward, based on fundamental scientific processes[1, 2]. Firstly, you would consult the literature (see Chapter 7) to get an idea of the size and scope of the injury problem. If no such information existed you would undertake a descriptive study (injury surveillance) to gather the necessary data on the magnitude and severity of sports injuries (see Chapters 5 & 6). Armed with this information you could target your preventive efforts at the most pressing injury problems. Once you have identified your 'target' you would again consult the literature to get an understanding of how the injuries of interest occur (the injury aetiology—see Part 3, Chapters 8–10). If the literature lets you down again, you would then conduct some further research to properly establish the various internal and external risk factors that lead to or 'cause' the injuries you have previously decided are worthy of preventing (see Chapter 9)[3, 4]. Now that you know the injury problem and you have a good understanding of the causal factors you can begin to turn your research talents to the process of selecting or developing injury-prevention measures, which of course will then need to be implemented and evaluated under both controlled and 'real-world' conditions (see Part 5, Chapters 13–16).

Again, in an ideal world, you would revisit the literature to see what effective interventions are available to address the risk factors of interest. If you are lucky enough to be focussing your attention on the prevention of fairly common and fairly severe injuries (such as lower limb or dental injuries) in a popular sport (such as running or football/soccer)[5], then your investigation of the literature might provide some clear guidance on interventions that have been shown to be effective in certain populations (youth, professionals, females, college students, etc.). However, in the 'real' world you will probably find that there is little information about effective interventions (i.e. those that have been demonstrated, using appropriate study designs such as randomized controlled trials, to successfully prevent injuries) in the literature [6] Indeed, most systematic reviews of sports-injury preventive interventions conclude, at least in part, with well-used phrases such as 'more high-quality studies are required'[7, 8], 'there is insufficient evidence'[9], or 'the evidence is inconclusive'[10].

Even when effective sports-injury preventive measures can be identified in the literature, it can be hard to know if they will work for you. For example, it can be difficult to know which components of the often multi-component programmes are the critical ones to ensure successful injury prevention. In addition, it can be difficult to glean from the available literature exactly what was evaluated – what was the intervention? How and where was it implemented, and who with? The successful transfer of effective interventions across settings and contexts is fraught with difficulties due to the complex interplay of social, political, organizational, and environmental factors[11]. Some potential context-related factors that can influence the transferability of effective interventions to new settings include the: target audience for the intervention (adults/youth/children, males/females, etc.); differences within and across sports (community/elite sport, culture, resources, etc.); and differences across national boundaries (administrative structures, policy implementation, culture, etc.).

Given all of the above, and the likelihood that most sports-injury prevention researchers and practitioners will find themselves having to come up with intervention ideas or, at the very least adapt and modify interventions that have been shown to effective or promising in contexts that are not directly relevant, the aim of this chapter is to help researchers approach this task in a way that is:

◆ Systematic

◆ Context relevant

◆ Evidence- and theory/first principle-based

A 5-step strategic approach to developing sports-injury preventive measures

The following is a step-by-step strategic approach to developing sports-injury preventive interventions. It draws on a number of more general public health, health promotion, injury prevention, and risk-management intervention-planning frameworks including the National Public Health Partnership Planning Framework[12], the Standards Australia Guidelines for Managing Risk in Sport and Recreation[13], and a systematic approach to injury intervention planning developed by Runyan and Freire[14]. It is impossible to discuss the development of sports-injury preventive measures without touching on issues such as injury epidemiology, risk-factor identification, and intervention implementation, which are covered in more depth in other parts of this book. However, the main focus of this chapter is on Step 5 (Deciding what to do – evidenced-informed and theory-based interventions to address identified sports-injury risks).

Although the steps below are presented in a linear and hierarchical way, they are not mutually exclusive nor are they necessarily progressive or consecutive. For example, under some circumstances it might be appropriate to consider the context into which an intervention is to be implemented (Step 2) simultaneously with, or even before, identifying relevant stake-holders and developing multi-disciplinary research partnerships (Step 1). In addition, communication (Step 1) is an on-going process that continues for the life span of any intervention[13].

Step 1: Tell people about it and get them on board – communication, consultation, co-ordination, and a multi-disciplinary approach

Preventing the injuries and managing the risks associated with participation in sport requires on-going communication, consultation, and co-ordination[13]. Given the multiple levels of influence on the successful implementation of injury prevention and public health interventions[15, 16], there will often be many people and organizations that need to be involved in identifying and developing interventions. Consistent with a 'bottom-up' approach to intervention development discussed later in this chapter, all of them should be informed and actively engaged as early as possible in the process. If effective interventions are to be developed and widely implemented, then researchers need to identify and co-ordinate the activities of key stakeholders who have an interest in the intervention and its consequences[17]. For example, sports administrators need to be committed to providing the organizational support necessary to successfully implement and evaluate an injury-prevention intervention in their setting. Facility-owners and managers can play a key role in developing and implementing interventions targeted at safe environments for sports participation and it is important that they are supportive of, and involved in selecting and planning such interventions. The same is true for equipment designers and manufacturers. Coaches, first aid providers, team managers, referees/umpires, and parents of junior participants are often the 'front line' in sports-injury preventive interventions. They need to know what is expected of them and how to fulfil their responsibilities. They are also an important source of information about the feasibility and sustainability of interventions to improve safety. Sports participants are the ultimate target, or 'end users' of sports safety efforts and it is vital that they are informed and actively engaged in the process of developing interventions that they will be required to comply with. The attitudes, knowledge, and behaviours of individual participants can significantly influence the success or otherwise of sports-injury preventive efforts[18, 19]. Other key stakeholders that might potentially be interested and influential in the successful development and implementation of sports-injury preventive interventions include: sports medicine peak bodies (such as the American College of Sports Medicine (ACSM) and Sports Medicine Australia); governmental and non-governmental injury-prevention agencies; local, regional, state/provincial, national, and international sports bodies; local, state/provincial, and national government health and sports departments; and schools, colleges, and universities.

Practical steps to communicate and consult with relevant stakeholders and co-ordinate the development and implementation of sports-injury preventive interventions can include:

- Establishing a research working group with representation from all relevant stakeholders;
- Promoting the research through sports and injury-prevention professional and industry networks;
- Seeking stakeholder opinions and input through regular presentations of the research as it is formulated and progressed;
- Publishing and publicly presenting and reporting intervention activity and evaluation findings (see Part 5);

As will be discussed later in this chapter, most frameworks that are used to inform the development of injury-prevention interventions are based on a socio-ecologic and a multi-disciplinary approach[20–22]. Therefore, it is worthwhile spending time at the planning stage thinking through the range of disciplines and research skills that might be required to successfully develop, implement, and evaluate an intervention. For example, depending on the nature of the proposed intervention, an intervention-planning team may benefit from the input of biomechanists, policy-makers, social and behavioural scientists, epidemiologists, evaluators, engineers, educators, designers, health promoters, and representatives of the intervention's target audience.

Step 2: Establish the context – understanding the bigger picture

Sports-injury preventive efforts, like other public health interventions, are unlikely to achieve sustained population benefits unless they are developed and implemented with a good understanding of the individual and organizational implementation context, even if they are based on sound evidence of efficacy[11, 23, 24]. People performing different roles (administrators, coaches, participants, referees/umpires, etc.) and organizations (state/provincial sporting organizations, regional associations, schools, community clubs, facility-owners and managers, insurers, etc.) will have different sports-safety responsibilities and different capacities, attitudes, and knowledge that will influence their ability and willingness to participate in sports-injury research and to implement and comply with interventions[25]. When developing a sports-injury preventive intervention, researchers need to understand what the individuals and organizations they plan to work with do (i.e. what they are responsible for, the activity they undertake and the service they deliver) and where they fit in the bigger picture. This will enable researchers to clearly establish the contribution that each individual or organization can make to improving safety and reducing the injury risks associated with participation in sport. For example, state/provincial sporting organizations might reasonably be responsible for providing leadership for safety in their sport at a state/provincial level. This might include: gathering and monitoring injury data to identify important issues that need to be addressed or to evaluate injury-prevention interventions; setting evidenced-based safety policies and guidelines that affiliated organizations are required to follow; and conducting research into effective and sustainable safety interventions. By contrast, a community club might be responsible for making sure all coaches are properly qualified and first-aid providers are in attendance at all games and training. Facility-owners and managers will be responsible for making sure that the playing environments are well maintained and safe for the purpose for which they are used. In turn, individual participants will be required to: abide by the rules of the sport; wear and maintain appropriate protective equipment; and maintain adequate levels of fitness to enable safe participation.

The following questions are useful to ask and answer when establishing the context into which an intervention is intended to be implemented:

◆ What is the external context or environment in which the intervention is to be implemented including: community attitudes; legal and statutory requirements; local by-laws, and governing-body policies?

◆ What is the internal or personal context including: organizational objectives, core activity, and operations; volunteer or professional nature of administration; available resources (financial, time, expertise, and competency); and safety culture?

◆ What are the legal and moral responsibilities?

◆ Is there appropriate organizational support (policies, resources, political, etc.) to successfully implement the intervention?

◆ What are other people and organizations responsible for? What are they doing? How can their activities be co-ordinated and integrated to ensure they facilitate successful implementation of the intervention?

◆ Who should the researchers inform about what they want to do?

◆ What safety standards apply to the individual or organization's operations?

◆ What are the capabilities of the organization?

◆ What safety strategies already exist in the organization?

Asking and answering such questions will enable researchers to understand more about the context in which they are operating and to set appropriate and achievable intervention goals and objectives.

Step 3: Identify the safety issues, concerns, and risks

Once the context in which the injury-prevention intervention is being conducted is understood, it is necessary to clearly define the injury problem. This will require developing a good understanding of the specific safety issues that should be addressed – who gets injured, how many, how severely, how frequently, what are the injury mechanisms, and what are the circumstances? (See Part 3) An enormous amount of work has already been done by a range of organizations (sports bodies, academic and research institutions, government departments, etc.) to identify the safety and injury issues and risks in many sports. The key to gathering relevant information is to know who to ask and where to look. The following practical steps will help to do this:

◆ Search the peer-reviewed literature and text books (see Chapter 7) – published systematic reviews, if available, can be particularly useful. Be aware that most published literature will provide only a general overview of safety issues and injury risks which may be of limited relevance or applicability to a specific context.

◆ Look at and ask for any available injury data – insurance claims; first-aid records; health-service data; governmental, non-governmental, and academic reports; etc.

◆ Ask people who are likely to know the issues or have concerns – coaches; players; first aid providers; parents; local medical service providers (hospitals, general practitioners, physiotherapists); etc.

◆ Conduct safety inspections and audits – of playing surfaces; facilities; equipment; qualifications; processes and procedures; injury histories and medical conditions of players; etc.

◆ Consult other relevant stakeholders – international, national, state/provincial and regional sports governing bodies; facility-owners and managers; etc.

◆ Ask the 'experts' – sports medicine and injury-prevention peak bodies; government departments responsible for sport, recreation and health; academic researchers; etc.

Once information or 'evidence' about the safety issues of concern has been gathered it is important to consider how much evidence there is, the quality of the available evidence and its relevance or applicability to the context established in Step 2[26, 27].

A useful framework for identifying the risk factor for sports injuries, particularly if little information is available in the literature, is Haddon's Matrix[28, 29]. Based on the idea that the transfer of energy is the underlying cause of all injuries[30] and incorporating the host, agent, and environment principles of infectious disease epidemiology[31], and the temporal (pre-event, event, and post-event) sequence of an injury, this matrix can be used to both conceptualize the risk factors associated with a given injury problem[17] (see Table 11.1 using lower-limb injuries in football/soccer as an example) and, as will be discussed later in this chapter, to generate potential intervention opportunities and strategies.

In the context of using Haddon's Matrix to conceptualize the risk factors for a given sports injury, the host can be interpreted as the sports participant who is injured; the agent as the energy (usually kinetic) or the mechanism through which the energy is transferred; and the environment as the physical, social, cultural, and policy setting or context within which the injury occurs.

Table 11.1 Identification of the risk factors for lower-limb injuries in football/soccer using Haddon's Matrix

Time sequence	Factor		
	Host (injured player)	Agent/Vehicle/Vector (game, other players, referee, etc.)	Environment (playing environment)
Pre-event	Poor player conditioning, and history of previous lower-limb injuries	Speed and congestion of the game	Playing surface not assessed for injury risk
Event	Lack of appropriate protective equipment (e.g. ankle supports and shin pads)	Illegal tackle from opposition player	Hard, uneven surface and limited turf cover
Post-event	Non-compliance with recommended rehabilitation protocol	Failure of referee to stop play to enable the injured player to receive first aid attention	Lack of appropriate first aid equipment

The outcome of Step 3 will be a list of injury risk factors that could potentially be addressed through intervention.

Step 4: Set priorities – short-term action and long-term planning

No researcher or research programme will be able to successfully tackle all the risk factors identified in Step 3 immediately. All research programmes operate with limited resources – people, finances, time, expertise, equipment, etc. – so it will always be necessary to make choices and prioritize intervention activities. Some issues will be more important to address than others and some will be easy to address with immediate action while others will require longer-term strategies. For example, repairing potholes in a playing surface might require an afternoon working bee while ensuring that all coaches are appropriately qualified will take more time to develop and implement the policy, raise the money to fund the required training, and deliver the training. Some practical considerations when setting safety priorities include:

◆ The 'frequency' of the risk – how often is the risk present or how likely is it that an injury will occur?

◆ The 'severity' of the likely injury – if the injury does occur, is it likely to be catastrophic, severe, moderate, or minor?

◆ What can be done about the issue? Is a simple, cost-effective solution available?

◆ The need to get some quick, short-term outcomes to maintain momentum and interest in the injury-prevention process.

◆ What injury risk factors are the community or other stakeholders interested in or capable of addressing?

◆ Legal and statutory requirements – will there be significant legal ramifications if nothing is done and an injury occurs? Is the risk 'reasonably foreseeable' and the solution 'practicable'?

Step 5: Decide what to do – evidenced-informed and theory-based interventions to address identified sports-injury risks

Identifying the important sports injuries to address; understanding the risk factors that contribute to these injuries; and knowing what to do about them are related, but separate steps in developing and implementing a strategic and pragmatic approach to sports-injury prevention. Irrespective of the nature of the injuries and the contributing risk factors, there are some general injury-prevention principles that can be applied to generate common sense solutions.

Andersson and Menckel[32] conducted a comparative analysis of injury-prevention conceptual frameworks and identified five key dimensions relevant to planning all injury-prevention efforts: time; the level at which the intervention is targeted; the degree of generality/specificity of the type of disease (which Andersson and Menckel considered became irrelevant when applied to a specific health issue like injuries); the direction of the intervention process; and the relationship between the injured individual (host), the mechanism of injury (agent, vehicle, or vector), and the environment in which the injury event occurs. These key dimensions of injury-prevention conceptual frameworks will now be discussed in relation to identifying and developing injury-prevention interventions in the context of sports injuries.

Time dimension

When developing sports-injury preventive measures it is useful to consider injuries as a logical sequence of events and intervention as interrupting the chain. One pertinent question to consider, therefore, is with regards to when to interrupt. Andersson and Menckel's[32] 'time' dimension is related to the temporal nature or 'natural course' of injury events. This dimension is most easily identified in the commonly used 'primary, secondary, and tertiary prevention' classifications originally derived from clinical medicine where:

- Primary prevention involves intervening to prevent or reduce the energy involved in the incident that leads to the injury
- Secondary prevention involves intervening immediately post the injury incident to reduce the severity of the injury through early detection and treatment (i.e. acute care and stabilization) and
- Tertiary prevention involves limiting the long-term consequences of the injury, promoting recovery, and reducing the likelihood of re-occurrence (i.e. post-acute care and rehabilitation)[21].

Haddon also applied the time-related concepts of pre-event, event, and post-event where opportunities to intervene in the causal chain exist before the injury event occurs (before the damaging transfer of energy), at the time of the injury event (the point of energy transfer), and after the injury event (once energy transfer has occurred)[29]. Further distinctions can be made in the pre-event phase where the focus of intervention can be on preventing the injury event from occurring, reducing the risk to an acceptable level, and building the capacity of the individual to cope with the consequences of the injury event[32].

Although there is a significant overlap between Haddon's 'event' time phase and 'secondary' injury prevention, they are not interchangeable. Strictly speaking, Haddon's event phase is focussed on the moment at which the energy is transferred from the agent to the host. It therefore incorporates the use of protective equipment or engineering modifications which reduce or dissipate the energy at the moment of exchange. Secondary prevention occurs immediately after the injury event and includes immediate first aid and medical attention. Tertiary injury prevention and Haddon's post-event phase both focus on interventions designed to minimize the consequences of the injurious event through rehabilitation and returning the injured individual to the 'pre-event' status. Clearly it can be difficult to delineate between the temporal phases of an injurious event, particularly if attempting to apply different conceptual models at the same time or where the injurious event is virtually instantaneous and the relationship between secondary and tertiary prevention is in fact a continuum.

If this 'time' dimension is applied to the injuries sustained during the tackle in rugby league, the primary prevention (or pre-event) strategies might include banning the tackle or restricting the tackle to certain types (e.g. no lifting or 'spear' tackles). Interventions targeted at the event phase would include coaching players in how to tackle (e.g. do not lead with the head) and be tackled (e.g. how to fall and land), and mandating the wearing of protective padding by all participant so as to reduce the risk of injury at the moment of energy exchange. Secondary injury prevention would include having appropriately trained first-aid personnel in attendance with access to the required equipment (e.g. neck braces and stretchers or spinal boards) – it should be noted that these interventions would be considered post-event interventions using Haddon's temporal classifications. Tertiary (or post-event) interventions would include post-first-aid treatment and rehabilitation (e.g. surgery, massage, physiotherapy) of the injured player. Again, it should be noted that these temporal delineations are somewhat arbitrary and some tertiary or post-event interventions could legitimately be categorized as pre-event or primary prevention if they also served to prevent the reoccurrence of injuries at a latter time.

As pointed out by Freire and Runyan, the first step in using Haddon's Matrix when brainstorming injury risk factors or potential interventions is to clearly define the temporal sequence of an injurious event[17]. For example, in the context of neck injuries sustained from 'spear' tackles in rugby league, it is possible to define the event as the moment the tackler lifts the tackled player beyond the perpendicular, or as the moment the tackled player makes head-first contact with the ground. If the event is defined as lifting, then preventing the lifting action is a pre-event strategy, ensuring the lifting motion does not go beyond the perpendicular is an event strategy and ensuring neck protection (assuming effective protective equipment is available) is worn is a post-event strategy. However, if the contact with the ground is considered the injurious event then preventing the lifting motion from going beyond the perpendicular becomes a pre-event strategy, ensuring neck protection is worn is an event strategy, and immediate first-aid including availability of appropriate lifting and neck-stabilizing equipment, is a post-event strategy.

Intervention-level dimension

The 'level at which the intervention is targeted' dimension incorporates the idea that injury-prevention interventions can be targeted at the micro/individual level (either those directly injured – e.g. sports participants, or a third party responsible for ensuring safety – e.g. coaches, administrators, referees/umpires); the meso/groups and organizations level (e.g. sporting teams or clubs and associations); the macro/community level; and society level. This dimension incorporates four common injury-prevention concepts that will be discussed in more detail in this section – the Three E's of injury prevention[33]; passive and active interventions[34]; an ecological approach to injury prevention[35–37]; and Haddon's 10 countermeasure strategies[38]. It should be noted that there is considerable overlap in these four concepts and application of any one will incorporate aspects of the other three.

The Three E's is a relatively unsophisticated approach to injury prevention which involves classifying and targeting intervention efforts into three groups—Education, Engineering/ergonomics/design, and Enforcement/policy/regulation/legislation. The education category includes both mass media/social marketing campaigns that attempt to change community awareness or acceptance of unsafe behaviours, and initiatives designed to generate behavioural changes among specific individuals. Examples of sports-injury-related mass media campaigns are the Fédération Internationale de Football Association (FIFA) Fair play component of 'The 11' programme developed by FMARC, the medical research centre of FIFA[39], and the New South Wales Sport and Recreation Sport Rage Program[40]. An example of an individually focussed sports-injury-prevention educational campaign is the New Zealand Football 'Soccer Smart' Program designed to change the behaviour of soccer coaches[41].

The engineering category of sports-injury preventive initiatives incorporates all efforts to modify the environment in which sports are conducted and the equipment that is used. Examples of this approach include modifying the design of baseball bases to prevent sliding injuries[42] and developing mandatory standards for American football helmets[43]. Other sports-safety initiatives that fall into this category include those related to the playing surface (e.g. ground hardness in the Australian Football League), and the padding and positioning of fixtures and fittings (e.g. padding on goal posts in rugby union, and the distance between the court and spectator seating in basketball). The engineering category is very closely related to the concept of passive injury prevention discussed later in this chapter.

The enforcement category of sports-injury preventive initiatives covers any attempts to improve safety and reduce the risk of injury through the development and enforcement of regulations, rules, policies, and legislation. This approach has been very successful in preventing automobile injuries through the introduction of legislation related to drunk driving, the lowering of speed limits in built-up areas, and the mandatory wearing of seat-belts[44]. An excellent example of an effective enforcement-related injury-prevention intervention in the sporting context is the changing of the scrummaging laws in rugby league and rugby union[45, 46].

Haddon coined the terms 'active' and 'passive' approaches to injury prevention in 1961[34] and distinguished between the two on the basis of *the amount of action on the part of individuals in the general population required for their efficacy.* Preventive strategies can be classified along a continuum from those that require continued, on-going behavioural change on the part of the individual to protect themselves (active), to those that involve structural, environmental, and engineering solutions requiring little action on the part of the individual being protected (passive). It has been argued that, in practice, it is nearly impossible to develop truly passive solutions to injury problems as some level of individual behavioural change or human adaptation is nearly always required to achieve injury reductions[15].

As a general rule, interventions based on education and increasing awareness tend to be more active, and those based on engineering and environmental solutions are more passive. Interventions using protective equipment are often mid-way along the active–passive continuum as they require the individual to wear or use the protective equipment, but once it is put on, it provides protection without requiring further individual action. In the context of sports-injury prevention, an example of a highly active intervention is educating coaches to change their coaching practices[41]. This intervention requires individual coaches to continue to implement the new practices on an on-going basis in order for their athletes to gain the associated injury-prevention benefits. At the opposite end of the continuum is the previously mentioned re-designing of baseball bases to ensure they do not remain in a fixed position when participants slide into them[42]. In this example, the individual player does not need to change their behaviour at all to reap the injury-prevention benefits of the intervention. However, even this type of intervention requires some level of behavioural change on the part of equipment manufactures and those responsible for purchasing and installing equipment at the individual team or club level. Fig. 11.1 illustrates how interventions can fall in between to the two extremes, using strategies to prevent ankle injuries associated with poor playing surfaces as an example. Compulsory ankle strapping is considered more 'passive' than voluntary ankle strapping because the individual player has less choice when the intervention is mandated by a powerful authority (e.g. coach, club- or sports-governing body).

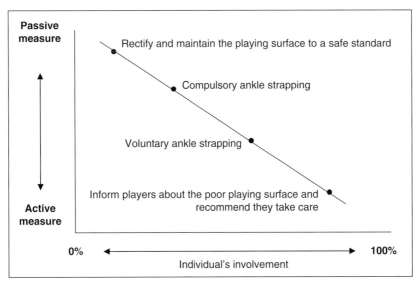

Fig. 11.1 The active and passive intervention continuum applied to strategies to prevent ankle injuries associated with poor playing surfaces.

It is generally acknowledged that the more passive an intervention is, the greater impact it will have on whole populations and the more effective it will be[21, 34, 47]. When no effective passive interventions are available then it has been recommended that efficacious active interventions should be mandated[34].

An ecological approach to injury prevention is based on the notion that individual behaviour is the result of interactions between people and their social and physical environment[35–37]. The underlying assumption in this model is that individuals will be unlikely to adopt and sustain desired behavioural changes unless their personal relationships and the social and physical environments in which they operate support and encourage the desired change. As a consequence, injury-prevention interventions can be potentially targeted at changing intrapersonal, interpersonal, institutional/organizational, community, and public policy factors that contribute to injurious incidents[36].

McLeroy et al., in their ecological model for health promotion[36], identify knowledge, attitudes, and skills of individuals as intrapersonal factors that can be addressed using educational, training, and mass media strategies. The primary outcome of interest when addressing intrapersonal factors is a change in the individual. Interpersonal influences on health and safety behaviours include social relationships and networks with significant others (friends, family, peers, etc.) which can be tackled through interventions targeted at changing social norms and modifying the social influences on the behaviour of individuals. Organizations and institutions are important sources of information, managers of environments, and transmitters of social norms and values. Setting-based changes and interventions can be used to support long-term individual behavioural change through strategies targeted at organizational culture, policies, management structures and processes, regulations, environments, incentives, etc. Communities can be defined either geographically/spatially (e.g. towns, suburbs) or though relationships and common interests (e.g. membership of groups and associations). Community-based interventions are those that are targeted at changing the facilities and environments in a given geographical location; building relationships between like-minded organizations to work in partnership and improve the efficiency of service delivery; or using community structures (schools, churches, local government, etc.) to deliver services and influence social norms. Broader public policy interventions included those that use advocacy, resource distribution, economics, regulations, and laws to influence individual behaviour.

The purpose of an ecological approach to injury prevention is to focus attention on the social and environmental causes of behaviour, and to identify interventions that target these[36]. It is therefore a useful model to apply when identifying and describing influencing factors, and when developing interventions[15]. Eime and colleagues have published one of the few studies based on applying an ecological model to the prevention of sports injuries[48]. In the context of preventing eye injuries in squash they developed and implemented a multi-level intervention targeted at individual, venue, and organizational factors that influence the wearing of protective eye-wear[49]. Table 11.2 shows how the ecological model can be applied to the example of preventing dental injuries in community football.

Proponents of an ecological approach to injury prevention believe that to successfully and sustainably reduce an individual's risk of injury, safety-promotion practitioners and researchers should focus on understanding and systematically changing the environmental and sociological factors that facilitate and support unsafe behaviour[37]. It is now generally acknowledged in the broader injury-prevention field that risky behaviours are most successfully changed through comprehensive, multi-level strategies that focus on intervening at several points of the ecological model and in multiple settings[49, 50].

Another of William Haddon's significant contributions to the field of injury prevention was his development of a hierarchy of 10 countermeasure strategies to reduce the damage caused by

Table 11.2 Strategies to prevent dental injuries in community football based on an ecological model

Level of intervention	Intervention strategy
Intrapersonal	◆ Mass media campaign encouraging football players to wear mouth guards
	◆ Availability of mouth guards in club colours
	◆ Provision of vouchers to players for a free dental consultation
Interpersonal	◆ Information to parents about the benefits of children wearing mouth guards
	◆ Coaches encouraging players to wear mouth guards
	◆ Senior players in community clubs acting as role models
	◆ Dentists encouraging football playing patients to wear mouth guards
Institutional/ Organizational	◆ Club policy requiring all players to wear mouth guards
	◆ Club partnership with local dentist to provide mouth guards at reduced prices
	◆ Club subsidized mouth guards for members
Community	◆ Regional association policy requiring clubs to ensure players wear mouth guards
	◆ Football referees empowered to enforce mouth guard policy
	◆ Co-operation between local schools and clubs with educational campaign and joint mouth guard policy
	◆ Local government sponsored dental health expo including training for first aid personnel in emergency treatment of dental injuries and subsidized mouth guards for members of local football clubs
Public policy	◆ Advocacy by dental association to have government legislation mandating the wearing of mouth guards in all contact sports
	◆ Insurance industry initiative providing reduced priced mouth guards to all policy holders
	◆ National football league policy requiring all professional players to wear mouth guards and act as role models
	◆ Lobbying of health insurance industry to have costs of getting mouth guards covered by policies

energy exchange[38]. The first of Haddon's 10 strategies is to prevent the creation of the energy; the second is to reduce the amount of energy created; the third is to prevent the release of the energy; the fourth is to modify the rate of spatial distribution of the energy; the fifth is to separate in space or time, the energy that is release and the person likely to be injured; the sixth is to create a mechanical barrier between the energy and the person to be protected; the seventh is to modify the basic structure of the hazard; the eighth is to strengthen the person who is likely to be injured; the ninth is to rapidly detect and evaluate any injury and prevent its continuation; and the tenth is to stabilize, care for, and rehabilitate the injured person. An example of the application of these 10 countermeasure strategies to the prevention of sports injuries is provided in Table 11.3.

Haddon argued that the prevention of 'loss' or damage was the important factor in selecting the level of intervention but generally, the larger the amounts of energy involved the higher up the countermeasure levels the intervention should be located[38]. An example of this principle is when preventing injuries due to snow avalanches in alpine areas where, once an avalanche has started it is almost impossible to prevent the associated losses. Therefore, the only acceptable

Table 11.3 Application of Haddon's 10 countermeasure strategies to the prevention of sports injuries

Countermeasure strategy	Example of an injury-preventive measure
1. Prevent the creation of the energy in the first place	Prevent the accumulation of snow that could cause an avalanche
2. Reduce the amount of energy created	Limit the power of racing cars
3. Prevent the release of the energy	Fit safety-catches to cross-bows
4. Modify the rate of spatial distribution of the energy	Reduce the angle of ski-slopes
5. Separate in space or time, the energy that is release and the person likely to be damaged	Enforce minimum distances between basketball courts and spectators
6. Place a mechanical barrier between the energy and the person to be protected	Face masks in ice hockey
7. Modify the basic structure of the hazard	Use cardboard corner posts in rugby union
8. Strengthen the person who is likely to be injured	Training and conditioning for footballers
9. Rapidly detect and evaluate any injury and prevent its continuation	Installing global positioning devices in all open ocean sailing boats
10. Stabilize, care for, and rehabilitate the injured person	Anterior cruciate ligament repair

interventions would be at level 5 or higher. In contrast, the development of appropriate mechanical barriers (level 6) such as airbags and energy-absorbent crash barriers may be very effective in reducing motor-racing injuries. Haddon recommended a systematic analysis of the harmful exchange of energy to identify the most appropriate mix of strategies to ensure maximum loss reduction while taking into consideration the associated costs and feasibility of implementing the identified countermeasures[38].

The direction of the intervention process

Sports-injury preventive interventions can be classified as operating in one of two directions–'top-down' and 'bottom-up'[51, 52]. Top-down interventions are those where the injury issues are identified by an 'outside' agency (or self-selected community leader) which then proceeds to establish the goals of the intervention, allocate resources, implement countermeasures, and evaluate effectiveness based on quantifiable outcomes and reductions in risk factors. Although top-down interventions may engage community organizations to deliver preventive programmes, they run the risk of lacking community support and local leadership, and are therefore less likely to be sustainable over the longer term[53]. In contrast, bottom-up interventions address safety issues that are defined as important by the community that are experiencing them, in ways that the community identify as appropriate and are based on principles of empowerment and capacity building. The role of the 'outside' agency in bottom-up interventions is predominately to respond to the needs of the community and to work with the community to develop strategies to resolve the community-identified issues[51]. Bottom-up interventions have the advantage of involving a variety of community members and organization in injury-prevention efforts thereby increasing the likelihood of community ownership of the problem and the solution. However, there is always the potential for bottom-up interventions to be easily de-railed by powerful local vested interests or a lack of local experience and expertise in designing and implementing effective interventions[53].

In the context of the prevention of sports injuries, a top-down approach might involve the following steps:

1. Local health service uses epidemiological data to identify a problem that it believes needs to be addressed in the community (e.g. large number of sport-related head injuries)

2. Local health-promotion service develops a suite of evidence-based interventions to prevent identified injuries (e.g. compulsory wearing of protective equipment)

3. Local health-promotion service works with sporting organizations, facility-owners, local media, protective equipment manufactures, and retailers to implement selected interventions (e.g. develop policies and strategies to improve access to and reduce costs of protective equipment)

4. Local health-promotion service conducts intervention evaluation (e.g. how many participants are wearing appropriate protective equipment, changes in incidence of sport-related head injuries recorded at local hospital and health centres).

An example of top-down sports-injury prevention research is the study into the effectiveness of protective headgear in junior rugby union conducted by McIntosh and colleagues[54].

A bottom-up approach might involve the following steps:

1. Local health-promotion service facilitates the sporting community to identify safety issues that are important and relevant to the sporting community (e.g. provides data, needs assessment skills training)

2. Sporting-community and local health-promotion agency work together to negotiate the design and management of evidence-based and contextually relevant interventions to be implemented

3. Local health-promotion service works to build the capacity of sporting-community to implement intervention (e.g. resource mobilization, leadership, programme management)

4. Sporting-community implements intervention with support of local health-promotion service

5. Local health-promotion service facilitates sporting community to conduct intervention evaluation (e.g. finding out what the community wants to know about the intervention and helping them develop the skills needed).

An example of bottom-up sports-injury prevention research is the study by Abbott and colleagues investigating the impact of risk-management training for community sports administrators on the safety policies, practices, and organizational infrastructure of community sporting organizations[55].

These two 'directional' approaches to sports-injury-prevention interventions – top-down planning and service provision, and bottom-up community empowerment and capacity building – do not need to be mutually exclusive. Their respective strengths and weaknesses can be used to complement each other if applied simultaneously in parallel design tracks[52, 56].

Host–agent–environment relationship

When identifying or developing strategies to prevent sports injuries it may be helpful to think in terms of strategies that are targeted at the sports participant (the host), the sporting activity itself (the agent) or the environment (physical, sociocultural, etc.) in which the sporting activity take place[57]. This classification-system complements the concepts of the three-Es and the ecological model discussed earlier in this chapter. Most education or intra- and interpersonal strategies target the host, while engineering, enforcement, organizational, and community strategies target the agent and the environment.

Sports-injury preventive measures that target the host include those that are designed to change individual player attitudes, knowledge, and behaviours. Examples of these are strategies to: encourage the use of protective equipment; raise awareness about risks; improve fitness and conditioning; encourage fair play; and improve skills and techniques. Measures that target the agent generally aim to reduce the amount of kinetic energy that is created and how much of it is transferred. This is often achieved by modifying the rules of the sport such as the de-powering of scrums in rugby union and rugby league, the banning of running in Lifeball (a modified version of netball specifically for older adults)[58], and penalizing tackles from behind in soccer. Equipment modifications, such as changing the weight and size of baseballs, improving the energy-absorption qualities of personal protective equipment, and lowering the height of barriers (hurdles, jumps, etc.) are also examples of interventions targeting the agent. Sports-injury preventive measures which target changing the environment can be narrowly focussed on reducing immediate injury risks (e.g. removing hazards from the playing surface) or extremely broad with the aim of reducing more distal, long-term injury-risk factors (e.g. changing safety culture, reducing racism, improving nutrition). Environmental measures include policy- and standards-based interventions such as: improving playing surfaces; implementing heat and lightning policies; and setting safety standards for environmental structures (e.g. portable soccer goal post and basketball ring/backboard standards). Other measures designed to influence sociocultural environmental risk factors include: alcohol policies; Fair Play rules and awards; coaching and first-aid accreditation; and return to play guidelines.

As has been documented extensively elsewhere, Haddon's Matrix – based on the host–agent–environment relationship and the pre-event, event, and post-event time sequence – can be a very useful framework for brainstorming potential interventions to address identified sports-injury risk factors[14, 17, 21, 56, 59]. An example of using Haddon's Matrix to identify potential interventions for reducing cycling injuries is given in Table 11.4.

Runyan has suggested the addition of a third dimension to Haddon's Matrix to facilitate making decisions about which of the potential countermeasures to actually implement[60]. This additional dimension is based on applying policy-analysis principles to develop a set of value criteria to assess each potential countermeasure. The value criteria should be developed and weighted by the decision-makers taking the intervention context into consideration. Runyan suggests a set of seven value criteria as a starting point for injury-prevention planners including: effectiveness;

Table 11.4 Identification of potential interventions to reduce cycling injuries using Haddon's Matrix

Time sequence	Factor		
	Host (injured cyclist)	Agent/Vehicle/Vector (bicycle, racing rules, event procedures, etc.)	Environment (racing track)
Pre-event	Provide safety training to cyclists	Maintain bicycles to appropriate standards	Design racing circuit to reduce cornering speed
Event	Wear protective equipment	Design bicycles with appropriate safety features	Allow sufficient run-off space around the edge of the race track
Post-event	Perform cool-down	Employ safety marshals to reduce risks to riders if an accident occurs	Access to emergency services

cost; freedom; equity; stigmatization; preference of affected community or individuals; and feasibility (technical, political, and resources)[60]. Another value that might be considered specifically relevant to the context of identifying and developing sports-injury preventive measures is the impact of the proposed countermeasure on the nature of the sport (e.g. will changing a rule also change the fundamental nature of the activity?). Both qualitative and quantitative information can be used to assess each countermeasure against the agreed value criteria although the type, amount, and quality of 'evidence' available to inform decision making will vary depending on the specific value criteria and countermeasure being considered. There are also inherent difficulties in comparing new and existing countermeasures and in considering options that span different settings (e.g. schools, community sport) and jurisdictions (local, national, international)[60]. When using the extended, three-dimensional Haddon's Matrix, Runyan recommends a 12-step process starting with using appropriate data to identify and understand the injury problem; then defining the three dimensions of the matrix; determining and weighting the relative importance of the values that will inform decision making; brainstorming to generate a list of potential countermeasures; gathering and using evidence and information to assess each countermeasure option; making decisions on countermeasures to implement; explaining the decision; and documenting the decision-making process[60].

Conclusion

This chapter has outlined a 5-step strategic approach to developing sports-injury preventive measures that are evidence and theory or first principle based. It is vital that researchers have a very good understanding of the injury aetiology and risk factors, and the context in which an intervention is to be implemented, before starting to think about identifying or developing interventions. Without this understanding it is unlikely that effective interventions that can actually be sustainably implemented will be identified or developed.

Building on the work of others is an excellent way to start the process of identifying and developing injury-prevention measures. By searching the published literature and communicating with other interested and influential stakeholders, researchers can identify what has worked to prevent injuries in other sports, in other contexts. However, applying interventions that have been demonstrated to be effective in other contexts is not straightforward. Careful consideration needs to be given to the quantity and quality of the evidence of effectiveness and the specific details of the intervention and the implementation context.

There are several well-established, systematic, and scientifically based injury-prevention and health-promotion frameworks that researchers can use to guide the process of identifying and developing sports-injury preventive measures. These frameworks encourage sports-injury preventive researchers to: think carefully about where in the injury 'chain' they should look to intervene; take a multi-strategic, multi-disciplinary approach; and to identify individual, organizational, and environmental opportunities for intervention.

References

1. Rivara FP (2003). Introduction: The scientific basis of injury control. *Epidemiol Rev*, **25**, 20–3.
2. van Mechelen W, Hlobil H, Kemper HC (1992). Incidence, severity, aetiology and prevention of sports injuries. A review of concepts. *Sports Med*, **4**(2), 82–99.
3. Meeuwisse WH (1994). Assessing causation in sport injury: a multifactorial model. *Clin J Sport Med*, **4**, 166–70.
4. Bahr R, Holme I (2003). Risk factors for sports injuries—a methodological approach. *Br J Sports Med*, **37**, 384–92.

5. Nichols AW (2008). Sports medicine clinical trial research publications in academic medical journals. *Br J Sports Med*, **42**, 909–12.

6. Chalmers D (2002). Injury prevention in sport: not yet part of the game. *Inj Prev*, **8**(suppl IV), iv22–iv25.

7. Aaltonen S, Karjalainen H, Heinonen A, Parkkari J, Kujala U (2007). Prevention of sports injuries: systematic review of randomized controlled trials. *Arch Intern Med*, **167**(15), 1585–92.

8. Junge A, Dvorak J (2004). Soccer injuries: a review of incidence and prevention. *Sports Med*, **34**(13), 929–38.

9. Fradkin A, Gabbe B, Cameron P (2006). Does warming up prevent injury in sport? The evidence from randomised controlled trials? *J Sci Med Sport*, **9**(3), 214–20.

10. Abernethy L, Bleakley C (2007). Strategies to prevent injury in adolescent sport: a systematic review. *Br J Sports Med*, **41**, 627–38.

11. Hawe P, Shiell A, Riley T, Gold L (2004). Methods for exploring implementation variation and local context within a cluster randomised community intervention trial. *J Epidemiol Commun H*, **58**, 788–93.

12. Shiell A (2000). *Deciding and specifying an intervention portfolio [planning framework—user guide]. National Public Health Partnership.* Available at http://www.nphp.gov.au/publications/phpractice/intervpf.pdf (accessed 10 February 2009).

13. Standards Australia (2004). *Guidelines for managing risk in sport and recreation HB 246–2004.* Available at http://www.saiglobal.com/shop/script/Result.asp?DegnKeyword=sport±and±recreation&Db=AS&SearchType=publisheronly&Status=all&Max=15&Search=Proceed (accessed 10 February 2009).

14. Runyan CW, Freire KE (2006). Developing interventions when there is little science, in Doll LS, Bonzo SE, Sleet DA, Mercy JA, Haas EN (eds) *Handbook of injury and violence prevention*, pp. 411–31. Springer, New York.

15. Gielen AC, Sleet D (2003). Application of behaviour-change theories and methods to injury prevention. *Epidemiol Rev*, **25**, 65–76.

16. Victorian Government Department of Human Services (2003). *Integrated health promotion resource kit.* Available at http://www.health.vic.gov.au/healthpromotion/downloads/integrated_health_promo.pdf (accessed 8 January 2009).

17. Freire K, Runyan C (2006). Planning models: PRECEDE-PROCEDE and Haddon matrix, in Gielen AC, Sleet DA, DiCelemente RJ (eds) *Injury and violence prevention: Behavioral science theories, methods, and applications*, pp. 127–58. Jossey-Bass, San Francisco.

18. Twomey D, Finch C, Roediger E, Lloyd D (2008). Preventing lower limb injuries—is the latest evidence being translated into the football field? *J Sci & Med Sport*, doi:10.1016/j.jsams.2008.04.002.

19. Finch CF, McIntosh AS, McCrory P, Zazryn T (2003). A pilot study of the attitudes of Australian Rules footballers towards protective headgear. *J Sci Med Sport*, **6**(4), 505–11.

20. Runyan CW (2003). Introduction: Back to the future—Revisiting Haddon's conceptualization of injury epidemiology and prevention. *Epidemiol Rev*, **25**, 60–4.

21. Stevenson M, Ameratunga S, McClure R (2004). The rationale for prevention, in McClure R, Stevenson M, McEvoy S (eds) *The scientific basis of injury prevention and control*, pp. 34–43. IP Communications Pty Ltd, Hawthorn East.

22. Martin JB, Green W, Gielen AC (2007). Potential lessons from public health and health promotion for the prevention of child abuse. *J Prev & Interven Comm*, **34**(1/2), 205–22.

23. Finch C (2006). A new framework for research leading to sports injury prevention. *J Sci Med Sport*, **9**(1–2), 3–9.

24. Van Tiggelen D, Wickes S, Stevens V, Roosen P, Witvrouw E (2008). Effective prevention of sports injuries: a model integrating efficacy, efficiency, compliance and risk taking behaviour. *Br J Sports Med*, **42**, 648–52.

25. Emery CA, Hagel B, Morrongiello BA (2006). Injury prevention in child and adolescent sport: whose responsibility is it? *Clin J Sport Med*, **16**(6), 514–21.

26. Rychetnik L, Frommer M, Hawe P, Shiell A (2002). Criteria for evaluating evidence on public health interventions. *J Epidemiol Commun H*, **56**, 119–27.

27. Peek-Asa CL, Mallonee S (2006). Interpreting evidence of effectiveness: How do you know when a prevention approach will work in your community?, in Doll LS, Bonzo SE, Sleet DA, Mercy JA, Haas EN (eds) *Handbook of injury and violence prevention*, pp. 383–415. Springer, New York.

28. Haddon W (1968). The changing approach to the epidemiology, prevention and amelioration of trauma: the transition to approaches etiologically rather then descriptively based. *Am J Public Health*, **58**(8), 1431–8.

29. Haddon W (1972). A logical framework for categorizing highway safety phenomena and activity. *J Traum*, **12**, 193–207.

30. Gibson JJ (1961). The contribution of experimental psychology to the formulation of the problem of safety—a brief for basic research, in Jacobs HH (ed) *Behaviour approaches to accident research*, pp. 77–89. New York Association for the Aid of Crippled Children, New York. Cited in Andersson R, Menckel E (1995). On the prevention of accidents and injuries: a comparative analysis of conceptual frameworks. *Accident Anal Prev*, 27(6), 757–68.

31. Gordon JE (1949). The epidemiology of accidents. *Am J Public Health*, April, 504–15.

32. Andersson R, Menckel E (1995). On the prevention of accidents and injuries: a comparative analysis of conceptual frameworks. *Accident Anal Prev*, **27**(6), 757–68.

33. Baker SP (1972). Injury control, accident prevention and other approaches to reduction of injury. In Sartwell PD (ed). *Prevention medicine and public health*. 10th edn. Appleton-Century-Crofts, New York. Cited in Pearn J, Nixon J, Scott I (2004). An historical perspective, in McClure R, Stevenson M, McEvoy S (eds) *The scientific basis of injury prevention and control*, pp. 5–17. IP Communications Pty Ltd, Hawthorn East.

34. Haddon W (1974). Strategy in preventive medicine: passive vs active approaches to reducing human wastage. *J Traum*, **14**(4), 353–4.

35. Bronfenbrenner U (1979). *The ecology of human development*. Harvard University Press, Cambridge, MA.

36. McLeroy KR, Bibeau D, Steckler A, Glanz K (1988). An ecological perspective on health promotion programs. *Health Educ Quart*, **15**(4), 351–77.

37. Hanson D, Hanson J, Vardon P, et al. (2005). The injury iceberg; an ecological approach to planning sustainable community safety interventions. *Health Promo J Aus*, **16**, 5–10.

38. Haddon W (1973). Energy damage and the ten countermeasure strategies. *J Traum*, **13**(4), 321–31.

39. Fédération Internationale de Football Association (FIFA). The 11. Available at http://www.fifa.com/aboutfifa/developing/medical/the11/index.html, accessed 5 March).

40. NSW Sport and Recreation (2006). *Stamp out sport rage—tips for coaches*. Available at http://www.dsr.nsw.gov.au/sportrage/ (accessed 17 January 2009).

41. Gianotti S, Hume PA, Tunstall H (2008). Efficacy of injury prevention related coach education within netball and soccer. *J Sci Med Sport*, doi:10.1016/j.jsams.2008.07.010.

42. Janda DH, Bir C, Kedroske BA (2001). Comparison of standard vs. breakaway bases: an analysis of a preventative intervention for softball and baseball foot and ankle injuries. *Foot Ankle Int*, **22**(10), 810–16.

43. Levy ML, Ozgur B, Berry C, Aryan HE, Apuzzo MLJ (2004). Birth and evolution of the football helmet. *Neurosurgery*, **55**(3), 656–62.

44. Martin JB, Green W, Gielen AC (2007). Potential lessons from public health and health promotion for the prevention of child abuse. *J Preven & Interven Com*, **34**(1/2), 205–22.

45. Quarrie KL, Cantu RC, Chalmers DJ (2002). Rugby union injuries to the cervical spine and spinal cord. *Sports Med*, **32**(10), 633–53.

46. Carmody DJ, Taylor TKF, Parker DA, Coolican MRJ, Cumming RG (2005). Spinal cord injuries in Australian footballers 1997–2002. *Med J Australia*, **182**, 561–4.

47. Peek-Asa C, Zwerling C (2003). Role of environmental interventions in injury control and prevention. *Epidemiol Rev*, **25**, 77–89.

48. Doll LS, Saul JR, Elder RW (2006). Injury and violence prevention interventions: an overview, in Doll LS, Bonzo SE, Sleet DA, Mercy JA, Haas EN (eds). *Handbook of injury and violence prevention*, pp. 21–32. Springer, New York.

49. Eime R, Owen N, Finch C (2004). Protective eyewear promotion: applying principles of behaviour change in the design of a squash injury prevention programme. *Sports Med*, **34**(10), 629–38.

50. Nation M, Crusto C, Wandersman A, et al. (2003). What works in prevention: principles of effective prevention programs. *Am Psychol*, **58**(6/7), 449–56.

51. Welander G, Svanström L Ekman R (2004). *Safety Promotion—an Introduction. (2*nd Ed)*. Karolinska Institute. Department Of Public Health Sciences, Division of Social Medicine. Stockholm. Available at http://www.phs.ki.se/csp/pdf/Books/Safety%20Promotion%20an%20Introduction%202004%20 Book%20incl%20pictures.pdf (accessed 10 February 2009).

52. Laverack G, Labonte R (2000). A planning framework for community empowerment goals within health promotion. *Health Policy Plann*, **15**(3), 255–62.

53. Treno AJ, Holder HD (1997). Community mobilization: evaluation of an environmental approach to local action. *Addiction*, **92**(Supplement 2), S173–S87.

54. McIntosh AS, McCrory P, Finch CF, Chalmers DJ, Best JP (2003). Rugby headgear study. *J Sci Med Sport*, **6**(1), 355–8.

55. Abbott K, Klarenaar P, Donaldson A, Sherker S (2008). Evaluating SafeClub: can risk management training improve safety activities of community soccer clubs? *Br J Sports Med*, **42**, 460–5.

56. Timpka T, Ekstrand J Svanstrom L (2006). From sports injury prevention to safety promotion in Sports. *Sports Med*, **36**(9), 733–45.

57. Gilchrist J, Saluja G, Marshall S (2006). Interventions to prevent sports and recreation-related injuries, in Doll LS, Bonzo SE, Sleet DA, Mercy JA, Haas EN (eds) *Handbook of injury and violence prevention*, pp. 117–34. Springer, New York.

58. Barnett L, Green S, van Beurden E, Campbell E, Radvan D (2009). Older people playing ball: what is the risk of falling and injury? *J Sci Med Sport*, **12**(1), 177–83.

59. Lett R, Kobusingye O, Sethi D (2002). A unified framework for injury control: the public health approach and Haddon's Matrix combined. *Injury Control and Safety Promotion*, **9**(3), 199–205.

60. Runyan CW (1998). Using the Haddon matrix: introducing the third dimension. *Inj Prev*, **4**, 302–7.

Chapter 12

The behavioural approach

Dorine Collard, Amika Singh, and Evert Verhagen

A crucial part of sports-injury prevention is understanding the injury risks and mechanisms of injury. As described in Chapter 8, a sports injury is the result of a complex interaction between internal risk factors, external risk factors, and an inciting event (mechanism of injury). Such factors are usually described biomechanical, biomedical, or physiological sense. However, whereas detailed descriptions of risk factors and mechanisms of injury may lead to potential efficacious preventive measures, this does not guarantee such measures are actually being used by the population[1]. Thus, when considering the real-life prevention of injuries one is actually talking about behavioural change. Accordingly, when establishing preventive measures one can take a more behavioural approach. One method to develop preventive measures that takes both behavioural and environmental determinants into account is the Intervention Mapping (IM) protocol[2]. IM captures the process of the development of a health-promotion programme in a series of six consecutive steps. IM maps the path from recognition of a need or problem to the identification of a behavioural solution, including the evaluation of this solution. The strength of IM lies therein that the end-users and others involved with the intervention programme are part of the developmental process. While originally designed for health-promotion programmes, the IM protocol can easily be used for injury-prevention programmes as well.

Following the IM protocol, before a start is made with the actual development of the intervention programme, the health problem needs to be assessed. This assessment should include related behaviours, environmental conditions, and their associated determinants for the at-risk populations. This initial problem-definition encompasses two components: (i) a scientific, epidemiological, behavioural, and social perspective of an at-risk group or community and its problems; and (ii) an effort to 'get to know' or begin to understand, the character of the community, its members, and its strengths. This starting point is more than a description of a health problem as commonly applied in sports medicine research; i.e. ankle sprains are the most common injuries. It is a description of a health problem, its impact on quality of life, behavioural and environmental causes, and determinants of behaviour and environmental causes. If a health or injury problem is approached in this way, in a sense the resulting intervention programme is built around the acting behaviours.

The practical use of the IM protocol and the choices that are made in practice can best be described trough a detailed example from within the field of sports-injury prevention. Therefore, the concept of IM is illustrated using the developmental process of a preventive programme targeted at the prevention of injuries in 10–12-year-old children through physical education classes. This programme has recently been evaluated in a cluster-randomized controlled trial[3]. This illustration might seem extensive in relation to the presented IM theory.

Intervention mapping: the theory

IM has been used to develop intervention programmes for various health problems, like nutrition, obesity prevention, sun protection, or human immunodeficiency virus (HIV) infection prevention. IM is based on the importance of planning interventions that are based on both theory and evidence, taking into account the social and physical environment that contributes to the health problem. Applying the IM protocol one is able to create programmes that are feasible and, most important, have a high likelihood of being effective.

The IM protocol consists of six steps (Table 12.1). The completion of the tasks within a step creates a product that is the guide for the subsequent step and results in a blueprint for the design, implementation, and evaluation of an intervention. Even though the application of the IM protocol is presented as a series of steps, the process is iterative rather than completely linear. One might move back and forth between the different steps as information that is obtained in a present step might inform and add information to previous steps.

Needs assessment

Assessing the health problem among the target population is the beginning of IM. In this step the health problem and its causes are analysed, and the priorities of the intervention are determined. During the Needs Assessment one answers the following questions: 'What is the health problem?' 'What is the target population?' 'What are the incidence and prevalence of the health problem?', 'Is there a subgroup of the population that has an excess burden from the health problem?', and finally 'In which setting can the population at risk be reached?'.

The Needs Assessment starts with the establishment of a planning group that includes potential programme participants. Their job is to plan the Needs Assessment and they need to investigate what is already known of the health problem and the target population and what further information is required. Second, using the PRECEDE–PROCEED model, the health problem and its causes are analysed[4]. This requires both primary and secondary data collection. Primary data refers to data obtained from surveys and interviews among participants of the target population, intermediaries, or stakeholders. Sources of primary data come in a wide variety, including questionnaires, telephone surveys, focus group interviews, etc. Secondary data are an important source to answer questions on the magnitude of the health problem. Useful secondary data can be obtained from e.g. health, governmental, and educational agencies. Hereafter, one needs to assess the strengths and capacities of the setting in which the intervention will take place. Proper insight into this setting leads to an optimized fit of the intervention to the intervention setting. Finally, the Needs Assessment is linked to the evaluation plan, by establishing the desired programme outcomes ('What will change as a result of the intervention?') – i.e. the overall programme objective.

Exemplary intervention

In the Netherlands 1.8 million injuries are reported through emergency departments each year. Sports are the main cause of these injuries. Sports-injury incidence in youth is much higher than in the adult population, and especially adolescents (12–16 years) were found to be at a high risk of injury[5]. Although there are a large number of children that participate in organized team sports, an increasing number of children is attracted to unorganized sports activities and individual sports[6]. Literature shows that most sports injuries occur during unorganized sports activities and leisure time, and that most commonly affect the lower extremities[7–9]. For this reason, activities aiming at preventing physical activity injuries in youth should focus not

Table 12.1 The six steps of the IM protocol

Step 1 Needs Assessment	◆ Plan needs assessment with PRECEDE model
	◆ Assess quality of life, behaviour, and environment
	◆ Assess capacity
	◆ Establish programme outcomes
Step 2 Matrices	◆ State expected changes in behaviour and environment
	◆ Specify performance objectives
	◆ Specify determinants
	◆ Create matrices of change objectives
Step 3 Theory-based Methods and Practical Strategies	◆ Review programme ideas with interested participants
	◆ Identify theoretical methods
	◆ Choose programme methods
	◆ Select or design strategies
	◆ Ensure that strategies match change objectives
Step 4 Programme	◆ Consult with interested participants and implementers
	◆ Create programme scope, sequence, theme, and list of materials
	◆ Develop design documents and protocols
	◆ Review available materials
	◆ Develop programme materials
	◆ Pre-test programme materials with target groups and implementers, and oversee materials production
Step 5 Adaptation and Implementation plan	◆ Identify adopters and users
	◆ Specify adoption, implementation, and sustainability performance objectives
	◆ Specify determinants and create matrix
	◆ Select methods and strategies
	◆ Design interventions to affect programme use
Step 6 Evaluation plan	◆ Describe the programme
	◆ Describe programme outcomes and effect questions
	◆ Write questions based on matrix
	◆ Write process questions
	◆ Develop indicators and measures
	◆ Specify evaluation design

exclusively on sports clubs, sports organizations, and sport federations. Since physical education (PE) classes are mandatory in Dutch schools, PE classes in secondary schools were deemed important settings for preventive activities within this age group of adolescents.

The programme objectives that are defined in step 1 come from a so-called 'needs assessment'. In this specific case, the needs assessment intended to detect and register the risk factors (different kinds of behaviours) of lower-extremity injuries in adolescents in the age range of 12–15 years. However, the target population of the study was changed to primary school children aged 10–12 years after focus-group interviews with PE teachers from secondary schools. The reason for this shift in focus will be explained in the following paragraphs.

In order to gain insight into the needs of this target population and to be able to design a feasible intervention programme focus-group interviews were held among secondary schoolteachers. There was general agreement among the interviewed PE teachers that there is a great diversity in physical fitness and motor control between 12- and 13-year-old children in the first grade of secondary schools, i.e. children moving from primary schools to secondary schools. The common opinion was that these inter-individual differences are an important contributing factor to injuries in the age group of 12–15 years. Although this common opinion cannot be supported by scientific literature, it showed that PE teachers were hesitant and not motivated to incorporate preventive measures in their PE classes while the problem of injuries in the target age group comes from a younger age. Furthermore, interviewed PE teachers responded that they already incorporate injury prevention in their regular PE classes since they had been thought to do so – another sign that low compliance can be expected from secondary school PE teachers when including an injury-prevention programme in their regular PE classes.

When the interviewed PE teachers were asked about the causes of the noted inter-individual differences and concerning possible solutions, it was argued by then that the proposed project should focus on primary schools. In primary schools, children receive regular PE classes for the first time. This first contact with regular PE is not always led by certified PE teachers, but is more often guided by the child's regular teacher due to economical reasons. Therefore, a preventive intervention in this setting will most likely achieve greater short-term results. Since PE classes in secondary schools are focussed on more sport-specific skills, and thus on more sport-specific injury prevention, it was postulated that a shift to primary schools would also achieve a greater long-term health gain.

Preparation of matrices of change objectives

Preparing the matrices of change objectives will provide the basis for the intervention by specifying who and what will change as a result of the intervention. Therefore, one needs to determine both the performance objectives at the individual level and those of the environmental agents.

As a start, one needs to identify the health-related behaviours in the target population. Examples of health-related behaviours are risk-reduction behaviours (e.g. the wearing of braces to prevent ankle sprains), health-promotion behaviours (e.g. the incorporation of specific preventive warm-up exercises by a coach), or self-management behaviours (e.g. the compliance to a home-based exercise programme). Additionally, changes in environmental conditions that are required to reach the overall programme objective need to be taken into account. The second task is to define the programmes' behavioural and environmental outcomes and to translate each of them into performance objectives. Performance objectives for behavioural outcomes answer the question; 'What does a member of the target population need to do to perform the health-related behaviour?' Performance objectives for environmental outcomes answer the question; 'What does someone need to do in order to accomplish the environmental outcome?' Once performance objectives are described, the most important and changeable determinants of the health-behaviour and environmental conditions can be selected. This selection should be based on the evidence from literature research. If there is no literature source to provide adequate information, one needs to consider data collection from the target population or other parties involved in the intervention. Finally, a first set of matrices can be created. At this stage one needs to define the different intervention levels and eventually subdivide the target population. The latter might be the case if subgroups of the target population differ substantially with regards to the performance objectives or determinants.

Table 12.2 Performance objectives and subsequent change objectives for the exemplary intervention programme

	Change objectives		
	Children will take fewer injury related risks	**Parents will create a safe environment outside PE classes**	**PE teachers will include injury prevention into their usual teaching routine**
Performance objective 1	Children learn the consequences of an injury	Parents learn the consequences of an injury	PE * teachers learn the consequences of an injury
Performance objective 2	Children learn which risk factors cause injuries	Parents learn which risk factors cause injuries	PE * teachers learn which risk factors cause injuries
Performance objective 3	Children gain insight into his/her own injury risk behaviour	Parents gain insight into the injury risks during the child's leisure-time physical activities	PE * teachers gain insight into the pupils' risk behaviour
Performance objective 4	Children form strategies to reduce his/her injury risk.	Parents form strategies to reduce the injury-risk during the child's leisure-time physical activities	PE * teachers form strategies to reduce the pupils' risk behaviour
Performance objective 5		Parents gain insight into the child's risk behaviour	
Performance objective 6		Parents form strategies to reduce the child's risk behaviour	

Exemplary intervention

In order to achieve the overall programme objective (prevention of lower-extremity injuries in 10–12-year-old children), several behavioural and environmental change objectives were defined that focussed on children, parents. and PE teachers. The underlying assumption of the risk-reducing behavioural change objectives was that, if an intervention reduces the risk factors it will reduce the incidence of sports injuries. Furthermore, the presence of support from important others, e.g. parents and teachers within the child's immediate interpersonal environment, may influence the performance of the injury-preventing behaviour[2].

The change objectives postulated for the preventive programme were (1) children take fewer injury-related risks; (2) parents create a safe physical activity environment for their children outside the PE classes; (3) teachers include injury prevention into their usual teaching routine. The performance objectives that accompany these change objectives are depicted in Table 12.2.

Selection of theory-based intervention methods and practical strategies

In this step, one moves from the stated change objectives to theoretical methods and practical strategies. A theoretical method is a general technique for influencing changes in the determinants of behaviour (or environmental conditions), whereas a practical strategy is a specific technique for the application of theoretical methods.

When developing an intervention programme, most commonly one commences with an idea of the look and feel of an intervention. Such ideas are driven by personal taste of the intervention-developer.

However, it is important to review the programme ideas with the intended target population and to keep their perspective in mind while selecting methods and translating methods into strategies. To do so, a linkage group consisting of both members of the target population and possible implementers of the intervention should be established. This linkage group may be derived from the planning group used at the Needs Assessment. In conjunction with this linkage group adequate theoretical methods influencing the determinants that need to be changed are identified and selected. This is done based on literature research and reviewing theories of change. During a creative process, the selected methods are then translated into practical strategies. Finally, it must be assured that the chosen strategies still match the change objectives that were determined in Step 2.

Exemplary intervention

Within the exemplary intervention the ASE (Attitude–Social influence–self-Efficacy) model was applied as a theory for behavioural change[10, 11]. The ASE-model is based on the theory of planned behaviour[12] and the social learning theory[13]. This model postulates that intention, the most proximal determinant of behaviour, is determined by three conceptually independent constructs – namely attitude, social influence, and self-efficacy. To change injury-preventive behaviour, one needs to improve attitude, social influence, self-efficacy, and intention. Although, increasing knowledge on injury prevention in children will not lead directly to behavioural change, knowledge is a basis for many different determinants of behaviour.

In the exemplary intervention programme the methods used included modelling, active learning, persuasive communication, and active processing of information. Strategies that were used for these methods included informative newsletters, awareness exercises, personal risk appraisal, posters with main information about injury prevention, and an interactive website. These programme ideas were reviewed by the intended target population and end-users. Teachers and children were informed on the programme ideas and look and feel of the intervention. Both teachers and children were positive about the programme ideas and believed that the programme would be feasible and effective. Teachers noticed that the programme should be easy to implement and time-efficient, otherwise the compliance with the programme would be very low.

Production of intervention components and materials

The programme intentions need to be translated into intervention materials. This step includes production, pre-testing, and eventually revision of these materials. The goal is that these materials are both creative and effective pieces of the intervention.

First, the target population and the end-users should be consulted with regards to their preferences for programme design. In focus-groups the experiences, associations, assumptions, etc. regarding the programme objective and performance objectives need to be explored. At this stage, one needs to consult potential implementers about barriers, promising strategies, and the setting in which the intervention might be implemented. This will help to answer the question 'What does adequate implementation require?' With information thus obtained, the scope and sequence of the programme can be created, as well as a theme of the intervention and a list of intervention materials. When developing a programme one must also decide on the intervention messages and how they are delivered. To determine this, one can to answer questions like 'What amount of time does the average person of the target group spend with certain media (television, reading newspaper and magazines, using mobile phones, etc.)?' and 'What preferences does the target population have to get information about the intervention topic?' Based on this information the production of the intervention materials can be prepared. If the budget allows for it, professionals can be hired for the development of the intervention materials (e.g. graphic designers, computer programmers, photographers). Finally, when the intervention materials are developed they need to be pre-tested. For the pre-testing it is important to select participants that have not been involved in the development of the programme.

Exemplary intervention

The exemplary preventive programme had to be a simple and ready-to-use programme that was to be implemented during one school year. The programme was not targeted at any specific type of sport and focussed on preventive measures in general in eight monthly modules.

Monthly newsletters were produced, both for children and parents. The newsletters aimed to increase knowledge and awareness about injury prevention. The monthly newsletters consisted of information about injury prevention, self-evaluation tests, and puzzles. By providing a monthly newsletter, new knowledge was imparted each month in a motivational way. Eight different posters accompanied the newsletters by highlighting the month's key messages. Posters were continuously displayed in the classroom in order to have maximum exposure.

Parallel to these eight monthly modules the course programme included a continuous exercise programme. This exercise programme consisted of exercises to be carried out during each PE class aimed at improving physical fitness (i.e. aerobic fitness, strength, speed, agility, flexibility) and co-ordination.

The intervention programme was accompanied by an interactive website containing general information on injury prevention for children, parents, and teachers. Children, parents, and teachers were able to view the newsletters online, and various instruction videos and photos were displayed to clarify for PE teachers how to teach the exercises. A teacher's manual contained all information about the intervention programme, including time schedule, explanation of the exercises, and topics of the newsletters.

The teachers who reviewed the programme ideas in step 3 of the IM protocol were asked for their comments on the programme components and materials. With the exception of some minor comments, teachers were satisfied with the programme components and materials. The exercises to improve motor fitness were pre-tested in two primary schools, involving three PE teachers. Teachers were asked specifically for their comments on the feasibility, intensity, and difficulty of the exercises and the clarity of the teachers' manual. Some exercises were perceived as being too difficult or too time consuming. Additionally, the teachers advised to deliver the exercises in a more competitive and playful way. Exercises were adapted as suggested by the PE teachers.

Adoption, implementation, and sustainability of the intervention

In step 5 of the IM protocol adoption and implementation performance objectives are formulated. In fact, in this step the procedures of step 2 are repeated, but now performance objectives result in change objectives that promote programme adoption and use. If effective preventive programmes are not adopted and sustained, they have no public health impact. Health-promotion frameworks that evaluate the public health impact of interventions could help to understand the implementation context. The RE-AIM Sports Setting Matrix is such a health-promotion framework and is specific to the community sports-setting-implementation context and could be used to guide the delivery of future sports-safety intervention[14] (also see Chapter 16).

The first task of this step aims to identify potential adopters and end-users of the intervention programme. Performance objectives for programme adoption and implementation are specified and, comparable to the health behaviours in step 2, one needs to identify the performance objectives of the end-users of the programme. The methods used for these tasks are the same as for step 2. Then matrices are created, in which the performance objectives and determinants for the adoption and implantation are linked. This results in the formulation of change objectives. The fourth task consists of the selection of adequate methods and strategies to address the objectives of change, applying the same methods as in step 2 (i.e. review relevant research and practical literature, additional data collection among potential adopters and implementers). Finally, an adoption and implementation plan is created. This is similar to the programme protocol designed in step 4, and includes the scope and sequence of activities, as well as staffing and budget issues.

Exemplary study

The exemplary intervention programme was designed to be a 'ready-to-use' programme. Therefore, it could be implemented directly in PE classes in primary schools. To ensure broad adoption and implementation of the programme, The Royal Association of Teachers of Physical Education (KVLO) and the Academy for Physical Education Teachers Education (ALO) were involved during the development of the intervention.

The performance objectives for the teachers were: (i) become aware of the availability of our sports injury prevention programme; (ii) adopt the programme into the usual teaching routine; and (iii) use the programme according to the developmental team's guidelines. By using the IM protocol in the development of the programme, the intervention was already tailored to the needs and wants of the PE teachers. By doing so, the practical and logistical issues of implementation were minimized. More importantly, teachers considered the aim of the intervention as useful and important. Other facilitating factors were ease of implementation, confidence in the ability to implement the programme, and the perception that both children and parents would appreciate the programme.

Generation of an evaluation plan

In the final step of the IM protocol an evaluation plan is developed. Basically, this final step consists of designing the actual effectiveness study that determines whether the preventive programme affects the outcome of interest (e.g. injury incidence). Keep in mind that when attempting to prevent injury through behavioural change, short-term effects of the intervention are likely to be changes in determinants (e.g. awareness, knowledge, self-efficacy) and that changes with regards to the actual health outcome may only be established on the long term.

The subsequent tasks within this final IM step lead up to the design of an evaluation study. One commences with formulating evaluation questions for the primary outcome measure, i.e. the health outcome ('What are the effects of the intervention on the health outcome?'). Second, evaluation questions are formulated based on the matrix of change objectives. These are often are considered mediators and moderators of the intended intervention effect (e.g. increasing awareness, knowledge, or self-efficacy as a required change objective for changes in a performance objective). Once evaluation questions are formulated, measurement instruments that provide the required outcome measures need to be selected. Health outcomes often can be measured objectively, e.g. weight or blood pressure. However, when evaluating changes in behavioural determinants or outcomes one is often restricted to methods of self-report. Ultimately, the study design can be finalized, an evaluation plan can be written and the developed intervention programme can be evaluated in an effect study.

Exemplary intervention

In short the primary research questions accompanying the exemplary intervention programme were 'What is the effect of the intervention programme on sports and physical activity injury incidence density and severity?' and 'What is the cost-effectiveness of this programme?' Due to the multifaceted nature of the intervention programme it was decided to incorporate a secondary research question on the programme's effect on knowledge, (determinants of) injury-preventing behaviour and motor fitness? The design of this particular study is described in full detail elsewhere[3].

In short, 40 primary schools (2210 children) participated in the study. Schools were randomly allocated to the intervention or control group, making the evaluation a cluster-randomized controlled trial. Throughout the school-year, the PE teacher recorded sports and PA injuries on a weekly basis. In case of an injury, the child completed an injury-registration form with the support of the teacher. The injury-registration form collected information on injury type, injury location, direct cause of the injury, and activity performed at time of injury. To determine time at risk for sports injuries, all children completed information on exposure time at baseline and follow-up. In order to evaluate the cost-effectiveness of the programme, parents of injured children received a cost-diary. The cost-diary registered all direct and indirect costs resulting from the sustained injury.

For the secondary outcome measures, children completed a questionnaire on knowledge and (determinants of) behaviour at baseline and follow-up. Knowledge about injury prevention was measured through nine multiple-choice questions on injury prevention in general. Behavioural determinants were assessed through the constructs' attitude, social influence, self-efficacy, and intention. Injury-preventing behaviour was defined as wearing appropriate protective equipment and footwear during PE classes, sports, and other physical activities. Finally, motor fitness was assessed with a fitness test. Supervised by a research assistant, groups of 3–4 children performed eight test items: i.e. bent-arm hang, 10 times 5-m run, plate tapping, leg lift, sit and reach, arm pull, standing high jump, and flamingo balance test. From this test, an overall score for motor fitness was derived.

Conclusion

In contemporary sports medicine, bluntly put, an injury risk factor is established and one studies what happens to the injury risk when the risk factor is reduced or expelled from sports. Due to the controlled nature of such studies the results of this approach can rarely be generalized to an actual sports setting, and are seldom adopted by a sports population. A better understanding of different acting behaviours and their relationship with injury risk is needed to truly be able to translate current knowledge to real-life injury prevention.

One should be aware that studies on real-life injury prevention still rely heavily on preventive measures that are established through biomedical and/or biomechanical research. A serious limitation in such an approach is that one expects that proven preventive measures can be adopted if the determinants and influences of sports-safety behaviours are understood. It is known from studies on lifestyle interventions that altering an individual's behaviour is the most difficult, if not impossible, task there is. One very promising method in constructing acceptable and evidence-based intervention programmes is the discussed IM protocol. IM maps the path from recognition of a need or problem to the identification of a behavioural solution. The strength of IM lies therein that the end-users and others involved with the intervention program are part of the developmental process. If a health or injury problem is approached in this way potential efficacious and truly effective intervention programmes can be developed.

References

1. Bahr R, Krosshaug T (2005). Understanding injury mechanisms: a key component of preventing injuries in sport. *Br J Sports Med*, **39**(6), 324–9.
2. Bartholomew LK, Parcel GS, Kok G, Gottlieb N (2006). *Planning health promotion programs, an intervention mapping approach*. Jossey-Bass.
3. DC Collard, M Chin A Paw, W van Mechelen, EALM Verhagen (2009). Primary school-based prevention of lower extremity PA injuries: Program development and study design of a randomized controlled trial. *Sports Med*, **39**(11), 1–13.
4. Green LW, Kreuter MW (2005). *Health program planning: An educational and ecological approach. 4 ed.* McGraw-Hill, New York.
5. Hildebrandt VH, Ooijendijk WTM, Hopman-Rock M (2007). *Trendrapport: bewegen en gezondheid 2004–2005*. TNO Kwaliteit van Leven, Leiden.
6. SCP (2003). *Rapportage Jeugd 2002*. Sociaal en Cultureel Planbureau, Den Haag.
7. Kahl H, Dortschy R, Ellsasser G (2007). [Injuries among children and adolescents (1–17 years) and implementation of safety measures. Results of the nationwide German Health Interview and Examination Survey for Children and Adolescents (KiGGS)]. *Bundesgesundheitsblatt Gesundheitsforschung Gesundheitsschutz*, **50**(5–6), 718–27.
8. Schneiders W, Rollow A, Rammelt S, Grass R, Holch M, Serra A, Richter S, Gruner E, Schlag B, Roesner D, Zwipp H (2007). Risk-inducing activities leading to injuries in a child and adolescent population of Germany. *J Trauma*, **62**(4), 996–1003.
9. Sundblad G, Saartok T, Engstrom LM, Renstrom P (2005). Injuries during physical activity in school children. *Scand J Med Sci Sports*, **15**(5), 313–23.
10. de Vries H, Dijkstra M, Kuhlman P (1988). Self-efficacy: the third factor besides attitude and subjective norm as a predictor of behavioural intentions. *Health Educ Res*, **3**, 273–82.
11. Kok G, de Vries H, Mudde A, Stretcher V (1991). Planned health education and role of self-efficacy:Dutch Research. *Health Educ Res*, **6**, 231–8.
12. Fishbein M, Ajzen I (1975). *Belief, attitude, intention and behavior: an introduction to theory and research*. Wiley, New York.
13. Bandura A (1986). *Social foundations of thought and action: a social cognitive theory*. Prentice Hall Englewood Cliffs, New York.
14. Finch CF, Donaldson A (2009). A sports setting matrix for understanding the implementation context for community sport. *Br J Sports Med*, published on February 6, 2009 as 10.1136/bjsm.2008.056069.

Part 5

Evaluating the efficacy and effectiveness of preventive measures

Chapter 13

Research designs for evaluation studies

Carolyn Emery

The focus of this chapter is to examine design, methodological, and analytical approaches to studies evaluating the effectiveness of prevention and treatment programmes in sports medicine. Evaluation studies are critical in sports medicine to assist health-care practitioners, sports and health administrators, legislators, athletes, coaches, parents, and the public in making informed decisions with regards to the prevention and treatment needs of the community in which we promote physical activity through recreation and sport. The results of such studies are often pivotal in decisions made to continue, discontinue, allocate, or reduce funds from given sport and health-care programmes.

Rossi et al.[1] classify evaluation research according to the focus on either process or outcomes. Formative evaluation studies are conducted to help form or shape a programme during the planning stages to optimize the outcome. In contrast, summative evaluation studies focus on the outcome in evaluating the effectiveness of a programme or policy after implementation. In sports medicine, an example of formative evaluation would be the development of a pre-season injury-prevention clinic in youth. The focus of formative evaluations may include process issues related to feasibility of recruitment, validation of pre-season functional measures that may predict injury, participant satisfaction, and cost of implementation. Summative evaluation, however, would be more focussed on the effectiveness of such a programme in identifying predictors of sports injury and ultimately in reducing the risk of sports injury in this population. In this chapter, primary consideration will be given to methods related to summative evaluation methods.

Research question

As with any research project or programme, identifying the problem to be addressed and developing the related research question are the critical first steps in the design of any evaluation study (also see Chapter 1). The initial problem statement may be broad. An example of this is 'The public health burden of Anterior Cruciate Ligament (ACL) injuries in female youth athletes is significant'[2]. It is critical to establish what the gaps in the knowledge are, prior to formulating the primary research question and associated optimal research design. Following a critical review of the literature examining the effectiveness of injury-prevention programmes in elite soccer players (also see Chapter 7), a research team may develop a primary research question as follows: 'What is the effectiveness of a team based physiotherapist delivered neuromuscular training program in reducing lower extremity injury rates in female youth soccer players?'[3] At this point, secondary research questions will often emerge. In this case, examples may include: 'What is the cost-effectiveness of a team based neuromuscular training programme in female youth soccer players?' and 'Is there a dose–response effect based on the reported adherence to a team based neuromuscular training programme in female youth soccer players?' Verhagen et al.[4] and Emery et al.[5] provide examples of similar research questions in the literature that provide economic evaluations alongside the evaluation of an injury-prevention programme in volleyball and youth basketball players, respectively.

Emery et al.[6] also provide an example of the examination of the dose–response effect of a balance-training programme in improvement of dynamic balance ability in high school physical education participants. In some instances the research question may relate to an interest in demonstrating that there is no difference between groups. For example, Grant et al.[7] set out to show there is no difference in functional outcomes following ACL reconstruction in a physiotherapist-guided home programme compared to a physiotherapist-supervised rehabilitation programme.

Portney and Watkins[8] describe three criteria to be considered in the development of any research question prior to pursuing a research plan. These include the importance, answerability, and feasibility of the question. In posing a research question related to evaluation in sports medicine, clearly the research should have an impact on the prevention or treatment of sports injuries and/or policies related to practice. If the research question is to be answerable, then the exposure (independent) and outcome (dependent) variables in question must be operationally defined and precisely measurable. In the case of injury prevention in sports, the outcome is typically 'sports injury' and the injury-definition should be clearly and operationally defined. Ideally, as more sport-specific consensus agreements are published examining definitions and methods in injury-prevention research, comparisons between studies will become more feasible. Examples of such critical consensus statements have been developed for rugby union and soccer[9, 10]. In the case of evaluation studies the independent variable is the intervention. The clarity of the both the intervention (and the comparison group) is also of utmost importance. The feasibility of the research question may relate to subject recruitment, community engagement, expertise, timelines, available funds, previous evidence, and ethical considerations.

It is critical to clearly identify efficacy versus effectiveness in defining the research question and designing an evaluation study. Efficacy refers to the benefit of an intervention under controlled and ideally randomized conditions, whereas effectiveness refers to the benefit of an intervention under 'real-world' conditions[8]. One must always, of course, consider the feasibility of delivery of clinical or community interventions beyond the context of the conditions and staff available during the evaluation study.

Research design

Arguably the strongest form of evidence in establishing whether a given intervention or treatment has the postulated effect, comes from a well-conducted randomized controlled trial (RCT). An RCT, which is a true experimental design, is the optimal research design to establish a cause–effect relationship[8]. Randomization tends to produce comparable groups with respect to known and unknown risk factors[11]. In a two-armed RCT, as typically found in the sports-injury prevention and sports medicine literature, subjects are randomly assigned to intervention (treatment) and comparison (control) groups. Well-conducted RCTs typically have the greatest influence on both practice and policy in health care[11]. Examples of this include the establishment of best practice neuromuscular training interventions, recommended in youth sports organizations based on the positive outcomes of RCTs in establishing the effectiveness of such programmes in youth sports such as team handball and soccer[3, 12]. Other RCT designs used in sports medicine include three-armed trials (i.e. typically one control group and two different intervention groups), factorial designs (i.e. two or more independent variables under consideration and subjects are randomly assigned to different combinations and/or levels of the variables), and repeated measures designs (i.e. a crossover design where subjects receive one treatment first and then crossover to the other treatment after a washout period, or there may also be a factorial component to such a crossover design). While a crossover design clearly controls for the potential influences of individual differences, there are also several disadvantages to such an approach.

For example, there may be carry-over effects from one intervention to the next, learning effects may influence the outcome over time, and the effects of time on baseline comparisons must be considered.

An RCT design is not always feasible in a clinical or community environment as it may be that is it not feasible or ethical to randomize participants. Quasi-experimental designs utilize similar methods to RCT designs; however, they may lack random assignment of subjects, a control group, or both[8]. For example, it may be increasingly difficult to randomize to a neuromuscular training prevention strategy or a true control group in sports such as soccer and European handball in light of the evidence currently available supporting the significant protective effects of such programmes[12–22, 27]. An example of a quasi-experimental study that significantly influenced practice in sports-injury prevention, is a 2-year follow-up study examining a neuromuscular training intervention to reduce the risk of ACL injuries in female youth soccer players[13]. In sports medicine, it is not uncommon to see one-group quasi-experimental designs. These may be a one-group pretest-posttest design (i.e. pre-experimental), repeated measures design over time, or time-series designs where there are multiple measures before and after the intervention[8]. Caution should be used in the interpretation of results from one-group designs without a control group, as one cannot be sure that changes in an outcome are not due to another independent factor (e.g. time) rather than the intervention itself. Multiple-group quasi-experimental designs may be similar to an RCT in that a control group exists but subjects are not randomly assigned to study groups. For example, subjects may self-select to study groups or participants may already exist in fixed groups where practice may dictate a given intervention. Historical cohorts (i.e. based on information from a study group defined in previous studies or through medical records) are sometimes used as the control group for comparison in the evaluation of injury-prevention strategies[28]. Further, if the intervention to be examined is not introduced by the researcher, but rather is already established, and a natural comparison group is also in place (concurrently or historically) an observational cohort study design may be the design of choice. In some cases the comparison group may be a historical cohort already established and followed with respect to the same outcome measure[14].

A quasi-experimental design, lacking random allocation of subjects to groups, is often limited by non-equivalent groups that may differ in many ways other than the intervention in question[8]. It is possible to control for some such differences in the analysis phase if such differences are expected potential confounders (e.g. gender, age, level of play, previous injury history) and measured at baseline. Limitations of some of the non-RCT evaluation studies in the field of injury prevention in sports, in addition to bias associated confounding variables and non-equivalency of study groups at baseline, also suffer from potential selection bias[13–17]. Selection bias occurs often in the absence of randomization, as group allocation may be predictable and the decision to enter a participant into the study may be influenced by the anticipated study-group assignment[11]. Evidence for such bias in overestimation of the preventative effect of neuromuscular training programmes in soccer implemented specifically to reduce lower-extremity injuries, can be described by combining the results of studies using non-RCT designs[13–17] (Fig. 13.1) and comparing to studies using RCT designs (Fig. 13.2)[3, 18–23]. A meta-analysis was conducted based on available outcomes to produce combined estimates of measure of effect using incidence rate ratios (IRR) based on a random-effects model for five studies using a non-RCT design (Fig. 13.1) and six studies using a RCT design (Fig. 13.2)[24]. All analyses were conducted in Intercooled Stata 10[26]. The size of the box in these figures represents the relative weights given to each study in calculating the overall summary measure. The weights depend on the standard errors of the rate ratio. The combined estimate for non-RCT studies examining a preventive effect of neuromuscular training in the reduction of lower-extremity injuries in soccer is 0.33 (95% CI: 0.16–0.65) and

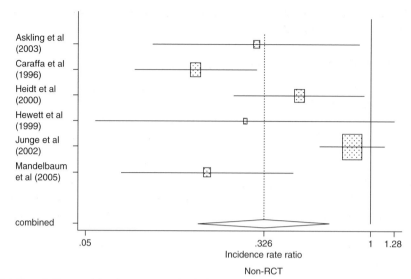

Fig. 13.1 Non-RCTs examining lower extremity (LE) neuromuscular injury-prevention strategies in soccer.

for RCT studies examining the same is 0.86 (95% CI: 0.72–1.03). The point estimates suggest a significantly greater protective effect in the non-RCT studies (67% reduction in injury rate) compared to the RCT studies (14% reduction in injury rate). In addition, the 95% CIs for the combined estimates indicate this protective effect to be significant only in the combined non-RCT studies. If the figures are examined descriptively it is clear that the RCT studies provide estimates of effect that are smaller and not significant based on the 95% CIs displayed graphically which

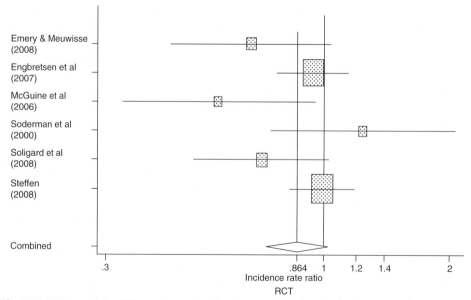

Fig. 13.2 RCTs examining LE neuromuscular injury prevention strategies in soccer.

cross IRR = 1.0 in all but one study. As such, this provides some evidence for the use of a RCT design where both feasible and ethical.

Study population and sampling methods

The generalizability of results of an evaluation study to a broader population (target population) depends on the precise inclusion and exclusion criteria (i.e. defining the sampling frame), the availability of potential study participants that meet those criteria, and the methods of sampling. For example, if a study relies on volunteers for recruitment, these individuals may significantly differ from non-volunteers on the outcome of interest and thus are not representative of the target population[11]. Ideally, probability sampling is used, where there is a process of random selection of study participants. Most commonly, simple random sampling methods are used where every individual has an equal probability of selection[8]. Random number tables, random digit dialing or computer-generated randomization are often used to generate a random list of individual participants. Stratified random sampling may also be employed to select a sample that reflects a similar distribution of study participants on particular characteristics that may be differentially distributed in the population (e.g. gender, level of play)[3, 5]. The number of strata is generally small and heterogeneity within stratum should be expected. Cluster sampling may also be considered if individuals naturally exist in groups (i.e. teams, families, clinics)[11]. The number of clusters is generally large and homogeneity within cluster should be expected. There are significant methodological implications of clustering to consider in the study design and analysis that will be discussed in this chapter[26].

As it is not always possible to obtain a random sample, non-probability sampling is often used. An example of non-probability sampling often employed in sports medicine research would be convenience sampling (i.e. using recruitment posters or websites requesting volunteers), consecutive sampling (i.e. recruiting consecutive patients attending a clinic), and snowball sampling (i.e. sampling through identification of additional participants through participants already recruited). In the case of non-probability sampling, one cannot assume that the sample will be representative of the target population.

It is critical that the sample size required to have adequate power to detect the desired effect size based on clinical significance is predetermined *a priori*. This sample size is typically based on the primary research question and primary outcome of interest as well as prior knowledge of the population (e.g. variance of the outcome in the population). There are numerous references that will facilitate the appropriate calculation of required sample size in the planning stages of the evaluation study at hand[11, 26–29]. Sample-size calculations must consider variable type (e.g. continuous, dichotomous) as well as other methodological details (e.g. paired data, cluster randomization, repeated measures, multiple comparisons, non-adherence, expected drop-outs).

If one is considering the implementation of a cluster RCT or other cluster design, it is important that there is clear justification for doing so, given the lack of statistical efficiency relative to an individual design including the same number of subjects[26]. A cluster design is often selected based on the significant risk of contamination between study groups if intervention-group allocation is at the individual level. In addition, interventions are often implemented at a cluster level (e.g. warm-up, training programme). This approach may enhance subject compliance to the intervention.

The loss of efficiency in a cluster-RCT or other cluster design arises because responses of individuals within a cluster are more similar than individuals in different clusters[26]. The responses of individuals within a cluster usually lack independence, which leads to decreased statistical power. Some of the reasons for greater similarities within a cluster in the field of sports medicine may include the fact that subjects frequently select the cluster to which they belong (e.g. selection of sports team may be related to socioeconomic status), important covariates may be similar within a cluster (e.g. practice facility, coaching style), and that there is on-going interaction among subjects within a cluster.

In some cases the rate of contamination may be large (e.g. team-training programme, policy related to sport rules and regulations) and individual randomization would not be an option. In other circumstances, the rate of contamination may be considerably smaller (e.g. brace prescription by medical practice setting) and individual randomization might be considered. In general, when cluster sizes are small and contamination is expected to be large, cluster randomization or study group allocation by cluster is favoured[26]. When clusters are large ($n > 100$), individual randomization is favoured unless contamination is expected to be so severe that it is not a practical alternative[26]. Not surprisingly, responses among subjects from smaller clusters (e.g. households) tend to be more similar than responses among subjects from larger clusters (e.g. communities)[26]. As such, it would be most efficient to randomize by smaller (e.g., team) rather than larger cluster (e.g. community). It is a possibility that there may be multiple levels of clustering to consider (i.e. classrooms within schools within the target population).

A common cluster type identified in sports medicine research is the sport team ($n = 10–20$), where risk of contamination is significant and cluster design is imperative. Selection of the unit of randomization will depend on statistical power, the need for independence in responses between different units of randomization, the need to avoid contamination, administrative and financial feasibility, the method of delivery of the intervention, and the anticipated effect of the intervention.

Randomization

In addition to producing study groups that are comparable with respect to known and unknown risk factors, random allocation removes investigator judgement or bias in participant study-group allocation, and validates assumptions for statistical tests[11]. There is the possibility of accidental bias if the randomization procedure does not produce balance on risk factors, but the chance of this for larger studies is small[11]. Restricting the sample based on a potentially significant confounding variable (e.g. gender) will ensure that there is not imbalance between study groups on this variable, but will also minimize the generalizability of study results beyond the gender being studied. For example, studies examining the protective effect of an ACL-injury-prevention strategy restrict recruitment to female athletes given the significantly greater risk of ACL injury in females[13, 25, 30]. Other studies may focus on male athletes, given the sport-specific nature of the intervention (i.e. American football)[31]. Stratified random sampling may also be used to increase the probability of group equivalency on the variables upon which the sampling is stratified (e.g. gender, level of play)[3, 5]. Caution should be given to the number of stratified variables. If too many stratified variables are used, it may actually increase the chance of imbalance between study groups. Block randomization or matching may also be considered to facilitate balance in the number of participants in each study group based on potential confounders[11]. Matching, however, limits the possibility of examining differential effects based on the level of the variable upon which matching was done. Cluster randomization is essential if individuals exist and enter a study in the context of a group (e.g. team, clinic, family, school, classroom).

Ideally, the randomization-sequence generation is done independent of the study investigators to ensure removal of investigator bias. Allocation concealment (i.e. method used to implement random allocation in which the sequence is concealed until the intervention is assigned) is ideal, again to minimize potential investigator bias[32]. One must also consider the possibility of selection bias associated with participant drop-out, particularly if the reasons for drop-out are related to the study outcome and/or drop-out rates are differential between study groups.

Baseline assessment

Baseline data in any evaluations study, be it a RCT or quasi-experimental design, is critical to allow for evaluation of baseline comparability of study groups before the commencement of the intervention. Such baseline comparisons, often critical in sports medicine, typically include other potential risk factors or prognostic factors (i.e. level of play, physiological measures, age, gender, maturation, socioeconomic variables, injury history). Baseline comparisons should not be examined through multiple comparisons statistically, but rather the point estimates and 95% CIs should be compared descriptively to avoid multiple-comparison issues. Baseline imbalances may be avoided by stratification at the time of randomization or controlled for in the analysis[11].

Meeuwisse et al.[33] developed a recursive model for research in injury prevention in sport which highlights the recursive and dynamic nature of risk and aetiology of injury (also see Chapter 8). This model highlights the fact that an initial set of risk factors (i.e. baseline measures) that are thought to precede an injury may have changed through repeated exposure to sport, whether such exposure produces adaptation, maladaptation, injury, or complete/incomplete recovery from injury[33]. A linear approach may not be appropriate, particularly if risk factors are not stable over time. The design should allow for intermittent follow-up measurements if baseline covariates are expected to change over time. In addition, analysis strategies must be selected that will allow for the inclusion of time-dependent covariates (e.g. generalized estimating equations or generalized linear mixed models).

Intervention

In developing a research question, concise operationalization of the intervention to be examined is necessary. This includes not only details related to the intervention at hand (i.e. components of a neuromuscular training programme), but precisely the method of delivery, length, and time-frame of a programme and definition of adherence. The comparison group may be a true control (i.e. no intervention, if this is deemed ethical in the context of current standard of practice) or may be an alternate intervention based on current standard of practice. If a true control group is the comparison group, interpretation of study results may also be limited. Any difference between groups may not be attributed to the components of the intervention alone, but may be attributed to time and/or interaction with study team (i.e. Hawthorne effect related to changes in perform-ance as a result of 'being studied'). One must also be aware of the potential bias that may accom-pany investigator interaction with a study participant in overcompensating for a potentially less desirable treatment regime[8]. A study participant may also respond to receiving a perceived less desirable treatment by compensation and extra effort to achieve positive results or conversely by a lack of effort to perform based on resentment related to receiving a less desirable treatment[8]. An approach to minimizing such potential threats to validity may include blinding subjects to details of the alternate intervention[3, 5, 34]. Another approach is to ensure the comparison group 'control intervention' mimics the 'study intervention' with respect to delivery, expected adherence, length, and timeframe and differs only on specific components under study[3, 5, 34]. In examining multiple-component interventions (i.e. orthotics plus exercise, balance training plus other agility training), interpretation of the results must also consider the interaction of the multiple components which may be additive, multiplicative, or subtractive.

Evaluation of adherence to study intervention is critical in the interpretation of study results. This may be self-reported by study participants, involved coaches, or, in some cases, evaluated by study personnel through intermittent observation or evaluated by a secondary or marker variable (i.e. measurement of balance ability in the context of a balance-training injury-prevention strategy)[3, 5, 6, 34]. If some measure of adherence is collected, then evaluation of a dose–response effect may be possible. In the context of intervention allocation, it is important to recognize not only the possibilities of nonadherence to an intervention but also contamination in the context of unintended uptake of an intervention by study participants (i.e. a control-group subject participating in 'intervention' component). The possibility of contamination may be minimised by blinding subjects to the specifics of the other study-group intervention or in the context of clusters (i.e. team, family, school, classroom, clinic), allocating study participants to groups by cluster not individually. Length of follow-up clearly needs to be consistent in the evaluation of group differences.

Outcome measurement

Clear operationalization of study-outcome definitions, including time to follow-up, is critical to the interpretation of study results. Concerns with regards to potential sources of measurement bias(es) should be considered in the planning stages of any evaluation study. Blinding evaluators to study-group allocation will minimize bias associated with measurement of outcomes of interest. The reliability and validity of all outcome measures under consideration is essential to reduce the effect of potential measurement bias. If a measurement is unreliable, then study groups will become more similar on the outcome measure of interest and treatment effect will be biased towards the mean[8]. By maximizing reliability of all outcome measures through calibration of all study instruments and pre-testing intra- and inter-rater reliability, measurement bias in this regards will be minimized.

Typically, an evaluation study is powered on the primary outcome variable of interest. In that regards, the sensitivity of a study is greater if the outcome variable of interest is measured at baseline and the change in this variable (i.e. VAS pain score, quality of life measure, blood pressure) becomes the outcome of interest with typically less variability that the actual score at follow-up[8]. In injury prevention in sport, the outcome is typically 'sport injury'. Critical consensus statements continue to be developed in this field, as have been developed for rugby union and soccer, to facilitate the comparisons between studies[9, 10].

In the collection of follow-up measurement the study design should include mechanisms to minimize the possibility of missing data and/or invalid data. Strategies may include validation and pre-testing of all study forms, adequate training, and standardization of data-collection and data-entry procedures, monitoring of data quality and data entry, and random data audits by an external data-monitoring committee[11]. In addition, adverse events should also be considered in the design of an evaluation study. These adverse events may be anticipated or not depending on the study intervention and availability of previous literature examining a similar intervention. This is why it is important to pre-test (i.e. pilot test) any new or adapted intervention in a small group of individual representative of the target population of interest in a larger study. An example of adverse events reported in an RCT examining the protective effect of neuromuscular training in reducing the risk of ankle-sprain injuries in elite volleyball players, was the increased risk of patellofemoral pain in the intervention group[4].

Validation and examination of the reliability of all study outcome measures is also critical. In injury-prevention research, validation of the injury-surveillance system implemented is critical[35]. In addition, such an injury-surveillance system must be adapted for use and validated in specific populations (i.e. community-based youth soccer programmes) as the feasibility and validity may differ from the population in which the system was originally developed and validated where there may have been a more controlled environment (i.e. varsity athletics with designated team physicians and therapists)[36].

Considerations for analysis

Appropriate selection of statistical analysis techniques in any evaluation study is critical in order to avoid misleading conclusions. A more detailed description of proper statistical techniques can be found in Chapter 14. In addition, Friedman et al.[11] provide guidance for statistical considerations in the analysis of data from clinical trials with a diversity of outcome measure types (i.e. dichotomous, continuous, repeated measures, clustering, time to event, count). Details related to various analysis techniques can be found in several statistics and biostatistics textbooks[26–29]. Multivariable analysis must be considered in order to adjust for covariate imbalance (i.e. potential confounding) at baseline or if examination and reporting of effect modification (i.e. varying level of effect based on the level of another covariate) is to be considered[11]. Stratified analysis in which the outcome or effect measure are considered by stratifying study-group participants into smaller more homogeneous groups based on another covariate (i.e. gender, age, previous injury). More sophisticated modelling techniques should also be considered to control for confounding and/or examine effect modification. Of course, sub-group analysis to examine effect modification (e.g. differential effect of intervention across another covariate such as gender) should be considered in the planning stages of an evaluation study as there are considerable sample-size implications. *Post hoc* analyses, sometimes referred to as 'data-dredging' or 'fishing', should be avoided due to the significant statistical implications of multiple comparisons[11]. For the same reason, analysis of multiple outcomes and interim analyses should be considered in the planning stages.

Analytical considerations related to withdrawals require consideration. Withdrawals (i.e. participants who have been randomized but are deliberately not included in the analysis) include subsequently determined ineligibility, non-adherence (i.e. dropouts or drop-ins related to contamination), poor quality or missing data and occurrence of competing events (e.g. death, injuries that do not meet the sports-injury definition such as motor-vehicle collision injuries). All of these will potentially lead to bias if not considered appropriately in the analysis. As a general rule, participants should be analysed according to the study group to which they are assigned[11]. This is often referred to as an 'intention to treat analysis'[8]. This may lead to a reduction in the power of the analysis given that some participants included in the analysis will not have had the optimal intervention based on the study group to which they were assigned. If this is expected, then sample size should include this predicted loss of power related to non-adherence[11]. Withdrawal related to subsequently determined ineligibility or drop-outs should be minimized in the study design by making every effort to establish eligibility prior to randomization and every effort to minimize loss to follow-up[11]. Withdrawal related to poor quality or missing data or extreme observations (e.g. outliers) must be considered. Intention-to-treat analysis may be considered in the case of missing data or extremely poor-quality data. If data is missing, the mechanism should be investigated as any technique to impute missing data is based on the assumption that the reason for the missing data is not related to the outcome. Missing data may be imputed using various techniques which include 'last observation carried forward', EM algorithm, bootstrapping, and multiple imputation[11, 37, 38]. Outliers should always be checked for physiological plausibility as well as for potential errors in recording or data entry. Decisions with regards to outliers may be made based on a comparison of results with and without inclusion of the outlier. If the results vary considerably based on inclusion of the outlier, then results should be interpreted with caution[11]. All major competing events (i.e. non-sports-related injury, death) require description in the results.

Cluster analysis

Cluster designs are clearly the design of choice in addressing many evaluation research questions in sports medicine and injury prevention where individuals often function in the context of a cluster (e.g. team, school, clinic). Despite the literature now available addressing appropriate design and analysis of cluster RCTs, there are only a few intervention studies in the field of injury prevention in sport which address clustering appropriately in the design and analysis[3, 6, 12, 31]. The 'CONSORT Statement: Extension to cluster randomisation trials' in the reporting of such study results is ignored in many studies[39]. Inappropriate individual-level analysis and poor reporting of cluster RCTs and other evaluation studies may lead to erroneous results and misleading conclusions, practice, and policy recommendations[40]. As such, Emery examined the implications of using a cluster RCT or other evaluation study design in which subjects are assigned to or naturally exist in clusters[40]. Emery uses an example from a study in which the effectiveness of an injury-prevention strategy in high school basketball was evaluated, to highlight the practical implications of appropriate cluster analysis of such designs and these will be summarised here[31].

The statistical measure of the degree of similarity within a cluster is known as the intra-cluster correlation coefficient (ρ) which may be interpreted in a similar fashion to a standard Pearson correlation coefficient between any two responses in the same cluster[26]. A positive ρ assumes that the variation between observations in different clusters is greater than the variation between observations in the same cluster. The intra-cluster correlation hence reflects the within cluster resemblance anticipated. If $\rho = 0$ then there is statistical independence between subjects within a cluster, and subjects within a cluster are no more similar than subjects between clusters. In the case that $\rho = 1$, there is complete dependence and all responses within a cluster are identical. The total information supplied by a cluster is no more than that supplied by a single member. To ensure similar power to a study randomizing individuals, the calculated sample size must be adjusted by a variance 'inflation factor' associated with the intra-cluster correlation (ρ). To achieve the equivalent power of an individually randomized RCT, the standard sample-size calculation needs to be inflated by this 'inflation factor' (IF) which is affected by both the degree of dependence within a cluster (ρ) and the average cluster size (n): IF $= 1 + (n-1) \rho$[26].

In large clusters such as a clinic or school, it is not uncommon to observe correlations as low as 0.01 and smaller[26]. However, given the average cluster size may be large, the sample-size adjustment may be significant. For example, if $\rho = 0.01$ and $n = 200$, the sample size must be tripled (IF $= 2.99$) to overcome the clustering despite the relatively small intra-cluster correlation[26]. If the cluster size is small (e.g. family of four) then the anticipated intra-cluster correlation would be anticipated to be larger (i.e. $\rho = 0.25$) and the sample-size inflation not as significant (IF $= 1.75$)[26]. Failure to take into account that individual responses within a cluster lack independence leads to an underestimation of p-values and incorrectly narrow confidence intervals. Given the need to interpret results at the level of individual subjects in most cases in sports medicine, there are numerous approaches to cluster adjusted analysis that may be considered. For example, in comparing event rates in two groups, the standard chi-square test can be adjusted for the clustering of responses within a cluster[26]. In order to account for the imbalance on baseline covariates, however, provided the number of clusters is sufficiently large, multiple regression methods may be used to increase the precision with which the intervention effect is estimated[26]. A Generalised Estimating Equation (GEE) extension of logistic regression developed by Liang et al.[41], which adjusts for the effects of clustering, may be considered.

An example examining the effectiveness of a neuromuscular training strategy in reducing the risk of injury in high school basketball players will be used to describe an appropriate approach to individual level analysis in the context of clustering by team[31]. A total of 920 high school basketball players (age range: 12–18) from 89 teams in Calgary and area were randomly allocated by school to the control ($n = 426$) and training groups ($n = 494$)[31]. All injuries occurring during basketball that required medical attention and/or caused a player to be removed from that current session and/or miss a subsequent session were then assessed and recorded through previously validated injury surveillance.

Injury rates (number of injuries per 1000 player hours) and 95% CI were calculated using a Poisson regression model, controlling for player hours and adjustment for clustering by team[31]. An extension of multivariable Poisson regression analysis which adjusts for covariates (e.g. gender, age, previous injury, endurance, strength, balance ability, leg-dominance) and clustering effects by team was done to estimate the relative risk of injury in the training group compared to the control group. This model was chosen in order to account for multiple, independent injury events in the same player (range: 0–3 injuries/player). Comparisons of injury rate (number of injuries per 1000 player hours) by study group, based on a cluster-adjusted Poisson regression analysis indicates a relative risk of 0.8 (95% CI: (0.57–1.11) ($p = 0.18$). Based on an inappropriate individual-level analysis, however, a Poisson regression analysis indicates a relative risk of 0.8 (95% CI: 0.63–1.0; $p = 0.05$). The similar comparison based on ankle-sprain injuries alone yields a RR = 0.71 (95% CI: 0.45–1.13) ($p = 0.15$) with the appropriate analysis adjusted for clustering by team and RR = 0.71 (95% CI: 0.51–0.99) ($p = 0.05$) based on an unadjusted individual level analysis. Based on an appropriate intent-to-treat analysis we found the training programme to be ineffective in reducing the risk of all injuries and ankle-sprain injuries in high school basketball players based on the wider confidence intervals. However, an inappropriate individual analysis suggests a protective effect in reducing all injury by 20% and ankle-sprain injury by 29% which are also statistically significant. Clearly the p-values are biased downwards and the 95% CIs considerably narrower in the incorrect analysis. This lack of consideration for inter-cluster variation would have lead to spurious scientific conclusions which overemphasized the effectiveness of the programme in reducing all injury and ankle-sprain injury in high school basketball players.

In this study, *a priori* sample size was estimated based on an expected injury rate of 30 injuries/100 players in the control group, a predicted intra-cluster correlation ($\rho = 0.006$) based on pilot RCT data and other adolescent behaviours, and potential drop-out/non-compliance (Ro = 0.05). Assuming a Type I error ($\alpha = 0.05$) and Type II error ($\beta = 0.10$), a total of 960 subjects were required to detect a risk reduction of 33%. The intra-cluster correlation coefficient calculated *post hoc* was greater than predicted ($\rho = 0.06$) and the effect size observed was only 20%. Thus, the appropriate 'inflation factor' [IF = $1 + (n - 1) \rho$] should have been 2.5 rather than 1.15. *Post hoc* power analysis suggests that 1984 players were required ($N = 248$ teams) to detect a 20% reduction in injury rate with statistical significance ($1 - \beta = 0.8$, $\sigma = 0.05$). Clearly this study was underpowered with the participation of 920 participants (89 teams). Unfortunately, the feasibility and cost associated with such a community cluster RCT of this magnitude preclude many researchers from considering such a design.

Despite the abundance of literature addressing appropriate methods for the design and analysis of cluster RCTs; the reported RCTs, non-RCT intervention studies, and observational studies in sports medicine and other primary-care settings that account appropriately for the effects of clustering remain in the minority[3, 6, 12, 31, 42–45]. In addition, there are very few trials which adequately report intra-cluster correlation values making it difficult in obtaining accurate estimates of intra-cluster correlation upon which to plan a future study. In the example related to an intervention in high school basketball, it is clear that underestimating the intra-cluster correlation coefficient can significantly under-power a study. As a result, the risk of finding spuriously significant findings and misleading conclusions will increase. Some of the strategies to improve the precision of estimates while appropriately considering clustering may include; establishing cluster-level inclusion criteria such that between-cluster variability will be reduced (e.g. geographic or socioeconomic restrictions), increasing the number of clusters rather than the cluster size where possible, maximizing compliance to treatment (e.g. training programme), minimizing losses to follow-up (particularly entire clusters), considering matching or stratification by important baseline variables that have previously been identified for example a risk factors for injury (e.g. gender, age, level of play), and obtaining adequate measurements on important covariates at baseline such that a multivariable approach to the analysis may be considered[40]. If, however, inferences are to be made at the cluster level, then an individual-level analysis may not be appropriate. For example, Kerry et al.[46] were interested in the effectiveness of guidelines for radiographic referral at the level of general practitioner practice and not at the level of the individual patient. It is important to note that only cluster-level inferences can be made using a cluster-level analysis, not inferences at an individual level.

Conclusion

It is critical that we understand the implications of the research design, methods, and analysis of evaluation studies in sports medicine to allow us to critically appraise and appropriately interpret the research that will lead us to clinical, community, and policy decisions that are informed by the evidence. Understanding and addressing the limitations of the design, methods, and analyses chosen in evaluation research is critical to the interpretation of a study's results. In addition, in conducting evaluation research in the field of sports medicine, it is imperative that the design, methods and analyses are rigorously planned in advance in order to offer the highest level of evidence appropriate for a given research question.

References

1. Rossi PH, Lipsey MW, Freeman HE (2004). *Evaluation: A systematic approach. 7th edition*. Sage Publications, Newbury Park, CA.
2. Hewett TE, Ford KR, Myer GD (2006). Anterior cruciate ligament injuries in female athletes. Part 2, a meta-analysis of neuromuscular interventions aimed at prevention. *Am J Sport Med*, **34**, 490–8.
3. Emery CA, Meeuwisse WH (2008). The effectiveness of a neuromuscular training program to reduce injuries in youth soccer. A cluster-randomized controlled trial. *Br J Sport Med*, **42**, 497.
4. Verhagen E, van der Beek A, Twisk J, Bouter L, Bahr R, van Mechelen W (2004). The effect of a proprioceptive balance board training program for the prevention of ankle sprains: a prospective controlled trial. *Am J Sports Med*, **32**(6), 1385–93.
5. Emery CA, Meeuwisse WH, McAllister JR (2006). A prevention strategy to reduce the incidence of injury in high school basketball: A cluster randomized controlled trial. *Clin J Sport Med*, **16**, 182.
6. Emery CA, Cassidy JD, Klassen T, Rosychuk RJ, Rowe BH (2005). The effectiveness of a proprioceptive balance training program in healthy adolescents. A cluster randomized controlled trial. *Can Med Assoc J*, **172**(6), 749–54.
7. Grant JA, Mohtadi NGH, Maitland ME, Zernicke RF (2005). Comparison of home versus physical therapy-supervised rehabilitation programs after anterior cruciate ligament reconstruction: a randomized clinical trial. *Am J Sports Med*, **33**, 1288–97.
8. Portney LG and Watkins MP (2007). *Foundations of clinical research; Applications to practice. 3rd edition*. Prentice HallUpper, Saddle River, New Jersey.

9. Fuller CW, Molloy MG, Bagate C, Bahr R, Brooks JHM, Donson H, Kemp SPT, McCrory P, McIntosh AS, Meeuwisse WH, Quarrie KL, Raftery M, Wiley P (2007). Consensus statement on injury definitions and data collection procedures for studies of injuries in rugby union. *Clin J Sport Med*, **17**, 177–81.

10. Fuller CW, Ekstrand J, Junge A, Andersen TE, Bahr R, Dvorak J, Hägglund M, McCrory P, Meeuwisse WH (2006). Consensus statement on injury definitions and data collection procedures in studies of football (soccer) injuries. *Clin J Sport Med*, **16**, 97–106.

11. Friedman LM, Furberg CD, DeMets DL (1998). *Fundamentals of clinical trials. 3rd edition*. Springer-Verlag, New York.

12. Olsen OE. Myklebust G. Engebretsen L. Holme I. Bahr R (2005). Exercises to prevent lower limb injuries in youth sports: cluster randomised controlled trial. *BMJ*, **330**(7489), 449–56.

13. Mandelbaum BR, Silvers HJ, Watanabe DS, Knarr JF, Thomas SD, Griffin LY, Kirkendall DT, Garrett W Jr. (2005). Effectiveness of neuromuscular and proprioceptive training program in preventing anterior cruciate ligament injuries in female athletes: 2-year follow-up. *Am J Sport Med*, **33**, 1003–10.

14. Heidt RS Jr, Sweeterman LM, Carlonas RL, Traub JA, Tekulve FX (2000). Avoidance of soccer injuries with preseason conditioning. *Am J Sports Med*, **28**, 659–62.

15. Caraffa A, Cerulli G, Projetti M, Aisa G, Rizzo A (1996). Prevention of anterior cruciate ligament injuries in soccer. A prospective controlled study of proprioceptive training. *Knee Surg Sport Tr A*, **4**, 19–21.

16. Hewett TE, Lindenfeld TN, Riccobene JV, Noyes FR (1999). The effect of neuromuscular training on the incidence of knee injury in female athletes. *Am J Sports Med*, **27**, 699–705.

17. Junge A, Rosch D, Peterson L, Graf-Baumann T, Chomiak J, Peterson L (2000). Prevention of soccer injuries: a prospective intervention study in youth amateur players. *Am J Sports Med*, **30**, 652–9.

18. Askling C, Karlsson J, Thorstensson A (2003). Hamstring injury occurrence in elite soccer players after preseason strength training with eccentric overload. *Scand J Med Sci Spor*, **13**, 244–50.

19. Engebretsen AH, Myklebust G, Holme I, Engebretsen L, Bahr R (2008). Prevention of injuries among male soccer players: a prospective, randomized intervention study targeting players with previous injuries or reduced function. *Am J Sports Med*, **36**, 1052–60.

20. McGuine TA, Keene JS (2006). The effect of a balance training program on the risk of ankle sprains in high school athletes. *Am J Sports Med*, **34**, 1103–11.

21. Soderman K, Werner S, Pietila T, Engstrom B, Alfredson H (2000). Balance board training: prevention of traumatic injuries of the lower extremity in female soccer players? A prospective randomized intervention study. *Knee Surg Sport Tr A*, **8**, 356–63.

22. Soligard T, Myklebust G, Steffen K, Holme I, Silvers H, Bizzini M, Junge A, Dvorak J, Bahr R, Andersen TE (2008). Comprehensive warm-up programme to prevent injuries in young female footballers: cluster randomized controlled trial. *BMJ*, **337**, a2469.

23. Steffen K (2008). Introduction, in Steffen K (ed) *Injuries in Female Youth Football. Prevention performance and risk factors. (Dissertation from the Norwegian School of Sport Sciences)*. Oslo Sport Trauma Research Centre, Oslo.

24. Deeks JJ, Altman DG, Bradburn MJ (2001). Statistical methods for examining heterogeneity and combining results from several studies in meta-analysis, in Egger M, Smith GD, Altman DG (eds) *Systematic Reviews in Health Care: Meta-analysis in Context*. BMJ Publishing Group, London.

25. Statacorp (2007). *Stata Statistical Software: Release 10.0*. College Station, TX: Stata Corporation.

26. Donner A, Klar N (2000). *Design and analysis of cluster randomization trials in health research*. Oxford University Press, New York.

27. Norman and Streiner (2001). *Biostatistics: the bare essentials*. B.C. Decker Inc., Toronto.

28. Altman DG (1991). *Practical statistics for medical research*. Chapman & Hall, London, UK.

29. Rosner BA (2006). *Fundamentals of biostatistics. 6th edition*. Duxbury Press, Boston.

30. Myklebust G, Engebretsen L, Braekken IH, Skjolberg A, Olsen O, Bahr R (2003). Prevention of ACL injuries in female handball players: a prospective intervention study over 3 seasons. *Clin J Sport Med,* **13**, 71–8.

31. Cahill BR, Griffith EH (1978). Effect of preseason conditioning on the incidence and severity of high school football knee injuries. *Am J Sports Med,* **6**, 180–4.

32. Moher D, Schulz KF, Altman D (2001). CONSORT Statement: Revised recommendations for improving the quality of reports of parallel-group randomized trials. *JAMA,* **285**, 1987–91.

33. Meeuwisse WH, Hagel BE, Emery CE and Tyreman H (2007). A Dynamic Model of Etiology in Sport Injury: The recursive nature of risk and causation. *Clin J Sport Med,* **17**(3), 215–19.

34. Emery CA, Rose MS, Meeuwisse WH, McAllister JR (2007). The effectiveness of an injury prevention strategy in high school basketball. A Cluster-Randomized Controlled Trial. *Clin J Sport Med,* **17**, 17–24.

35. Meeuwisse W, Love E (1997). Athletic Injury Reporting: Development of universal systems. *Sports Med,* **24**(3), 184–204.

36. Emery CA, Meeuwisse WH, Hartmann S (2005). Risk factors for injury in adolescent soccer. Pilot implementation and validation of an injury surveillance system. *Am J Sports Med,* **33**, 1882–91.

37. Dempster AP, Laird NM, Rubin DB (1977). Maximum Likelihood from Incomplete Data via the EM Algorithm. *J Roy Stat Soc B,* **39**(1), 1–38.

38. Little RJA, Rubin DB (1987). *Statistical analysis with missing data.* John Wiley & Sons, New York.

39. Campbell MK, Elbourne DR, Altman DG (2004). CONSORT group. CONSORT statement: extension to cluster randomised trials. *BMJ,* **328**, 702–8.

40. Emery CA (2007). Considering cluster analysis in sport medicine and injury prevention research. *Clin J Sport Med,* **17**(3), 211–14.

41. Liang KY, Zeger SL (1986). Longitudinal data analysis using generalized linear models. *Biometrika,* **73**, 13–22.

42. Simpson J, Klar N, Donner A (1995). Accounting for cluster randomization; a review of primary prevention trials, 1990–1993. *Am J Public Health,* **85**, 1378–83.

43. Butler C, Bachmann M (1996). Design and analysis of studies evaluating smoking cessation interventions where effects may vary between practices or practitioners. *Fam Pract,* **13**, 402–7.

44. Rooney BL, Murray DL (1996). A meta-analysis of smoking prevention programs after adjustment for errors in the unit of analysis. *Health Educ Quart,* **23**, 48–64.

45. Eldridge SM, Ashby D, Feder GS, Rudnicka AR, Ukoumunne OC (2004). Lessons for cluster randomized trials in the twenty-first century: a systematic review of trials in primary care. *Clin Trials,* **1**, 80–90.

46. Kerry S, Bland JM (1998). Analysis of a trial randomized in clusters. *BMJ,* **316**, 549.

Chapter 14

Statistics used in effect studies

Andrew Hayen and Caroline F. Finch

This chapter describes some of the statistical methods used in studies of sports-injury-prevention effectiveness. Such studies aim generally to determine whether or not a trialled injury-prevention measure (or intervention) does actually prevent the injuries that it targets. There are a number of important features of typical sports-injury intervention trials that affect the appropriate statistical methods that need to be chosen. Many modern randomized trials[1–4], e.g. compare injury rates in two or more groups that are allocated to either received the intervention being tested or to act as a control group. Additionally, some other studies of effect have compared injury rates before and after the introduction of an intervention or programme in a community to determine if the programme has been effective[5]. These studies are often referred to as ecological study designs, where the setting of intervention is not able to be fully controlled. Whilst this chapter particularly focusses on statistical methods of the analysis of trials where the outcome of interest is an injury rate, the general approaches also apply to other trials where the outcome of interest may be a precursor to injury reduction *per se*, such as the adoption of a preventive measure such as protective equipment[6, 7].

In both cases, statistical methods that are appropriate to the analysis of rates must be used. The calculation of rates requires an estimate of exposure time, which in sports-injury studies is typically the amount of time (in hours) that players participate in matches or games and/or undertake training. Sometimes other measures, such as the number of games played or training sessions attended, are used. Other measures may include player registrations. Statistical methods that can be used to compare rates across two or more study arms, such as rate ratios, are discussed in this chapter. More advanced regression methods are also discussed.

Several recent studies[1–4, 6, 8] have used cluster or group randomization – often teams or clubs – rather than individual-player randomization. This clustering needs to be taken into the analysis, because two players within the same team tend to be more similar than two players from different teams. The chapter therefore concludes with a discussion of methods for analysing injury-rate data from cluster-randomized trials in sports-injury prevention.

Examples

A number of examples are used throughout this chapter. Some background information about the studies is given below.

Spinal injuries in New Zealand rugby

A study compared the number and rate of spinal injuries in New Zealand before and after the introduction of a nation-wide injury-prevention programme that was introduced in 2001[5]. The number of serious spine-related injuries (scrum-related and other injuries) and estimates of player numbers are given in Table 14.1. The number of players in 1996 and 1997 was unknown, and the average number of players from 1998 to 2000 was used for the player numbers in these years.

Table 14.1 Number of rugby union players and injuries by type of injury and year, New Zealand, 1996–2005

Year	Number of players (thousands)	Scrum injuries	Other injuries	Total injuries	Injury rate per 100 000 players	95% CI
1996	127	3	1	4	3.1	0.9–8.1
1997	127	0	1	1	0.8	0.0–4.4
1998	122	0	2	2	1.6	0.2–5.9
1999	130	4	1	5	3.8	1.2–9.0
2000	129	2	3	5	3.9	1.3–9.0
2001	120	0	2	2	1.7	0.2–6.0
2002	122	0	1	1	0.8	0.2–4.6
2003	121	0	2	3	1.7	0.5–7.2
2004	129	1	1	2	1.6	0.2–5.6
2005	138	0	1	1	0.7	0.0–4.0

Adapted from Quarrie et al.[5]

Soccer example

A prospective study compared injury rates during game and practice sessions between 19 high-skilled and 36 low-skilled soccer players[9]. Information on the type of play was also collected. The number of injuries and exposure time are given in Table 14.2.

Padded headgear in rugby

A cluster randomized controlled trial of headgear was conducted with players allocated to either a control arm (usual behaviour) and two intervention arms (standard and modified headgear)[2]. Data on head injuries sustained during games are presented in Table 14.3.

Injuries in female floorball players

A Finnish study examined the effects of neuromuscular training and leg injuries in female floorball players[3]. In total, there were 457 players of whom 256 (from 14 teams) were in the intervention group (neuromuscular training) and 201 were in the control group (also from 14 teams). The number of non-contact leg injuries and exposure data are presented in Table 14.4.

Table 14.2 Injury and exposure by skill levels for 55 soccer players

Type of sport activity	Injuries	Exposure (hours)	Rate per 1000 h (95%CI)
Game			
High-skilled	15	759	19.8 (11.1–32.6)
Low-skilled	21	1015	20.7 (12.8–31.6)
Practice			
High-skilled	14	3440	4.1 (2.2–6.8)
Low-skilled	7	1231	5.7 (2.3–11.7)

Adapted from Poulsen et al.[9]

Table 14.3 Injury and exposure data for rugby headgear study

Intervention (headgear)	Players	Clusters (teams)	Exposure (hours)	Head injuries	Rate (per 1000 h)	95% CI
Control	1493	63	10 040	82	8.2	6.5–10.1
Modified	1474	60	10 650	96	9.0	7.3–11.0
Standard	1128	46	8170	56	6.9	5.2–8.9

Adapted from McIntosh et al.[2]

Injuries in Australian Football players

A study is being conducted to reduce knee injuries in Australian Football players through exercise. [10] The study will be randomized at a team level, and it aims to see whether football-related knee injuries are reduced through the use of a coach-led exercise programme versus usual behaviour. This example will be use to discuss sample sizes in this chapter.

Incidence rates

The incidence rate is generally defined as the number of new cases of the outcome of interest per unit of person-time at risk. In the context of sports injury, the number of new cases will usually be the number of new (or incident) injuries, and the person-time at risk, or exposure time, will usually be the number of hours of participation in the sporting activity. However, often such information is not available, and other measures, such as the number of player registrations per year, can be used[5].

Throughout this chapter, the symbol Y will be used to denote the number of injuries, and T will represent a unit measure of exposure, however it is defined in the particular study. The injury rate is then defined as $R = Y/T$.

Counts, and consequently rates, are typically modelled using the Poisson distribution, allowing the calculation of confidence intervals. The Poisson distribution is the natural distribution to handle outcomes such as the number of sports injuries and other variables that are counts. The Poisson distribution is described in the work by Kirkwood and Sterne[11].

For statistical reasons, rates are typically best analysed on the natural logarithmic scale. Throughout this chapter the mathematical notation log is used for the natural logarithm (often also written as ln). The standard error of the log rate is given by $\sqrt{1/Y}$.

A $100 \times (1 - \alpha)\%$ confidence interval for the log rate is given by $\log(R) \pm z_{\alpha/2} \times \sqrt{1/Y}$ [11]. The confidence interval for the rate can then be derived by exponentiating the lower and upper limits of the confidence interval for the log rate. The lower limit of the confidence interval is then $\exp\left(\log(R) - z_{\alpha/2}\sqrt{1/Y}\right)$ and the upper limit is $\exp\left(\log(R) + z_{\alpha/2}\sqrt{1/Y}\right)$.

The confidence interval given above is based on an approximation. When the number of counts is small, it is also possible to obtain 'exact' confidence intervals for rates; these are based

Table 14.4 Injury and exposure data for Finnish floorball study

Trial arm	Players	Clusters (teams)	Exposure (hours)	Non-contact leg injuries	Rate (per 1000 practice and playing hours)	95% CI
Intervention	256	14	32 327	20	0.6	0.4–1.0
Control	201	14	25 019	52	2.1	1.6–2.7

Adapted from Pasanen et al.[3]

on a relationship between the Poisson and chi-squared distributions[12]. An exact confidence interval does not rely on approximations like the confidence intervals presented above.

The lower and upper limits for a $100 \times (1 - \alpha)\%$ confidence interval are given by $\dfrac{\chi^2_{2Y,\alpha/2}}{2T}$ and $\dfrac{\chi^2_{2(Y+1),1-\alpha/2}}{2T}$.

Note that α is the significance level of a test, so if $\alpha = 0.05$, then $1 - \alpha = 0.95$ and we have 95% conference limits. If confidence intervals per 1 000 hours, say, are desired rather than per hour then the lower and upper limits can both be multiplied by 1000.

Example

The total number of serious spinal injuries in the New Zealand rugby union study for the period 1996 to 2005 was 25, and there were 1 265 000 player years of exposure. The injury rate is $R = \dfrac{25}{1265000} = 0.00002$ or 0.00002 injuries per player per year or 2.0 injuries per 100 000 players per year.

The 95% confidence interval for the log of the rate is given by $\log\left(\dfrac{25}{1265000}\right) \pm 1.96 \times \sqrt{1/25} =$ $-10.83 \pm 1.96 \times .39$, or -11.59 to -10.07. Taking antilogs and multiplying by 100 000 gives a 95% confidence interval of $\exp(-11.59) \times 100\,000 = 1.3$ to $\exp(-10.07) \times 100000 = 2.9$. Therefore, the 95% confidence interval is 1.3 to 2.9 injuries per 100 000 players per year.

For scrum-related injuries, there were 10 injuries over the period 1996 to 2005, and the rate was 0.8 injuries per 100 000 players per year. The 95% confidence interval was 0.4 to 1.5 injuries per 100 000 players per year.

An exact confidence interval can also be calculated. The lower limit of the 95% exact confidence interval for the serious spinal injury rate is $\dfrac{\chi^2_{2\times25,0.025}}{2\times1265000} \times 100,000 = \dfrac{32.4}{2\times1265000} \times 100,000 = 1.3$ injuries per 100 000 players per year. The upper limit is $\dfrac{\chi^2_{2\times(25+1),0.025}}{2\times1265000} \times 100,000 = \dfrac{73.8}{2\times1265000} \times$ $100,000 = 2.9$ injuries per 100 000 players per year. Therefore the 95% exact confidence interval is 1.3–2.9 serious spinal cord injuries per 100 000 players per year. Note that in this case the two forms of confidence intervals give the same result. Typically the results of the two methods are fairly similar.

For scrum-related injuries, the 95% exact confidence interval is 0.4–1.5 serious spinal cord injuries per 100 000 players per year.

Comparison of rates

This section aims to describe how two rates can be compared. Two measures can be used One based on the difference between the two rates, and the other on the ratio of two rates. The difference in rates is sometimes preferred as a measure of comparing two groups because it has an easier interpretation. Combined with its confidence interval, it says how many more (or less) injuries there are per hour of exposure in the intervention group than in the control group.

In this section, we assume that we have two groups that we wish to compare, and that the number of injuries in the groups are Y_1 and Y_2, that the rates in the groups are R_1 and R_2 and that the exposure times in the groups are T_1 and T_2.

Difference in rates

The difference in rates between the two groups is $R_1 - R_2$ and the standard error of the difference is $\sqrt{R_1/T_1 + R_2/T_2}$. Therefore a $100 \times (1 - \alpha)\%$ confidence interval for the differences is given by $R_1 - R_2 \pm z_{\alpha/2} \times \sqrt{R_1/T_1 + R_2/T_2}$ (when $\alpha = 0.05$, $z_{\alpha/2} = 1.96$). If this confidence interval contains the value zero (0), it can be concluded that the two rates are not significantly different. If the confidence limits are both negative (less than 0), then it can be concluded that $R_2 > R_1$. Conversely, we could conclude that $R_2 > R_1$, if both the lower and upper confidence limits are bigger than 0.

Ratio of rates

The rate ratio is simply the ratios of the rates in the two groups. The rate ratio is sometimes called the incidence rate ratio. It is given by $RR = \dfrac{R_1/T_1}{R_2/T_2}$. To obtain a confidence interval for the rate ratio, it is necessary to consider the log of the rate ratio. The standard error[11] of the log of the rate ratio is $se\big(\log(RR)\big) = \sqrt{\dfrac{1}{Y_1} + \dfrac{1}{Y_2}}$. A $100 \times (1 - \alpha)\%$ confidence interval for the log of the rate ratio is given by $\log(RR) \pm z_{\alpha/2} \sqrt{\dfrac{1}{Y_1} + \dfrac{1}{Y_2}}$.

Exponentiating the lower and upper endpoints gives the confidence interval for the rate ratio. If the confidence interval contains the value 1, then it can be concluded that the two rates are not statistically different, i.e. $R_1 = R_2$. If the confidence limits are both less than 1, then it can be concluded that $R_2 > R_1$. Conversely, we could conclude that $R_1 > R_2$, if both the lower and upper confidence limits are less than 1.

Hypothesis test for a rate ratio

The null hypothesis is that the rates in the two groups are equal, or equivalently that the rate ratio is 1. This can be tested using a z-statistic $z = \dfrac{\log(RR)}{se\big(\log(RR)\big)}$, which is then compared against a standard normal distribution to obtain p-values[11].

While the rate ratio is often harder to interpret than the difference in rates, it is usually easier to use for statistical modelling. In addition, the regression techniques considered later in this chapter are based on rate ratios rather than differences in rates.

Example

The New Zealand rugby union study aimed to compare differences in the overall rate of injury from 1996–2000 with that in 2001–2005. There were 17 injuries in 1996–2000 and eight in 2001–05. This appears to be a reasonably large reduction. The total number of player years for 1996–00 was 635 000 and 630 000 for 2001–05.

The difference in the rate of injuries per 100 000 players per year for the two groups is $(8/630000 - 17/635000) \times 100000 = -1.4$. In other words, there are 1.4 fewer injuries per 100 000 players per year from 2001–05 compared to 1996–2000.

The standard error of the difference is 0.79 injuries per 100 000 players per year, which gives a 95% confidence interval from −3.0 to 0.1 injuries per 100 000 players per year. The interpretation of this is that with 95% confidence, there were between 3.0 fewer injuries and up to 0.1 more injuries per 100 000 players per year in 2001–05 than from 1996–2000. Thus the introduction of the preventive programme in 2001 had no significant effect on overall spinal injuries.

For scrum-related injuries, the difference in rates was −1.3 with a 95% confidence interval of −2.2 to −0.3 injuries per 100 000 players per year. In other words, there were 1.3 fewer injuries per 100 000 players per year in 2001–05, and with 95% confidence there were between 0.3 and 2.2 fewer injuries per 100 000 players per year. Thus, the introduction of the preventive programme in 2001 did appear to have a significant reduction on the rate of scrum-related injuries.

The rate ratio for 2001–05 versus 1996–2000 is $RR = \dfrac{8/630000}{17/635000} = 0.47$. The standard error of the log of the rate ratio is $\sqrt{1/8 + 1/17} = 0.43$. A 95% confidence interval for the log rate ratio is then $\log(0.47) \pm 1.96 \times 0.43$ or −1.59 to 0.09. Exponentiating the lower and upper limits gives a 95% confidence interval for the rate ratio as 0.20–1.10.

With 95% confidence, the injury rate from 2001 to 2005 was as much as 80% lower than that between 2001 and 2005, but may have been up to 10% higher.

For scrum-related injuries, the rate ratio is 0.11, with 95% confidence interval of 0.11–0.88.

To test the hypothesis that the spinal injury rates in 2001–05 and 1996–2000 are equal, the test-statistic is $z = \log(0.47)/0.43 = -1.73$, which gives a p-value of 0.08, indicating that there is no strong evidence that the rates are different between the two time periods.

For scrum-related injuries, the test statistic is $z = \log(0.11)/1.05 = 2.08$, which gives a p-value of 0.04, indicating evidence that the rate of scrum-injuries were lower in 2001–05 compared with 1996–2000.

Confounding

Confounding arises when an observed difference in outcomes is actually due to some factor other than the intervention being assessed. For example, in a two group comparative trial, one group (e.g. team of players) may be older with more years of playing experience than the comparison group and may have a lower injury rate solely because of this, rather than due to the intervention they received. Confounding is less likely to be an issue in randomized controlled trials than in other studies of effectiveness, such as pre-post designs, since in randomized controlled trials both known and unknown confounders should be equally distributed across the arms of the trial because of the randomization.

Example

In the soccer data, the rate of injuries in high-skilled players is 6.9 injuries per 1000 h and in low-skilled players it is 12.5 per 1000 h; the rate ratio (low- vs. high- skill) is 1.81 (95% CI: 1.08–3.03). There is evidence that the injury rate is higher. However, examination of Table 14.2 and Table 14.5 suggests that type of play (either game or practice) is a possible confounder. For both skill-levels, injury rates are much higher in games than in practice sessions. Secondly, the proportion of time spent in practice games is much higher in the high-skill players than the low-skill players and this confounds the exposure measure. We use this example to illustrate two approaches to adjustment for confounding.

Mantel–Haenszel methods

Mantel–Haenszel methods enable the estimation of the rate ratio that adjusts for confounding. In the soccer example, game type is a potential confounder with two levels or strata (game or practice). Mantel–Haenszel methods can be used to adjust for a confounder with more than two

Table 14.5 Rates of injury and confidence interval by skill level and type of play for 55 soccer players

Type of play	Rate per 1000 h (95% CI)
Game	
High-skilled	19.8 (11.1–32.6)
Low-skilled	20.7 (12.8–31.6)
Practice	
High-skilled	4.1 (2.2–6.8)
Low-skilled	5.7 (2.3–11.7)

From Poulsen et al.[9]

levels, but if there is more than one potential confounder of interest, Poisson regression would be used instead.

The soccer injury dataset may be stratified into S 2×2 tables, where S is the number of levels of the stratifying variable. Each 2×2 table is of the form depicted in Table 14.6[11].

The Mantel $\times$ Haenszel method weights the stratum specific rate ratios to produce a combined rate ratio[11]. In the soccer example, it weights the rate ratios of low- to high-skilled players in the game and practice strata. The total exposure in each stratum can be written as $T_i = T_{1i} + T_{2i}$ and the total number of events as $Y_i = Y_{1i} + Y_{2i}$. The weight for each stratum is $w_i = \dfrac{Y_{2i} \times T_{1i}}{T_i}$. The Mantel–Haenszel rate ratio is given by $RR_{\text{Mantel–Haenszel}} = \dfrac{\sum_i w_i RR_i}{\sum_i w_i}$[11]. The standard error is again best calculated on a log-scale. It is given by $se\log RR_{\text{Mantel–Haenszel}} = \sqrt{\dfrac{\sum_i Y_i \times T_{1i} \times T_{2i} / T_i^2}{\left(\sum_i w_i RR_i\right) \times \sum_i w_i}}$[11].

Note that one weakness of the Mantel–Haenszel method is that it allows only for the control of one categorical confounder, such as level of play or sex, e.g. it cannot handle a potential confounder such as age in years or multiple confounders.

Examples

The rate ratio of low- to high-skilled players for games is $(21/1015)/(15/759) = 1.05$. For the practice stratum, the rate ratio is $(7/1231)/(14/3440) = 1.40$. The weight for the game stratum is $(15 \times 1015)/(759 + 1015) = 8.58$; for the practice stratum it is $(14/1231)/(3440 + 1231) = 3.69$. Thus, the Mantel–Haenszel rate ratio is $RR_{\text{Mantel–Haenszel}} = \dfrac{(8.58 \times 1.05 + 3.69 \times 1.40)}{(8.58 + 3.69)} = 1.15$.

The interpretation of this is that the injury rate is about 15% higher in the low-skilled players than in the high-skilled players, after adjusting for type of play; a 95% confidence interval for the rate ratio is 0.68–1.97, indicating that this is not a significantly higher injury rate.

Table 14.6 Structure of each 2×2 table in a Mantel–Haenszel test

Stratum i	Injuries	Exposure	Rate
Group 1	Y_{1i}	Y_{1i}	$R_{1i} = Y_1/T_{1i}$
Group 2	Y_{2i}	Y_{2i}	$R_{2i} = Y_2/T_{2i}$

Adapted from Kirkwood & Sterne[11].

The hypothesis test that the combined rate ratio = 1 has test statistic 0.25, which gives a p-value of 0.6 when compared to a chi-squared distribution with 1 degree of freedom. There is no evidence of a difference in injury rates between low- and high-skilled players once type of play is controlled for. This result is consistent with the confidence interval interpretation in the previous paragraph.

Poisson regression

The regression approach to sports-injury research allows greater flexibility than the approaches that have been considered so far. As with the previous methods, it allows the comparison of groups but it is also able to control for multiple confounding, including continuous confounders.

A key idea[11] behind the Poisson regression model is that the rate ratio defined earlier may be rewritten as: rate in exposed group = rate in baseline group × rate ratio.

The baseline group can often be thought as the unexposed group, or as the referent group, against which other groups are compared. Alternatively, on a log scale, which is used for the purposes of fitting the model in statistical software, this may be written as: log rate in exposed group = log(rate in baseline group) + log(rate ratio).

More generally, Poisson regression fits models of the form $\log (\text{rate}) = \beta_0 + \beta_1 x_1 + ... + \beta_p x_p$. The p independent or predictor variables $x_1,...,x_p$ can be either continuous or discrete variables.

Poisson regression is a special case of a generalised linear model, and some computer software (e.g. SAS) fits Poisson regression models using this more general type of model. When fitting a Poisson regression using generalized linear models, the exposure time for each group is entered into the model as an offset.

The significance of the terms in a model can also be assessed in Poisson regression. Many computer programmes will give a p-value based on a Wald-test for variables in the model[11].

Example

For the New Zealand rugby union data, a Poisson regression model is fitted to the data for all spinal injuries, in which the period 1996–2000 is the baseline, and the exposed group is the period 2001–05. The results are displayed in Table 14.7.

From the output, we can see that the rate ratio for the period from 2001–05 is exp(−0.746) = 0.47. The rate for the period 1996–2000 is exp(−10.258) × 100,000 = 3.5 injuries per 100 000 players per year, and it is exp(−10.258 − 0.746) × 100,000 = 3.5 × 0.47 = 1.7 injuries per 100 000 players per year in for the period 2001–05. Finally, taking antilogs of the confidence interval above gives a 95% confidence interval from 0.20 to 1.10. This is the same as found previously with the same data. Note that the p-value of 0.08, which is based on a Wald-test, indicates that the difference between periods is not significant.

Table 14.7 Poisson regression output for NZ rugby union data

	Coefficient	Standard error	Z	P > |z|	95% CI Lower	Upper
2001–05	−0.746	0.429	−1.74	0.08	−1.59	0.094
Constant*	−10.258	0.243	−43.41	0.000	−11.0	−10.1

*corresponds to the baseline in this example
NZ: New Zealand

Example

We can also fit a Poisson regression model to the soccer data to control for confounding. The model is fit with two predictor variables: skill level and type of play. The output, displayed as rate ratios, is displayed in Table 14.8.

The rate ratio and 95% confidence interval for low- versus high-skilled players from the Poisson regression are almost identical to those generated from the Mantel–Haenszel estimates. This is the rate ratio in which one type of play has been controlled for. In addition, it is clear that practice play has a much lower rate of injury than game play, as shown in Table 14.2 (after controlling for skill level). If skill level is removed from the model, the rate ratio for practice versus game is 0.22.

Example

A Poisson regression model was fitted to the rugby headgear data, with the control group as the referent group. The results are displayed in Table 14.9.

Neither of the modified or standard headgear arms is significantly different to the control arm. It is also of interest to see whether there is variation in rates among the three arms of the trial. A computer package can be used to perform a Wald test to see if the rates vary. The test statistic is 2.65, which gives a p-value of 0.27 when compared with a chi-squared distribution with two degrees of freedom. Note that there are two degrees of freedom because the variable trial arm has three levels. Also, the individual p-values given in Table 14.9 compare the specific groups (modified and standard) individually against the control arm, which is the reference group in the regression.

Clustering

Clustering is a common problem in sports-injury research[13]. In a cluster-randomized trial, teams or clubs are typically randomized to intervention arms, rather than individual players. Because players from the same team tend to be more similar than players from different teams, data within each cluster are likely to be correlated. This correlation needs to be taken into account when analysing cluster-randomized trials and other studies where players are recruited on the basis of their teams. The reason for this is that estimates of variances, such as standard errors, are likely to be too small if clustering is not accounted for. There are many different approaches to analysing cluster randomised trials. In this chapter, three methods will be discussed.

Robust standard errors

One of the simplest ways to account for clustering is to use robust standard errors in the regression model. Methods based on robust standard errors use between-cluster information. Robust standard errors tend to be larger than standard errors that ignore clustering, although their use

Table 14.8 Poisson regression output for soccer data

	Rate ratio	z	P>|z|	95% CI	
				Lower	Upper
Low skill	1.16	0.52	0.603	0.67	1.99
Practice	0.23	−5.07	<0.0001	0.13	0.41

Table 14.9 Results of Poisson regression model for rugby headgear data

	Rate ratio*	z	P > |z|	95% CI	
				Lower	Upper
Modified	1.10	0.66	0.512	0.82	1.48
Standard	0.84	−1.01	0.312	0.60	1.18

*relative to the control group

will not affect parameter estimates – e.g. they will not affect the rate ratio itself, but will affect the width of its confidence interval. The number of clusters that need to be used should be reasonably large (30 or more)[11].

Generalized estimating equations

Generalized estimating equations provide one way of obtaining valid inferences for clustered data. Models that use generalized estimating equations are sometimes called marginal models. These models only make assumptions about the average response and do not make further assumptions about the distribution of the responses. Generalized estimating equations also make it possible to fit models that do not assume that individuals within a cluster are independent. This approach uses the method of robust standard errors as part of its model fitting.

Example

Table 14.10 gives the rate ratios and confidence limits for the rugby headgear study ignoring and accounting for clustering; the results adjusting for clustering are from McIntosh et al.[2]

   While the rate ratios are the same ignoring and accounting for clustering (note that this only applies to the modified data in Table 14.10), the confidence interval is much wider when clustering is accounted for. The robust standard error of the log rate ratio for modified headgear is about 0.23, whereas the standard error that ignores clustering is about 0.15. There is also a large number of clusters in the study (169 teams in total), which meets one of the conditions for the use of robust standard errors.

Multilevel models and random-effects models

Random effects models are also known as mixed, multilevel, or hierarchical models. In sports-injury studies, individuals (at the lowest level of the hierarchy) are typically part of a sports team, which can be thought of as the second, or a higher, level. It is possible to have further levels in the model, such as club or geographical district.

Table 14.10 Rate ratios and confidence limits for rugby headgear study ignoring and accounting for clustering

	Ignoring clustering			Accounting for clustering		
	Rate ratio*	95% CI		Rate ratio*	95% CI	
		Lower	Upper		Lower	Upper
Modified	1.10	0.82	1.48	1.10	0.71	1.72
Standard	0.84	0.60	1.18	0.23	0.51	1.38

*relative to control group

The simplest random-effects model allows the average rate to vary randomly across clusters (hence the name random effects). One desirable feature of random effects models is that they allow both cluster and individual level covariates to be estimated. For example, individual covariates might include a player's weight and playing position, while team-level covariates might include the playing grade of the team.

Example

For the analysis of the Finnish floorball study, a random-effects model was fitted to the data (this analysis was described by the authors as a 'two-level Poisson regression' model)[3]. For the outcome of non-contact leg injuries, the rate ratio – without adjusting for confounders or clustering – was 0.31 with a 95%CI of 0.17–0.58. When a random-effects model adjusting for confounders and clustering was fitted, the rate ratio was 0.34 (95%CI: 0.20–0.57)[3]. Covariates in the model were both at the individual level (age, body mass index, floorball experience, playing position, and number of orthopaedic operations) and the cluster level (league and previous incidence of injuries)[3].

Intra-cluster correlation coefficient

The intra-cluster correlation coefficient (ICC) is a measure of the degree of clustering. It is defined as the ratio of the between cluster variance to the total variance. It is zero when there is no clustering, and 1 if there is no within cluster variability. In the latter case, all of the observed variation is due to the clustering.

Values of the intra-cluster correlation will vary depending on the outcome of interest. For example, the ICC was almost zero (0.004) for knee-ligament injuries but was 0.059 for ankle-ligament injuries in the Finnish floorball study[3]. In the handball study[1], ICCs varied from 0.043 to 0.071.

Implications for sample size

Clustering can have a large impact on the sample size required to conduct a study, and needs to be considered when designing an effectiveness study.

Sample-size calculations of cluster randomized trials are typically based on those for individually randomized trials, but are adjusted to account for clustering. For an individually randomized trial, suppose that the rate in the control groups R_1 and that it is desired that the rate in the intervention group will be R_2 The anticipated rate in the control group can usually be estimated from previous descriptive studies on the incidence of the injury and sport being examined.

For a two-sided test with significance level α and power of $100(1-\beta)$% the exposure-time required in both groups is $(z_{\alpha/2}+z_\beta)^2 (R_1+R_2)/(R_1-R_2)^2$ [14]. For a test with $\alpha=0.05$, $z_{0.025}=1.96$. If the desired power is 90%, $\beta=0.1$ and $z_\beta=1.28$; for desired power of 80%, and $\beta=0.2$ and $z_\beta=0.84$.

If it is planned to design a cluster trial, and if the true ICC is ρ and the average cluster size is $\bar{m}$ then the necessary sample size (exposure time) is;

exposure time required from individually randomized trial $\times (1+(m-1)\rho)$.

The term $(1+(m-1)\rho)$ is often called the inflation factor or the design effect[13, 15]. Note that if individuals are randomized, then the average cluster size is 1, and so the inflation factor is 1.0.

The inflation factor can have large implications for required sample sizes. For example, in the design of the handball study[1], the trial was designed with a cluster size of 15 and $\rho=0.07$ giving an inflation factor of approximately 2. In other words, the required sample sized for the cluster-randomized trial of the 915 players per group, was twice that of an individually randomized trial.

Emery [15] discusses the design of a trial to reduce ankle-injuries in high-school basketball[8]. The trial was designed assuming $\rho = 0.006$ and $\bar{m} = 26$, which gives an inflation factor of 1.15. However, the actual ICC calculated from the analysis of the trial was $\rho = 0.06$, meaning that the inflation factor was 2.5[15].

It is important that ICCs are reported in cluster-randomized trials, so that future researchers are able to estimate the potential effects on sample size based on realistic data[8, 15]. This will allow future researchers to design studies that have sufficient power to detect clinically important effects of interventions on the incidence of sports injuries.

However, even with good estimates of ICCs, it is always sensible to estimate the sample size under a range of values for the ICCs. Additionally, ICCs should also be reported for other study types that involve clustering, such as ecological studies (e.g. [6]).

Example

Suppose that the rate of injuries among soccer players is 0.1 per player per year, and it is hoped that an exercise programme can reduce the rate by 50% to 0.05 injuries per player per year. Researchers wish to conduct a trial with significance level of $\alpha = 0.05$ and power of 90%. If the study is individually randomized, the required sample size is $(1.96 + 1.28)^2 \times (0.1 + 0.05)/(0.1 - 0.05)^2 = 631$ player-years per trial arm.

If the trial is cluster randomized, assuming 11 players per team and $\rho = 0.05$, the inflation factor is 1.5, giving a required sample size of 946 player-years. In other words, 86 teams per trial arm would need to be recruited.

If, however, $\rho = 0.01$, the inflation factor is 1.10, giving a required sample size of 694 player years. In other words, 64 teams per trial arm would need to be recruited.

Coefficient of variation

An alternative approach to estimating sample sizes in cluster-randomized trials is based on the coefficient of variation[14]. For a sports-injury intervention, the coefficient of variation can be thought of as the standard deviation of the team rates divided by the mean of the team rates.

The coefficient of variation can be used to calculate sample sizes for cluster-randomized trials. Let y denote the total number of hours of follow-up per cluster or team, and k denote the coefficient of variation. For example, y might denote the number of game hours multiplied by the number of players in a team for an entire season. The number of clusters required is given by $1 + (z_{\alpha/2} + z_\beta)^2 \left[(R_1 + R_2)/y + k^2 (R_1^2 + R_2^2) \right] (R_1 - R_2)^2$ [14]. Note that this formula gives equivalent sample sizes to the formula above when the coefficient of variation is zero (except for the 1 in the formula)[14].

The paper [14] gives details on how to calculate the coefficient of variation from data. It can be obtained from a cohort study that has information on injury rates by team.

Example

A study is being conducted to reduce knee injuries in Australian Football players through exercise[10]. The study will be randomized at a team level. Data from a previous study indicates that the rate of all injuries in Australian Football players is about 60 injuries per 1 000 playing hours and that about one-third of these are knee injuries, so that the incidence of knee injuries is about 20 per 1 000 playing hours[10, 16]. It is hoped that the exercise programme will reduce injuries by 35%.

Ignoring any clustering, to have 80% power to detect the reduction in injuries by 35% and with significance level $\alpha = 0.05$ of the number of hours of exposure in intervention and control arms needed is $(1.96 + 0.84)^2 \times (0.02 + 0.013)/(0.02 + 0.013)^2 = 5286$ hours. The number of hours of exposure that each team contributes per season is 600 game-hours; this is based on 18 players per team, matches lasting for 100 minutes, and 20 games within a season. Therefore 8.8 teams per arm of the trial will be needed, but this ignores team-based clustering.

An estimate of the coefficient of variation for injuries in Australian Football is $0.35[16,10]$. Therefore the number of clusters or teams required per arm of the trial is $1 + (1.96 + 0.84)^2 \times \left[(0.02 + 0.013)/600 + 0.35^2(0.02^2 + 0.013^2) \right] (0.02 - 0.013)^2 = 21$. The design effect in this case is about 2.38; this partly reflects the large team sizes of 18 in Australia Football.

Conclusion

This chapter has focused on the analysis of randomized trials and intervention studies in sports research. These studies aim to reduce the incidence of sports-related injuries through the use of interventions.

The methods described in the chapter have focussed on the statistical analysis of rates, and the comparison of rates between two or more groups. The chapter has developed analyses in increasing order of sophistication. The first described were analyses of a single rate. The comparison of rates between two or more groups was discussed, such as would arise in an individually randomized study. Mantel–Haenszel methods and Poisson regression methods, which allow for adjustment for potential confounders, were discussed next. Finally, methods that allow for the analysis of clustered data, including cluster-randomized trials, have been discussed.

This chapter has focussed on injury rates as the outcome rather than other measures such as player behaviour, knowledge, or attitudes. The general approaches used here also largely apply to these other sorts of trials, although these studies may use statistical techniques such as logistic regression in their analysis because the outcome variable may be a proportion rather than a rate. However, these types of studies also require appropriate adjustment in analyses to handle clustering, such as clustering or team or club. An example of such a trial, with cluster assessment, is the study of Eime et al.[6].

This chapter has also emphasized the importance of reporting of measures such as intra-cluster correlations for studies with clustering by team or club. The need for such data is particularly important when designing future cluster-randomized trials, which need good estimates of clustering to ensure adequate sample sizes to detect the hypothesized differences.

References

1. Olsen O-E, Myklebust G, Engebretsen L, Holme I, Bahr R (2005). Exercises to prevent lower limb injuries in youth sports: cluster randomised controlled trial. *BMJ*, **330**(7489), 449–56.
2. McIntosh AS, McCrory P, Finch CF, Best JP, Chalmers DJ, Wolfe R (2009). Does padded headgear prevent head injury in rugby union football?. *Med Sci Sports Exerc*, **41**(2), 306–13.
3. Pasanen K, Parkkari J, Pasanen M, Hiilloskorpi H, Makinen T, Jarvinen M, Kannus P (2008). Neuromuscular training and the risk of leg injuries in female floorball players: cluster randomised controlled study. *Br J Sports Med*, **42**, 502–5.
4. Finch C, Braham R, McIntosh A, McCrory P, Wolfe R (2005). Should football players wear custom fitted mouthguards? Results from a group randomised controlled trial. *Inj Prev*, **11**(4), 242–6.
5. Quarrie KL, Gianotti SM, Hopkins WG, Hume PA (2007). Effect of nationwide injury prevention programme on serious spinal injuries in New Zealand rugby union: ecological study. *BMJ*, **334**(7604), 1150–3.

6. Eime E, Finch C, Wolfe R, Owen N, McCarty C (2005). The effectiveness of a squash eyewear promotion strategy. *Br J Sports Med,* **39**, 681–5.

7. Iversen MD, Friden C (2008). Pilot study of female high school basketball players' anterior cruciate ligament injury knowledge, attitudes, and practices. *Scand J Med Sci Sport,* DOI: 10.1111/j.1600-0838.2008.00817.x.

8. Emery CA, Rose MS, McAllister JR, Meeuwisse WH (2007). A prevention strategy to reduce the incidence of injury in high school basketball: A cluster randomized controlled trial. *Clin J Sport Med,* **17**(1), 17–24.

9. Poulsen TD, Freund KG, Madsen F, Sandvej K (1991). Injuries in high-skilled and low-skilled soccer: a prospective study. *Br J Sports Med,* **25**(3), 151–3.

10. Finch C, Lloyd D, Elliott B (2009). The preventing australian football injuries with exercise (PAFIX) study: a group randomised controlled trial. *Inj Prev,* **15**, e1.

11. Kirkwood BR, Sterne JAC (2003). *Essential medical statistics. 2nd edition.* Blackwell, Oxford.

12. Ulm K (1990). Simple method to calculate the confidence interval of a standardized mortality ratio (SMR). *Am J Epidemiol,* **131**(2), 373–5.

13. Hayen A (2006). Clustered data in sports research. *J Sci Med Sport,* **9**(1–2), 165–8.

14. Hayes RJ, Bennett S (1999). Simple sample size calculation for cluster-randomized trials. *Int J Epidemiol,* **28**(2), 319–26.

15. Emery CA (2007). Considering Cluster Analysis in Sport Medicine and Injury Prevention Research. *Clin J Sport Med,* **17**(3), 211–14.

16. Finch C, Costa AD, Stevenson M, Hamer P, Elliott B (2002). Sports injury experiences from the Western Australian sports injury cohort study. *Austr NZ J Publ Heal,* **26**(5), 462–7.

Chapter 15

Cost-effectiveness studies

Judith Bosmans, Martijn Heymans,
Maarten Hupperets, and Maurits van Tulder

A variety of preventive, diagnostic, and therapeutic interventions is commonly used in sports medicine. An increasing number of randomized trials has evaluated the effectiveness of these interventions. Sports injuries have a huge financial impact on society, because of the costs of the interventions and the costs associated with production loss due to work absenteeism and disablement as a result of sports injuries[1, 2]. It is important to obtain insight into the efficiency or cost-effectiveness of sports medicine interventions. Economic evaluations may help policy-makers in their decision to include an intervention in the public health insurance system and they may help health professionals and patients to make decisions in clinical practice. A more efficient use of limited financial resources results in optimal care for more individuals. As yet, only a few full economic evaluations in the field of sports medicine have been published[3]. This chapter discusses the theory and methodology underlying economic evaluations in sports medicine in an attempt to improve the quality of future economic evaluations in this field.

What is an economic evaluation?

An economic evaluation can be defined as the comparative analysis of two or more alternative interventions in terms of both their costs and consequences[2]. The main tasks involved in any economic evaluation are identifying, measuring, valuing, and comparing these costs and consequences. Economic evaluations can be subdivided into partial evaluations and full evaluations. Most economic evaluations are partial evaluations, in which only the costs (cost of illness study) or costs and effects (cost-outcome description) of one intervention are described, or in which the costs of two or more interventions (cost analysis) are compared. Only with full economic evaluations – in which the costs and effects of two or more interventions are compared – can questions about efficiency be answered. This chapter focusses on full economic evaluations performed alongside randomized controlled trials.

The four most commonly used methods of full economic evaluations are: cost-effectiveness, cost-utility, cost-minimization, and cost–benefit analysis. The designs of these studies are similar, the main difference is the type of outcome measure that is used to determine efficiency. In a cost-effectiveness analysis the outcomes of the alternative interventions are expressed as disease-specific effects (e.g. pain, functioning, severity of injury). In a cost–utility analysis, the outcomes of the interventions are expressed in a measure that combines quality and quantity of life (health-utility measure). The most well-known example of such a measure is the quality-adjusted life-year (QALY). In a cost-minimization analysis the clinical effects of the alternatives are considered to be equal and, therefore, only the costs of the interventions are compared. The relative simplicity of this analysis may seem attractive. However, Briggs and O'Brien showed that only when a study has been specifically designed to show the equivalence of treatments, a cost-minimization analysis is appropriate[4]. In a cost–benefit analysis both costs and effects of the interventions are expressed in monetary units. An intervention is considered efficient if the benefits outweigh the costs. However, measuring clinical benefits in monetary units presents substantial difficulties.

Design of an economic evaluation

An economic evaluation can be conducted alongside a randomized controlled trial or be based on a decision-model. Decision-models are particularly suited to modelling chronic diseases, where it is not possible to prospectively measure long-term outcomes. For example, if you want to evaluate the cost-effectiveness of a lifestyle programme for obese children to prevent chronic diseases (e.g. diabetes or cardiovascular disease) in the long term, you might need to follow these children for the rest of their life. Economic evaluations in the area of sports-injury medicine will usually focus on short-term effects and be conducted alongside randomized controlled trials. In this case, the term 'piggy-back' economic evaluation is often used. Advantages of this approach are that (i) having patient-specific data on both costs and effects is attractive for analysis and internal validity and (ii) given the large fixed costs in performing a randomized controlled trial the marginal costs of collecting economic data may be modest[3]. However, there are a number of issues that have to be taken into account when linking an economic evaluation to a randomized controlled trial. The most important of these issues are considered below. All concepts are illustrated using a recent randomized controlled trial evaluating the cost-effectiveness of an unsupervised proprioceptive balance-board training programme as compared to usual care to prevent ankle sprain recurrences in people who had sustained a lateral ankle sprain up to 2 months prior to inclusion[5].

Perspective

Different perspectives can be adopted in an economic evaluation. The perspective chosen determines what costs and effects are considered in the economic evaluation and to what extent the data can be generalised to other settings. Possible perspectives for an economic evaluation are the societal perspective, the health-care insurer's perspective, the health-care provider's perspective, or the company's perspective. The societal perspective is the broadest, meaning that all relevant costs and effects are considered, regardless of who pays or who benefits from the effects. Which perspective is chosen depends on the costs and outcomes that are relevant for the decision-maker. However, in general the societal perspective is recommended[2, 6]. When a narrower perspective is required, presenting results from both the societal perspective and the narrower perspective is recommended.

Choice of control treatment

To determine the cost-effectiveness of an intervention a comparison should be made with one or more alternatives. In an economic evaluation from a societal perspective the question to be answered is: 'What is the cost-effectiveness of replacing existing sports medicine practice with the intervention under study?' To answer this question, the intervention under study should be compared with existing clinical practice. Comparison of the new intervention with an intervention that is not considered part of existing clinical practice can lead to misleading results. For example, comparison of a new painkiller for a tennis elbow with no treatment will make the new painkiller seem more cost-effective than it is in reality, because 'no treatment' does not resemble existing clinical practice. However, many studies in the field of sports medicine are concerned with preventing sports injuries. In these cases, 'doing nothing' will be the appropriate control treatment.

In intervention research, doing nothing is only seldom the relevant control treatment. Placebo is not considered a relevant control treatment, because this does not represent an acceptable treatment option in clinical practice. Therefore, an economic evaluation incorporating a placebo as control treatment is not informative to decision-makers in judging the cost-effectiveness of a new intervention in comparison with existing sports medicine practice.

The unsupervised proprioceptive balance-board training programme in the exemplary ankle-sprain trial was given in addition to usual care. After the ankle sprain all participants received usual care by choice of the athletes consisting of self-treatment and/or treatment by health-care providers according to existing clinical guidelines. At the end of usual care when participating in sports was again possible, participants allocated to the intervention group received the training programme aimed at preventing recurrent ankle sprains[5].

Identification, measurement, and valuation of effects

An important design-issue in economic evaluations is the choice of effect measures. Since economic evaluations are often performed alongside a randomized controlled trial, the primary outcomes of the trial should also be used in the economic evaluation, i.e. in the cost-effectiveness analysis. Generally, some or all of the following outcome measures are included in trials concerning sports injuries: pain intensity, physical functioning, number of prevented (re)injuries, recovery, and work disability. The choice for a particular primary outcome measure may vary across studies and depends on the type of sports injury at issue.

Quality of life refers to the emotional, social, and physical well-being of people and, therefore, is one of the main economic benefits of treatment. Quality of life is measured with specifically designed instruments. Disease-specific instruments focus on aspects of health status that are specific to an individual disease. Examples of disease-specific instruments are the Arthritis Impact Measurement Scale[7] and the Asthma Quality of Life Questionnaire[8]. An advantage of using disease-specific instruments is that they are sensitive to changes in the patient's health state; a disadvantage is that they give a restricted view on quality of life and cannot be used to compare interventions for different diseases. Generic quality-of-life instruments aim to give a comprehensive overview of the health-related quality of life of a patient and can be applied across different patient groups and diseases. Examples of such instruments are the SF-36[9] and the Nottingham Health Profile[10]. An important disadvantage of both generic and disease-specific instruments is that they do not produce a single quality-of-life score but provide scores on a number of different domains, i.e. a health profile. In contrast, preference-based instruments can be used to transform health states rated by patients into an index score. These values are called utilities and are anchored by 0 ('death') and 1 ('perfect health')[11]. Scores less than 0 are possible when a specific health state is considered worse than death. Brazier et al. recently developed a preference-based instrument, the SF-6D, using 11 questions from the SF-36[12]. In economic evaluations, the EQ-5D is probably the most widely used preference-based instrument; it consists of five domains (mobility, self-care, usual activity, pain/discomfort, and anxiety/depression) with three levels (no problems, some problems, and major problems)[13]. The EQ-5D has been translated into many languages and there are several value sets that are used to generate values for all possible 243[35] health states available (http://www.euroqol.org).

After obtaining the utilities, Quality Adjusted Life Years (QALYs) can be calculated by multiplying the utility of a particular health state with the time (in years) spent in this health state. The main advantage of QALYs is that both quality and quantity gains of an intervention are combined in one outcome measure. As stated before, QALYs are the main outcome in cost–utility analyses.

The primary outcome in the exemplary ankle-sprain trial was the number of recurrent ankle injuries in both groups within 12 months after the initial sprain. Secondary outcomes were the severity of the re-injury and the aetiology of the re-injury. This study focussed on the prevention of ankle-sprain recurrences, which probably does not have a substantial impact on quality of life. Therefore, quality of life was not included as an outcome measure in this economic evaluation.

Identification, measurement, and valuation of costs

One of the most important issues in the design of an economic evaluation is to decide which costs should be included in the economic evaluation and how these costs should be measured and valued. A societal perspective implies that all relevant costs are included. Costs are often subdivided into direct health-care costs, direct non-health-care costs, indirect health-care costs, and indirect non-health-care costs[14, 15]. Direct healthcare costs are costs of health care service use directly related to the disorder under study, such as costs of general practitioner care, computed tomographic (CT) scans, painkillers, and physiotherapy. Direct non-health-care costs are costs of care outside the formal health-care system that are directly related to the disorder under study. Examples of these costs are costs of over-the-counter medication, travel expenses to receive medical care, and informal care by family and friends. Indirect health-care costs include costs during life years gained, e.g. costs of treating unrelated heart problems after a life-saving operation after head trauma. These costs are hard to estimate and are often not incorporated in economic evaluations. In economic evaluations of sports medicine interventions, these indirect health-care costs will often not be relevant, because most interventions will not lead to an increase in life expectancy. Indirect non-health-care costs are costs of productivity-loss due to absenteeism from paid or unpaid work and to presenteeism (being present at work but working at a reduced capacity). These indirect costs often make up the largest part of total costs, especially in relatively healthy populations like those included in sports medicine trials. A different classification of costs has been proposed more recently: health-sector costs, patient/family costs, costs of productivity-loss, and costs in other sectors[2]. Since both classifications contain all possibly relevant costs, the choice for one of the classifications should not lead to differences in total societal costs, and, consequently, should not have any impact on the final results of the economic evaluation.

Clinical guidelines and descriptions of the care-process for the disorder under study can provide important information for deciding which costs should be included in an economic evaluation. Table 15.1 lists the costs that were included in the ankle sprain trial. Only direct health-care and indirect non-health-care costs were included in the trial; direct non-health-care and indirect health-care costs were not included.

Costs are estimated by multiplying health-care utilization with the appropriate prices. It is recommended that researchers report health-care-utilization data and costs separately. In this way readers can extrapolate the results to their own setting.

There are several ways in which health-care utilization can be measured. Health-care providers might be expected to give the most accurate and detailed information on health-care use by using their administrative systems. However, it seems realistic to assume that a patient with a sports-injury visits more than one health-care provider (e.g. general practitioner, physical therapist, orthopaedic surgeon) which means that many health-care providers should be approached for information[16]. Obtaining data from health-care insurers may be another potentially attractive method, but they are often unable to provide detailed resource-use information[17]. In addition, health-care insurers are often unable to report health-care utilization related to a specific disease or disorder. For example, health-care insurers may have registered the total number of visits to a physiotherapist in a specific year, but not the number of visits related to the ankle-sprain episode.

Table 15.1 Cost categories included in the exemplary ankle-sprain trial

Cost category	Price (€)
Direct health-care costs	
Intervention (per player)	27.50
General practitioner (per visit)	21.36
Physical therapist (per visit)	24.06
Sports physician (per visit)	68.17
Medical specialist (per visit)	71.92
Alternative therapist (per visit)	34.65
X-ray/cast (per unit)	43.58
Emergency room (per visit)	147.01
Drugs*	-
Medical devices	
Tape (per roll)	3.82
Brace (per unit)	86.49
Crutches (rent per week)	19.11
Indirect non-health-care costs	
Absenteeism from paid work (per hour)#	-
Absenteeism from unpaid work (per hour)	8.78

*Price depending on type of drug; #Price based on mean income of the Dutch population according to age and gender.

Moreover, neither health-care providers nor insurers can provide information on patient costs, costs of informal care, and productivity-loss. Especially in sport injuries, these costs may be an important part of the total costs. Therefore, in most studies patients themselves should be approached to obtain the necessary cost-information. Methods of self-report by patients include questionnaires, cost-diaries, and interviews. Questionnaires are less labour-intensive and, thus, more feasible than cost-diaries and interviews. However, questionnaires and interviews usually rely on momentary recall and, therefore, may be prone to recall bias; cost-diaries are completed prospectively over time, resulting in reduced recall error and more valid results. On the other hand, cost-diaries may be too burdensome for elderly or seriously ill patients[16, 17]. Van Den Brink et al. recently found only small differences between cost-diaries and questionnaires and concluded that questionnaires may replace cost-diaries for recall periods of up to 6 months[16].

The method that is eventually chosen depends very much on the patient population and disorder under study. In the exemplary ankle-sprain trial, participants who sustained a re-injury were asked to keep a cost-diary including the items listed in Table 15.1 to track health-care utilization and productivity-loss associated with the re-injury. Participants completed the cost-diary for the entire period from the re-injury until full recovery.

The next step is to value the resource-use data using appropriate cost prices. If the economic evaluation is conducted from a societal perspective the cost prices should reflect the opportunity-costs. This means that resources should be valued as the benefit foregone from not using these resources for their best alternative use[2, 6, 18]. Five alternative ways to obtain valid cost prices are distinguished: (i) prices derived from national registries; (ii) prices derived from health economics literature and previous research; (iii) standard costs; (iv) tariffs or charges; and (v) calculation of unit costs. An important advantage of using prices from national registries or previous research is that it is relatively easy to collect the data. However, only a limited set of prices may be available and it is often unclear how prices have been determined. The use of charges has the advantage that they are available for an extensive list of health-care services; an important disadvantage is that charges usually do not reflect the actual cost price, because they are based on negotiations. Estimation of unit costs is time consuming and should only be used for health-care services that have a substantial impact on the total costs and for which standard costs are not available. Standard costs are national average prices of health-care services and should be used when available to facilitate comparison of different studies from the same country[15].

Two approaches are used to calculate lost-productivity costs due to absenteeism from paid work: the Human Capital Approach (HCA) and the Friction Cost Approach (FCA). The first of these approaches assumes that productivity-loss occurs from the moment of absence until full recovery or, in the absence of recovery, until the moment of death or retirement and uses the real wages earned by patients to value absenteeism[19]. The HCA does not take into account the fact that for short-term absences production-loss is compensated for by the employee on his return to work or that for long-term absences the sick employee is replaced[2]. The FCA is based on the principle that production-loss is restricted to the time period needed to replace a sick employee (friction period). National mean wages according to age and gender are used to value the productivity-loss[20].

In the exemplary ankle-sprain trial, standard costs were used to value health-care-services utilization[15]. To calculate costs of absenteeism from paid work the friction-cost approach was used with a friction period of 4 months and using the mean age- and sex-specific income of the Dutch population[15, 20]. A friction period of 4 months is currently the recommended friction period in The Netherlands. The duration of the friction period may vary over time and from county to country. To value absenteeism from unpaid work, such as study and domestic work, a shadow price of €7.94/h was used. This shadow price reflects the hourly wage of a legally employed cleaner. Prices that were applied in the economic evaluation are included in Table 15.1.

Statistical analysis

In a full economic evaluation the costs and effects of two or more interventions are compared. The first step in the statistical analysis of an economic evaluation is to analyse costs and effects separately. The second step is to analyse the relation between the cost and effect differences between the treatments. In this chapter we will not discuss the statistical techniques that can be used to analyse the effects. For analysing costs and cost-effectiveness specific statistical techniques are needed. These are presented below.

Analysis of costs

For policy-makers the most informative measure of cost data is the arithmetic mean, because they can use the mean to estimate the total budget that is needed to treat all people with a certain disorder or sports injury (total budget = mean cost × number of patients)[21, 22]. The most commonly used statistical test to compare means between two groups is the independent t-test. However, cost-data typically have a highly skewed distribution as shown in Fig. 15.1. There are two reasons for this skewed distribution: (1) costs are bounded by zero meaning that costs cannot be negative and (2) most patients incur relatively low costs, while there is also a long right-hand tail that is caused by a small number of patients that incur high costs. This skewed distribution means that the normality assumption underlying the t-test is violated. Frequently used approaches

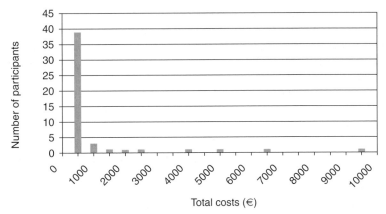

Fig. 15.1 Distribution of total costs in the exemplary ankle-sprain trial in participants with a re-injury.

to analyse cost-data are *t*-tests after log transformation or non-parametric tests such as the Mann–Whitney U-test. However, these methods do not compare the mean costs between the treatment groups and, therefore, are not suitable to analyse cost-data[21–23]. Non-parametric bootstrapping is considered the most appropriate method to analyse differences in costs; when using this method there is no need to make assumptions about the shape of the cost-distribution; instead, the observed distribution of the cost-data is used. Bootstrapping uses re-sampling to estimate an empirical sampling distribution of the statistic of interest.

Table 15.2 shows the mean (standard deviation) direct, indirect, and total costs in intervention and control participants with complete follow-up in the exemplary ankle-sprain trial. It can be seen from the large standard deviations in relation to the mean costs that the cost-distribution is very skewed. Direct costs in the intervention group were somewhat higher than in the control group. This is caused by inclusion of the costs of the balance-board training programme in the direct costs. Indirect and total costs in the intervention group were significantly lower than in the control group.

Incremental cost-effectiveness ratio

The differences in costs and effects between two interventions can be related to each other in an Incremental Cost-Effectiveness Ratio (ICER) which is calculated as $ICER = (C_i - C_c)/(E_i - E_c) = \Delta C/\Delta E$, where C_i = mean costs in the intervention group, C_c = mean costs in the control group, E_i = mean effects in the intervention group, and E_c = mean effects in the control group.

The ICER represents the additional cost of one extra unit of effect by an intervention compared to the next best alternative intervention, e.g. the additional costs of a balance-board training

Table 15.2 Mean (SD) costs in intervention and control participants with complete follow-up with mean differences (95% confidence interval)

Cost category	Intervention (*n* = 242)	Control (*n* = 243)	Difference (95% CI)*
Direct costs	31 (22)	18 (77)	13 (–1 to 21)
Indirect costs	6 (44)	123 (794)	–117 (–278 to –49)
Total costs	37 (60)	141 (827)	–104 (–271 to –27)

*95% confidence interval obtained by bootstrapping with 5000 replications.

programme in comparison with usual care to prevent one ankle-sprain recurrence. To be able to interpret an ICER, information is needed on the size and direction of the cost and effect differences[25]. Consider the following example: ICER = €250 per injury prevented by the intervention compared to usual care. This ICER can mean that the intervention costs €250 more to prevent one injury extra in comparison with usual care, but also that the intervention costs €250 less and results in one prevented injury less in comparison with usual care.

In the exemplary ankle-sprain trial, 10 (4%) participants in the intervention group and 39 (16%) participants in the control group (cases with complete follow-up) had a recurrent ankle sprain. Total costs were €37 in intervention participants and €141 in control participants. This leads to an ICER of €11 per percentage point which should be interpreted as: 1% improvement in the rate of recurrences of ankle sprains in the intervention group is associated with €11 lower costs in comparison with the control group. The number needed to treat to prevent one ankle sprain is 8.4, thus the prevention of one recurrent ankle sprain is associated with €876 lower costs.

Cost-effectiveness plane

To facilitate the interpretation of the ICER, the cost-effectiveness plane (CE plane) can be used[26]. In the cost-effectiveness plane the difference in effects between the two treatments is plotted on the horizontal axis and the difference in costs on the vertical axis resulting in four quadrants (Fig. 15.2). The origin represents the control treatment and the slope of the line through the origin and the plotted point estimates of ΔC and ΔE (point A) is equal to the incremental cost-effectiveness ratio. The four quadrants in the CE plane are described as follows:

- South-east quadrant (SE): the intervention is more effective and less costly than the control treatment and is considered dominant to the control treatment; the intervention should be adopted in favour of the control treatment.

- North-west quadrant (NW): the intervention is less effective and more costly than the control treatment and is dominated by the control treatment; the control treatment is preferred to the intervention.

- North-east quadrant (NE): the intervention is more effective and more costly than the control treatment; whether the intervention is adopted in favour of the control treatment depends on whether the ICER falls below the 'ceiling ratio' of the decision-maker (the maximum amount of money the decision-maker is willing to pay to gain one unit of effect extra). This ceiling ratio is indicated as λ in Fig. 15.2. In this case the intervention should be adopted in favour of the control treatment because the slope of the line through A (€250 per injury prevented) is smaller than λ (€400 per injury prevented).

- South-west quadrant: the intervention is less effective and less costly than the control treatment; whether the intervention is adopted in favour of the control treatment again depends on the value of the ceiling ratio (λ). The intervention is adopted if the ICER is larger than λ.

Uncertainty around ICERs

Because the ICER is a ratio, there is no mathematically tractable formula for the variance of the ICER, and confidence intervals cannot be estimated. There has been considerable debate on appropriate methods to estimate uncertainty surrounding the ICER and non-parametric bootstrapping is now considered the standard method to estimate this uncertainty[24, 27]. Samples of the same size as the original data are randomly drawn with replacement from the original

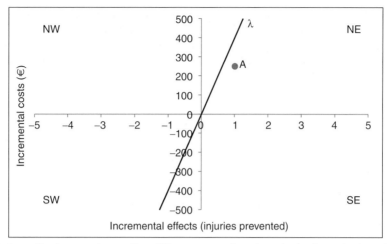

Fig. 15.2 Cost-effectiveness plane: effect differences are plotted on the horizontal axis and cost differences on the vertical axis. NE = north-east, SE = south-east, SW = south-west, and NW = north-west.

intervention and control data separately; next the ICER for this bootstrap replication is calculated. This process is repeated a large number of times to generate an empirical distribution of the ICER. At least 1000 bootstrap samples are needed, but with the fast computer speeds nowadays we recommend using 5000 samples[24, 27]. Each of the bootstrapped cost and effect differences from the bootstrapping process can be plotted on the CE plane. The point estimate of the ICER is always based on the observed cost and effect differences.

The CE plane in Fig. 15.3 shows the uncertainty around the ICER found in the ankle-sprain trial (complete cases). The CE plane shows that the intervention is more effective in preventing ankle-sprain recurrences than the control treatment and that the intervention is associated with lower costs than the control treatment.

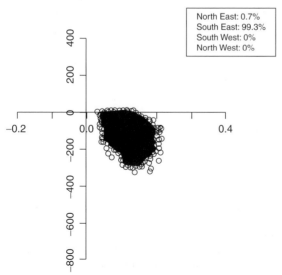

Fig. 15.3 Cost-effectiveness plane from the exemplary ankle-sprain trial. Costs are expressed in € and effects in the absolute number of ankle sprain recurrences prevented.

Decision uncertainty: cost-effectiveness acceptability curves

The traditional decision rule in economic evaluations is that the new intervention is adopted in favour of the control treatment if the ICER is smaller than the maximum amount of money the decision-maker is willing to pay to gain one unit of effect extra (ceiling ratio or λ). A decision-maker who is faced with the decision whether or not to reimburse a new intervention will be interested in the probability that the new intervention is cost-effective in comparison with the control treatment (e.g. usual care). This probability can be identified from the CE plane by determining the proportion of bootstrapped cost–effect pairs that fall to the south and east of a line with slope λ through the origin[28, 29]. However, the problem with λ is that its exact value is unknown. A solution is to vary λ between its logical bounds: zero and positive infinity. The probability that the intervention is cost-effective in comparison with the control treatment can be plotted against a range of λs in a cost-effectiveness acceptability curve (CEAC). Thus, the CEAC shows a decision-maker the probability that the intervention is cost-effective, in comparison with the control treatment, for various ceiling ratios. A policy-maker will decide to reimburse a new intervention if the probability of cost-effectiveness is considered high enough at a specific ceiling ratio. In this way the CEAC shows a decision-maker the probability that, if he decides to reimburse the new intervention, this will be the correct decision[2, 30].

Fig. 15.4 shows the CEAC for the exemplary ankle-sprain trial. This curve shows that for all possible values of the ceiling ratio the probability that the intervention is cost-effective in comparison with the control treatment is (almost) 1. Of course, this corresponds with the larger effects and smaller costs found in the intervention group as compared with the control group in this trial.

Net-benefit approach

To overcome the problems associated with the interpretation of ICERs Stinnett et al. proposed a simple rearrangement of the traditional cost-effectiveness decision rule[25]. According to the traditional decision rule a new intervention is deemed to be cost-effective in comparison with the control treatment if ICER < λ or $\Delta C/\Delta E < \lambda$. This formula can be rearranged to the alternative decision rule $\lambda \Delta E - \Delta C > 0$. Herein, $\lambda \Delta \dot{E} - \Delta C$ is called the net monetary benefit (NMB) of the new intervention in comparison with the control treatment. The new intervention should replace the control treatment when NMB is positive. The advantage of NMB is that it is a linear expression with a tractable variance and a much better behaved sampling distribution than the ICER [24, 47]. Because NMB relies on the value of λ and λ is generally unknown, NMB should be calculated for

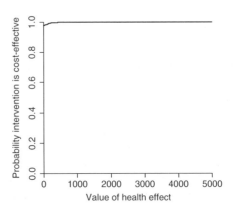

Fig. 15.4 Cost-effectiveness acceptability curve for ankle-sprain recurrences prevented.

various values of λ. NMB can also be used to estimate a CEAC. The points of the CEAC can be plotted by calculating for each value of λ the probability that NMB is positive[31]. The resulting CEAC will be the same as the one obtained based on the joint density of the cost and effect differences[24, 27].

Missing data

Even in the most carefully conducted randomized controlled trial there are likely to be data missing. Patients can (temporarily) drop out of a study or there may be occasional missing values on the resource level. When dealing with a data-set with incomplete data it is important to investigate the mechanism of the missing data. The data may be missing completely at random (MCAR) meaning that the missing values are not related to any other values (observed or unobserved). However, often the missing values will be related to the values of other observed variables. In this case, data are missing at random (MAR). If the missing values are related to values of unobserved variables, the data are missing not at random (MNAR)[32]. A complete case analysis is often used to deal with missing data in economic evaluations. This, however, reduces the power of the study and may bias the results if subjects with missing values are not a random subset of the complete study sample[33]. Simple imputation methods, such as mean imputation, conditional mean (regression) imputation, and last observation carried forwards do not give an adequate estimate of the missing values because the uncertainty surrounding the imputed estimates is not taken into account[33, 34]. Recent guidelines for economic evaluations recommend to impute missing data using multiple imputation techniques [35] that do take the imprecision caused by imputation of missing values into account[32]. One should realize that imputation does not improve the internal validity of an economic evaluation. A large proportion of missing data should be regarded as a fatal flaw in any study and efforts should be made to ensure low rates of missing values.

In the exemplary ankle-sprain trial, complete follow-up was available on the number of recurrent ankle sprains. However, 14 (25%) cost-diaries were missing in the intervention group and 23 (26%) in the control group. Multiple imputation according to the Multivariate Imputation by Chained Equations (MICE) algorithm was used to handle the missing data[36]. The cost difference in the pooled data sets after multiple imputation was −€103 (95% CI: −253 to −23) and the pooled effect difference 11% in the advantage of the intervention group. Fig. 15.5 shows the cost-effectiveness plane and cost-effectiveness curve for the pooled data sets. In this study with percentages of missing data of around 25%, the results of the complete case and imputed data analyses were very similar just like the study conclusions. Note, however, that this will not always be the case. If results between the complete case and the multiple imputed data analyses substantially differ, strong conclusions and recommendations are not justified.

Sensitivity analysis

Statistical methods for handling uncertainty relate only to uncertainty due to sampling variation. However, there will also be uncertainty that is associated with the assumptions and decisions made in performing the economic evaluation. To address this uncertainty sensitivity analysis is used, which involves systematic examination of the influence of uncertainties in the variables and assumptions employed in an economic evaluation on the estimated results[37]. The first step in performing a sensitivity analysis is to identify the uncertain parameters. In principle, all variables are potential candidates for a sensitivity analysis. Therefore, researchers should give arguments why certain variables were included in the sensitivity analysis and why others not. The second step is to specify the plausible range for the uncertain parameters. Methods for doing this are literature review, expert opinion, or using a specified confidence interval around the mean.

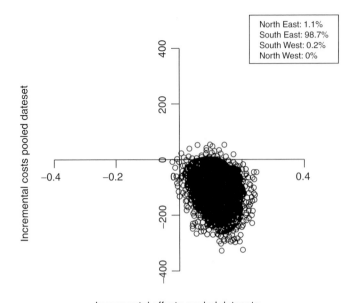

Fig. 15.5 Cost-effectiveness plane from the exemplary ankle sprain trial. Costs are expressed in €
and effects in the absolute number of ankle sprain recurrences prevented.

The third step is to perform the sensitivity analysis[3]. There are three main types of sensitivity
analysis[37]:

- One way sensitivity analysis: here the impact of each uncertain variable is examined separately
  by varying it across a plausible range of values while holding all other variables constant.
- Extreme scenario analysis: each variable is simultaneously set to its most optimistic or pessi-
  mistic value to generate a best- or worst-case scenario.
- Probabilistic sensitivity analysis: values of uncertain variables are allowed to vary simultaneously according to predefined distributions in a large number of Monte Carlo simulations.

To facilitate the interpretation of the results of the sensitivity analysis it is useful to present CEACs
for the different scenarios tested in the sensitivity analysis. For example, Miller et al. presented
both the main analysis and two different ways of dealing with missing data in one CEAC[38].

Critical assessment of economic evaluations

One of the most important questions when reading an economic evaluation is probably whether
the results are useful in a specific setting or not. To be able to answer this question it is necessary
that methods and results of an economic evaluation are reported in a transparent manner; there are
several reporting formats for economic evaluations[35, 39]. Checklists for the critical appraisal of
published papers can also be used as an instrument to improve the quality of a paper describing an
economic evaluation. One of these checklists is the CHEC-list[40]. This core set of items to critically
assess economic evaluations has been developed using a Delphi method among a group of international experts. Readers may use this CHEC-list to assess the risk of bias in published economic
evaluations. It may also be used to assess the quality of economic evaluations included in systematic
reviews and as a tool for authors to make economic evaluations more transparent, informative, and

Table 15.3 The CHEC-list for assessing the risk of bias of economic evaluations

1. Is the study population clearly described?
2. Are competing alternatives clearly described?
3. Is a well-defined research question posed in answerable form?
4. Is the economic study design appropriate to the stated objective?
5. Is the chosen time horizon appropriate in order to include relevant costs and consequences?
6. Is the actual perspective chosen appropriate?
7. Are all important and relevant costs for each alternative identified?
8. Are all costs measured appropriately in physical units?
9. Are costs valued appropriately?
10. Are all important and relevant outcomes for each alternative identified?
11. Are all outcomes measured appropriately?
12. Are outcomes valued appropriately?
13. Is an incremental analysis of costs and outcomes of alternatives performed?
14. Are all future costs and outcomes discounted appropriately?
15. Are all important variables, whose values are uncertain, appropriately subjected to sensitivity analysis?
16. Do the conclusions follow from the data reported?
17. Does the study discuss the generalizability of the results to other settings and patient/client groups?
18. Does the article indicate that there is no potential conflict of interest of study researcher(s) and funder(s)?

comparable. The CHEC-list is presented in Table 15.3. The focus of the CHEC-list is on economic evaluations alongside randomized controlled trials. Other methodological criteria are relevant when assessing the risk of bias of other designs, e.g. modelling studies or scenario-analyses. Clinicians, researchers, and policy-makers can use the CHEC-list to critically read a report of an economic evaluation and consequently be better able to value its merits.

Conclusion

The aim of this chapter was to provide insight into the design and analysis of economic evaluations in the field of sports medicine. Although mostly not life threatening, sports injuries are associated with high costs due to health-care utilization and disability. Therefore, it is important to have information on both costs and effects of interventions to treat or prevent sports injuries. Economic evaluations can provide this information by identifying the most efficient preventive or therapeutic interventions. However, if economic evaluations are to be used in the decision-making process by clinicians, policy-makers, or patients, it is of utmost importance that they provide valid and reliable information.

Most economic evaluations are conducted alongside a randomized controlled trial. In these cases the economic evaluation should be fully integrated into the randomized controlled trial and be equally carefully designed as the clinical trial. In particular, when designing the economic evaluation special attention has to be paid to the perspective of the economic evaluation, the identification, measurement, and valuation of costs and effects, the sample size, and the length of follow-up. When analysing the results of an economic evaluation specific statistical techniques are required to deal with the skewed cost distribution and the ICER.

References

1. Parkkari J, Kujala UM, Kannus P (2001). Is it possible to prevent sports injuries? Review of controlled clinical trials and recommendations for future work. *Sports Med*, **31**(14), 985–95.

2. Janda DH (1997). Sports injury surveillance has everything to do with sports medicine. *Sports Med*, **24**(3), 169–71.

3. Verhagen EA, van Tulder M, van der Beek AJ, Bouter LM, van Mechelen W (2005). An economic evaluation of a proprioceptive balance board training programme for the prevention of ankle sprains in volleyball. *Br J Sports Med*, **39**(2), 111–15.

4. Briggs AH, O'Brien BJ (2001). The death of cost-minimization analysis? *Health Econ*, **10**(2), 179–84.

5. Hupperets MD, Verhagen EA, van Mechelen W (2008). The 2BFit study: is an unsupervised proprioceptive balance board training programme, given in addition to usual care, effective in preventing ankle sprain recurrences? Design of a randomized controlled trial. *BMC Musculoskelet Disord*, **9**, 71.

6. Gold MR, Siegel JE, Russel LB, Weinstein MC (1996). *Cost-Effectiveness in Health and Medicine*. Oxford University Press, New York.

7. Meenan RF, Mason JH, Anderson JJ, Guccione AA, Kazis LE (1992). AIMS2. The content and properties of a revised and expanded Arthritis Impact Measurement Scales Health Status Questionnaire. *Arthritis Rheum*, **35**(1), 1–10.

8. Juniper EF, Guyatt GH, Epstein RS, Ferrie PJ, Jaeschke R, Hiller TK (1992). Evaluation of impairment of health related quality of life in asthma: development of a questionnaire for use in clinical trials. *Thorax*, **47**(2), 76–83.

9. Ware JE, Jr., Sherbourne CD (1992). The MOS 36-item short-form health survey (SF-36). I. Conceptual framework and item selection. *Med Care*, **30**(6), 473–83,

10. Hunt SM, McEwen J, McKenna SP (1985). Measuring health status: a new tool for clinicians and epidemiologists. *J R Coll Gen Pract*, **35**(273), 185–8.

11. Guyatt GH, Feeny DH, Patrick DL (1993). Measuring health-related quality of life. *Ann Intern Med*, **118**(8), 622–9.

12. Brazier J, Roberts J, Deverill M (2002). The estimation of a preference-based measure of health from the SF-36. *J Health Econ*, **21**(2), 271–92.

13. Brooks R (1996). EuroQol: the current state of play. *Health Policy*, **37**(1), 53–72.

14. McIntosh E, Luengo-Fernandez R (2006). Economic evaluation. Part 1: Introduction to the concepts of economic evaluation in health care. *J Fam Plann Reprod Health Care*, **32**(2), 107–12.

15. Oostenbrink JB, Koopmanschap MA, Rutten FF (2002). Standardisation of costs: the Dutch Manual for Costing in economic evaluations. *Pharmacoeconomics*, **20**(7), 443–54.

16. van den Brink M, van den Hout WB, Stiggelbout AM, Putter H, van de Velde CJ, Kievit J (2005). Self-reports of health-care utilization: diary or questionnaire? *Int J Technol Assess Health Care*, **21**(3), 298–304.

17. Goossens ME, Rutten-van Molken MP, Vlaeyen JW, van der Linden SM (2000). The cost diary: a method to measure direct and indirect costs in cost- effectiveness research. *J Clin Epidemiol*, **53**(7), 688–95.

18. Palmer S, Raftery J (1999). Economic Notes: opportunity cost. *BMJ*, **318**(7197), 1551–2.

19. Tranmer JE, Guerriere DN, Ungar WJ, Coyte PC (2005). Valuing patient and caregiver time: a review of the literature. *Pharmacoeconomics*, **23**(5), 449–59.

20. Koopmanschap MA, Rutten FF (1996). A practical guide for calculating indirect costs of disease. *Pharmacoeconomics*, **10**(5), 460–6.

21. Thompson SG, Barber JA (2000). How should cost data in pragmatic randomised trials be analysed? *BMJ*, **320**(7243), 1197–200.

22. Doshi JA, Glick HA, Polsky D (2006). Analyses of cost data in economic evaluations conducted alongside randomized controlled trials. *Value Health*, **9**(5), 334–40.

23. Barber JA, Thompson SG (2000). Analysis of cost data in randomized trials: an application of the non-parametric bootstrap. *Stat Med*, **19**(23), 3219–36.

24. O'Brien BJ, Briggs AH (2002). Analysis of uncertainty in health care cost-effectiveness studies: an introduction to statistical issues and methods. *Stat Methods Med Res*, **11**(6), 455–68.

25. Stinnett AA, Mullahy J (1998). Net health benefits: a new framework for the analysis of uncertainty in cost-effectiveness analysis. *Med Decis Making*, **18**(2 Suppl), 68–80.

26. Black WC (1990). The CE plane: a graphic representation of cost-effectiveness. *Med Decis Making*, **10**(3), 212–14.

27. Briggs AH, O'Brien BJ, Blackhouse G (2002). Thinking outside the box: recent advances in the analysis and presentation of uncertainty in cost-effectiveness studies. *Annu Rev Public Health*, **23**, 377–401.

28. Van Hout BA, Al MJ, Gordon GS, Rutten FF (1994). Costs, effects and C/E-ratios alongside a clinical trial. *Health Econ*, **3**(5), 309–19.

29. Fenwick E, Marshall DA, Levy AR, Nichol G (2006). Using and interpreting cost-effectiveness acceptability curves: an example using data from a trial of management strategies for atrial fibrillation. *BMC Health Serv Res*, **6**, 52.

30. Fenwick E, O'Brien BJ, Briggs A (2004). Cost-effectiveness acceptability curves – facts, fallacies and frequently asked questions. *Health Econ*, **13**(5), 405–15.

31. Lothgren M, Zethraeus N (2000). Definition, interpretation and calculation of cost-effectiveness acceptability curves. *Health Econ*, **9**(7), 623–30.

32. Donders AR, van der Heijden GJ, Stijnen T, Moons KG (2006). Review: a gentle introduction to imputation of missing values. *J Clin Epidemiol*, **59**(10), 1087–91.

33. Briggs A, Clark T, Wolstenholme J, Clarke P (2003). Missing… presumed at random: cost-analysis of incomplete data. *Health Econ*, **12**, 377–92.

34. Oostenbrink JB, Al MJ (2005). The analysis of incomplete cost data due to dropout. *Health Econ*, **14**(8), 763–76.

35. Ramsey S, Willke R, Briggs A, Brown R, Buxton M, Chawla A, Cook J, Glick H, Liljas B, Petitti D, Reed S (2005). Good research practices for cost-effectiveness analysis alongside clinical trials: the ISPOR RCT-CEA Task Force report. *Value Health*, **8**(5), 521–33.

36. van Buuren S, Oudshoorn CGM (2000). *Multivariate Imputation by Chained Equations*. TNO, Leiden.

37. Briggs AH, Gray AM (1999). Handling uncertainty in economic evaluations of healthcare interventions. *BMJ*, **319**(7210), 635–8.

38. Miller P, Chilvers C, Dewey M, et al (2003). Counselling versus antidepressant therapy for the treatment of mild to moderate depression in primary care: economic analysis. *Int J Technol Assess Health Care*, **19**(1), 80–90.

39. Drummond MF, Jefferson TO (1996). Guidelines for authors and peer reviewers of economic submissions to the BMJ. The BMJ Economic Evaluation Working Party. *BMJ*, **313**(7052), 275–83.

40. Evers SM, Goossens ME, de Vet HC, van Tulder MW, Ament AJ (2005). Criteria list for assessment of methodological quality of economic evaluations: Consensus on Health Economic Criteria. *Int J Technol Assess Health Care*, **21**(2), 240–5.

Chapter 16

Implementing studies into real life

Caroline F. Finch

Advances in real-world sports injury prevention will only be achieved if research efforts are directed towards understanding the implementation context for injury prevention, whilst continuing to build the evidence-base for the efficacy and effectiveness of interventions[1]. Throughout earlier chapters of this book, guidance has been given on the design, conduct, and analysis of research studies leading to intervention development and evaluation. The Translating Research into Injury Prevention Practice (TRIPP) Framework, as shown in Fig. 16.1, provides a useful conceptualization of how that research fits into broad strategies to prevent sports injuries[1, 2]. Previous sections of this textbook have described research corresponding to the first four TRIPP stages, with some consideration of factors likely to impact on stage five. This chapter is concerned mostly with research needed to address TRIPP stages five and six, which correspond to intervention implementation and effectiveness research. These stages are particularly important for injury prevention because understanding the barriers and facilitators to the widespread adoption and sustainability of prevention measures is vital to ensuring effective and sustainable sports injury prevention.

Effectiveness versus efficacy

Research studies for demonstrating the preventive potential of sports injury interventions can be broadly categorized into two types:

(1) Efficacy research where the preventive effect of the intervention is assessed under ideal and tightly controlled conditions. The highest form of this research evidence is from randomized controlled trials (RCTs), though other experimental designs can also contribute knowledge. The high level of control is necessary to ensure large effect sizes, corresponding to the preventive capacity of the intervention under study. Such studies correspond to TRIPP stage four. The vast majority of sports injury prevention trials are efficacy studies.

(2) Effectiveness research where the preventive effect of the intervention is assessed under everyday circumstances. This implies little or no control over how the intervention is implemented, though in practice, this may be hard to ensure. The goal of effectiveness studies is to determine the extent to which the intervention actually prevents injuries when delivered as it would be used in real-world sporting practice. Broader implementation research studies measure factors such as how the intervention was delivered as well as how it was complied with and used. This focus is necessary because if efficacious interventions are not widely adopted, complied with, and sustained as on-going practice, then it is very unlikely they will have any significant or long-lasting injury-prevention impacts. These studies correspond to TRIPP Stage 6. To date, very few effectiveness or implementation studies have been published.

TRIPP Stage	Research need	Research process
1	Count and describe injuries	Injury surveillance
2	Understand why injuries occur	Prospective studies to establish aetiology and mechanisms of injury
3	Develop 'potential' preventive measures	Basic mechanistic and clinical studies to identify what could be done to prevent injuries
4	Understand what works under 'ideal' conditions	Efficacy studies to determine what works in a controlled setting (e.g. RCTS)
5	Understand the intervention implementation context including personal, environmental, societal and sports delivery factors that may enhance or be barriers	Ecological studies to understand implementation context
6	Understand what works in the 'real-world'	Effectiveness studies in context of real-world sports delivery (ideally in natural, uncontrolled settings)

Fig. 16.1 The Translating Research Into Injury Prevention Practice (TRIPP) Framework. Highlighted sections correspond to implementation- and effectiveness-research needs
Reproduced from Finch and Donaldson[2] with permission from BMJ Publishing Group Ltd.

The differences between the design and conduct of efficacy and effectiveness studies have been discussed by a number of authors[1, 3–6]. Table 16.1 summarizes the key features of these study types and highlights some of the particular challenges that arise in the conduct of implementation studies.

Intervention-implementation study designs

As explained above, intervention-effectiveness studies have less control than more experimental or RCT designs because their aim is to assess the impact of real-world constraints and influences on intervention outcomes. Broadly speaking, the best design for intervention studies depends on two factors – the unit of intervention delivery and the unit of analysis – this is shown in Fig. 16.2. Ecological designs are discussed further in Chapter 5, RCTs in Chapters 2 and 13, and quasi-experimental designs in Chapter 13. These chapters also discuss the limitations of these study designs, especially when conducted in the absence of adequate controls or randomization, when assessing cause-and-effect relationships.

There has been increasing debate over recent years as to the most appropriate study designs for implementation studies[7–10]. Whilst the clear benefits of RCTs for assessing direct causal relationships do not apply in intervention studies, it is also worth pointing out that causal inferences are not the major focus of implementation studies. For this reason, designs such as quasi-experimental designs and interrupted time-series analyses can be useful, particularly at the population or broad community level when RCTs are impractical. Moreover, the stringent control often required in RCTs can preclude them from being able to fully assess key determinants of intervention-effectiveness or implementation factors that need to be assessed in the absence of such control to mimic the real world. Nonetheless, implementation studies should still aim to include randomization of delivery units to control and intervention groups.

Examples of implementation studies

Some examples of studies that have assessed some aspects of intervention implementation are summarized below, to demonstrate the range of interventions and study designs that have been

Table 16.1 A comparison of the key features in the design- and conduct-effectiveness and efficacy-intervention studies

Component	Efficacy studies	Effectiveness studies	Considerations for the design and evaluation of interventions in implementation studies
Study design	Rely on highly controlled studies for best evidence, including RCTs and other experimental designs (e.g. controlled laboratory-based study).	Whilst RCTs can be adopted, their level of control may preclude full assessment of relevant implementation factors. Other study designs include quasi-experimental designs, interrupted-time series, ecological studies, etc.	Effectiveness studies are best when they still involve randomisation of units to intervention-implementation groups. Control groups add strength to all studies and can reduce the risk of ecological fallacy.
Intervention delivery	Under the strict control of the research team according to a well-defined protocol that must be adhered to. People who deliver the intervention are usually employed by the research team.	The intervention and/or accompanying resources (e.g. educational brochures) are provided to others to deliver or implement (e.g. coaches, sports clubs, etc.). People who deliver the intervention are not employed by the research team.	This means that the motivation and commitment of the deliverers, as well as their usual practices, need to be assessed and considered. It is recommended that potential barriers and enablers of the desired behaviors of those intended to deliver the intervention are assessed before any full-scale implementation of the study and before the final package format is finalised.
Study participants, intervention allocation and targeting	Under the strict control of the research team according to a well-defined protocol that must be adhered to. This then leads to analysis according to intention-to-treat principles. Usually specific individuals that meet specific inclusion/exclusion criteria (i.e. a relatively homogeneous set of individuals) are targeted and included in the evaluation.	An allocation plan is determined by the research team but the actual allocation is undertaken by others in the real-world setting. The intervention is delivered to all members of a defined group or population (i.e. a heterogeneous group).	There will be different levels of uptake of the intervention that need to be monitored across all stages of the implementation process. Where possible, reasons for why there is/is not uptake should be assessed at each stage.
Sample size and length of study	These studies require adequate numbers of study participants to ensure power and follow-up over large amounts of time.	Studies are often of shorter duration but involve many more study participants than are involved in efficacy RCTs.	Shorter-duration studies can show immediate behavioral/knowledge-change effects but longer studies will be needed to show sustainability and maintenance of these changes into the future.

(continued)

Table 16.1 (continued) A comparison of the key features in the design- and conduct-effectiveness and efficacy-intervention studies

Component	Efficacy studies	Effectiveness studies	Considerations for the design and evaluation of interventions in implementation studies
The intervention protocol and setting constraints	The intervention protocol is rigidly structured and must be adhered to by all staff involved in the study. It needs to be based on intensive, specialized interventions that cannot be modified and developed specifically with the specific target population in mind. The goal is not to assess generalizability across settings.	Whilst the starting point is a formal protocol, it is important that this is flexible enough to allow adaptations to suit the particular application context. Interventions need to be able to be adaptable to different settings, ideally with some capacity for further modification of their implementation during the study if/when significant delivery issues are identified. A major goal is to assess the extent to which the intervention can be useful in different settings.	Engagement of key stakeholders in the development of the delivery plan should help to minimize the need to modify the intervention during the evaluation. Pilot testing of the intervention and delivery plan should be undertaken and community feedback should be sought.
Staffing, local infrastructure, and funding issues	These studies are very labour intensive and require full funding for staff to both deliver the intervention and to collect evaluation data. These staff are employed by the research team and require significant support funding, particularly for the intervention delivery. Usually only involves a limited number of staff with specific training in the study protocol.	Staffing for intervention delivery is usually the responsibility of the real-world agencies/individuals. Some support for this may come from research funds, but it expected to be minimal. Usually involves a variety of different people, with different training experiences. The evaluation data is often collected by researchers (to ensure some independence from the intervention delivers) and this would be funded by the researchers.	Stakeholder engagement and buy-in for the intervention and its development should be obtained from the outset. The intervention programmes are more likely to be successful if these groups are involved at all stages as equal partners to the researchers during any implementation trial and evaluation.

reported in the literature. This list has been chosen to cover a range of different safety interventions and because of the specific implementation-evaluation issues they raise.

Example 1: Randomized controlled trial of soft-shell headgear and custom-fitted mouth-guards in Australian Football

An RCT was designed as a four arm factorial trial – soft-shell headgear only, custom-fitted mouth-guard only, soft-shell headgear + custom-fitted mouth-guard, and control (usual behaviour) – to

UNIT OF DELIVERY	UNIT OF ANALYSIS	STUDY DESIGNS

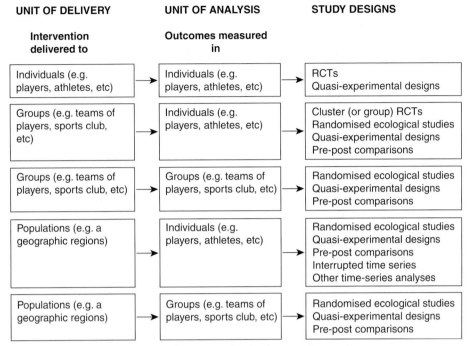

Fig. 16.2 Summary of study designs for intervention-implementation studies.

determine the effectiveness of these forms of protective equipment in preventing orofacial injuries in Australian Football players[11]. Players from randomized teams were provided with the headgear and/or mouth-guard depending on which study arm they were allocated to, and encouraged to use this protective equipment throughout one playing season. In addition to the players' injury outcomes, information was collected about the extent to which players actually wore their allocated protective equipment during both games and training sessions[12]. This assessment of intervention-uptake found extremely low numbers of players actually wore the soft-shell headgear; because of this it was not possible to assess its effectiveness in the trial, but the factorial design used for intervention allocation meant that formal hypotheses about the preventive potential of the custom-fitted mouth-guards could still be tested[11]. This example highlights the importance of only conducting effectiveness studies with interventions which are likely to have good levels of acceptance, and hence compliance, by the trial participants. In Australian football, the culture of the sport is such that mouth-guards are regarded as useful but headgear is considered unnecessary by most players and coaches and this accounted for the intervention-uptake levels.

Example 2. Small-scale RCT of FIFA's 'The 11' training programme in young football players

A small-scale RCT was conducted within one local football (soccer) club in New Zealand[13]. Twenty-four players were recruited, with half of them allocated to a control group and the remainder to an intervention group. These latter players were required to undertake nine of the 10 exercises using the exact FIFA guidelines (www.fifa.com) on 5 times a week for 6 weeks. One weekly session was supervised, with the remaining sessions conducted at home with assistance from parents. Players in both groups underwent a battery of physical performance tests before and after the intervention and the players from the intervention group also completed a post-intervention survey that asked questions about the following aspects of the exercise pro-gramme: enjoyment, frequency of execution, perceived benefits of participation, intention to continue/adhere, and feedback on specific exercises. No injuries occurred over the 6-week period and compliance to the intervention was 73% players. Importantly, most players from the inter-vention group considered the exercise programme to be beneficial but also rated it as not enjoy-able in the prescribed format. The authors concluded that some modification to the FIFA guidelines would be necessary to ensure high levels of adherence and enjoyment with them by young players before full injury prevention and performance outcomes could be achieved. This example shows that even when an intervention is developed and shown to be efficacious in one athlete group (in this case older soccer players for the FIFA 11), it may not necessarily be suitable for direct use in another context or athlete group, even children engaged in the same sport.

Example 3. Pre–post evaluation of responses to a brain and spinal cord injury-prevention video aimed at ice hockey players

A Canadian study aimed to evaluate knowledge transfer and behavioural outcomes following the viewing of a safety video by 11–12-year-old ice hockey players[14]. The Smart Hockey video was developed by experts and included a component on concussion. Thirty-four teams of players from one district league were randomly allocated to either a control or intervention group, in which coaches were asked to show the video to their players at mid-season. The timing of inter-vention delivery was to allow for some pre-assessment of some factors as a baseline for the inter-vention evaluation. Players from both groups had their knowledge levels surveyed both at mid-season and 3 months later; the intervention group was also surveyed 5 min after viewing the video. The players shown the video had higher, and significantly improved, knowledge scores than the control players compared to their baselines. Whilst the major outcome of this study was knowledge change in the players, because the intervention was delivered by the coaches, the authors also collected qualitative data from them about how the video could be improved and their views on how coaches influence head injuries in their players. Some coaches refused to show the video to their players and this was related to their own negative attitudes and behaviours. On the other hand, coaches who did agree for them to be included in the intervention had a personal history of concussion or direct knowledge of a player having sustained a concussion. These results demonstrate that factors such as how and why interventions are/are not delivered are likely to have an effect on intervention effectiveness, even if the intervention has been shown to have clear injury-prevention benefits.

Example 4: Randomized ecological evaluation of a squash eye-wear promotion strategy

An awareness-raising and knowledge-information squash protective eye-wear promotion-strategy was developed from behavioural theory principles and prior research[15]. The aim was to increase knowledge about appropriate eye-wear and self-reported use of this. Two distinct geographical regions in Melbourne, Australia, were defined and all squash venues within each region identified. The regions were randomly allocated to either having a sample of their squash venues receiving the promotion strategy or not (i.e. control)[16]. The unit of analysis was therefore a public squash venue and four such venues were involved in each study arm/region. A pre- and post-implementation controlled ecological assessment of the effectiveness of the promotion strategy was undertaken. Intervention-effectiveness outcomes assessed in the selected squash venues in each study arm at both time points included players' protective eye-wear knowl-edge levels and their self-reported eye-wear-use behaviours. Other intervention-implementation factors were assessed after the 4-month intervention period in both the intervention and control venues and included: players' recall of seeing the promotional materials; players' recall of the safety slogans; and the numbers of sales and episodes of hiring of protective eye-wear at each venue. The intervention was associated with a significantly increased level of player knowledge about inappropriate eye-wear at the intervention venues. Specific components of the intervention (e.g. stickers, posters, the availability and prominent placement of the eye-wear) were all found to contribute to players adopting favourable eye-wear behaviours in the intervention venues. This example shows that collecting information about the desired injury-prevention outcome, as well as some intervention-delivery factors, can be used to identify which particular components of an intervention are most likely to have led to the desired changes in injury-prevention behaviours.

Example 5. Controlled pre-, post-, and follow-up evaluation of a risk-management training programme aimed at soccer clubs

An Australian study delivered injury-risk-management training to 32 soccer clubs and used data collected through a sports safety audit tool to compare their policy, infrastructure, and overall safety scores before and after the training and at the 12 months follow-up[17]. The same measures were also obtained at the same time points from 44 clubs that had not participated in the training programme. Neither the control nor intervention clubs were randomly selected. The evaluation found that the training programme assisted clubs in developing and improving a number of processes relating to good risk-management practice. A particular strength was the inclusion of a 12-month follow-up period so that some assessment of sustainability of the intervention outcomes could be assessed. Interestingly, the longer-term evaluation also showed a trend towards adoption of some key safety processes, such as having a specific safety budget, requiring some time to develop. This example shows that assessing intervention-sustainability is different to just assessing immediate change due to an intervention. It also demonstrates how implementation studies can focus on desirable outcomes in groups responsible for sports safety and not just individual athlete outcomes.

Example 6. Interrupted time-series analysis of population level impact of a mouth-guard regulation on dental injuries

Since 1997/1998, mouth-guards have been made compulsory for all New Zealand Rugby union players. An interrupted time-series examination of the effect of this regulation was assessed using country-wide dental injury insurance-claim records over the period 1995–2003[18]. This study capitalized on the availability of a unique national population database that recorded information on all sports injury insurance-claims as the measure of injury numbers and outcomes. By comparing the number of dental injury claims after the full introduction of the regulation with those in the years immediately preceding it, the study demonstrated a 43% reduction in these claims associated with rugby union. This is an interrupted time-series study because the annual numbers of claims are split into two sections, one before and one after the law was introduced. The authors were careful to stress that whilst they tried to minimize most sources of bias, there could still have been some ecological fallacy in their results because they did not have accurate mouth-guard-wearing-rate data over the evaluation period, precluding any direct link between reduced injury claims and increased mouth-guard use. Moreover, accurate figures on the numbers of rugby union players were not available and so they could not rule out the possibility that some of the observed reduction in rates could be due to fewer players playing the sport. However, the example shows the value of routinely collected population-level injury data in assessing the broad public health impact of sports injury prevention programmes.

Example 7. Time-series analysis comparison of observed and predicted population-level injury-claim numbers

Using the same population database that was used in the previous example, the effect of a new international scrum law on neck and back injuries was assessed at the population level in rugby union players in New Zealand[19]. By combining injury-claim numbers with numbers of registered players, the authors constructed a population-level statistical model relating the scrum-related neck- and back-injury claims-rate to the calendar year. Using data from five successive years, 2002–06, they predicted the number of such claims that would be expected in subsequent years assuming the same trend in injury rates would occur. The International Rugby Board introduced a new scrum law on 1 January 2007 and the effect of this on injury claim-rates was assessed by comparing the observed number of scrum-related neck- and back-injury claims to that predicted by the model trend before that date. A limitation of this evaluation was that it had only one time point after the law introduction, but there was a suggestion of an effect, with the observed rate being less than that predicted, though not significantly so. Nonetheless, this example does serve to demonstrate how routinely collected data and statistical prediction models can be used to monitor the effects of nation-wide interventions.

Example 8. Quasi-experimental, non-randomized, evaluation of a safe community programme

In Sweden, considerable effort has been invested in the development of safe community programmes whereby broad-based evidence-informed safety programmes are delivered to entire communities[20]. One study evaluated the outcomes of a community sports safety-promotion programme incorporating principles of local safety rules in relation to protective equipment use and educational programmes relating to fair play and novice participants[21]. A quasi-experimental design was used because the safe community programme was implemented in a well-defined geographic region. Another geographically defined region of Sweden was chosen as the control and routinely collected injury-morbidity data rates were compared in the two regions. The implementation of the population-based programme was over 1987–88. For evaluation purposes, the pre-implementation period was taken as 52 weeks from 1 October 1983 to 30 September 1984 and the post-intervention period was from 1 January 1989 to 31 December 1989. As the two study groups were not randomly selected, an examination of some socio-demographic factors (e.g. age and gender distributions, sports club membership) was also undertaken. Overall, there was a reduction in the total population rate of sports injury cases treated at health-care units in the intervention group, but this trend was not significantly different to that in the control communities, suggesting that there may have been a concurrent decline in sports injuries across the whole country. Moreover, the fact that this was a quasi-experimental design means that adequate adjustment for other potential factors impacting on injury rates could not be assured. This example shows the difficulty in interpreting the results from quasi-experimental designs, especially when it is not possible to also measure extraneous factors that could impact on sports injury rates.

Example 9. Quasi-experimental evaluation of a multifaceted injury-prevention programme, using historical controls

A multi-component injury-prevention programme was evaluated for its effect on injury and physical injury outcomes in a group of United States army soldiers[22]. This study used data from an army-based clinical injury surveillance system in a Cox regression analysis to compare the time to first injury in 2 559 trainee soldiers before the programme was implemented to that in 1 283 trainee soldiers after the programme. The evaluation found a significant reduction in relation to time-loss injury associated with the programme but could not ascertain which components of the programme most contributed to the injury reductions. This example highlights a major problem with the evaluation of many multifaceted injury-prevention programmes in that it is often not possible to determine which of the individual programme components or interventions contribute to the injury reductions or required safety-behaviour changes.

Towards a theoretical basis for implementation studies

Overall, there have been very few published studies of aspects of sports injury-prevention implementation. When studies have considered implementation issues, this has typically been as a minor component of an effectiveness study. The selected examples above highlight some of the complexities involved in conducting implementation research in real-world settings. It is also apparent from just these few examples that not every study has evaluated all aspects of intervention-implementation. For example, only two of the examples above reported whether or not the intervention target groups actually adopted, or complied with, the intervention. Some studies only reported injury outcomes without also examining the required intermediary behavioural change, such as exercise adoption or protective equipment use, necessary to firmly link those reductions to the preventive measures. Only two of the examples above recognized that individual safety-behaviour change was also influenced by other factors such as the form of the intervention delivery and the person delivering it as well as who collected information on this aspect.

There is no doubt that there is a complex relationship between desired injury-reduction benefits and how interventions are packaged, delivered, and promoted[20]. It has been argued that the conduct of well-designed of large-scale intervention-effectiveness trials has been hampered because of a lack of intervention models and theoretical considerations in their design, implementation, and evaluation and that the field will only develop if it begins to incorporate these[3, 10, 23–27]. Moreover, as also noted in Chapters 11 and 12, there are many different types of implementation and intervention-delivery approaches that can be considered to support prevention efforts, either in isolation of jointly. These range from educational/behavioural change strategies [28–32] to environmental modifications [28, 29] to making policy/law changes [28–31] to public awareness/advocacy [28, 31] and stake-holder engagement[28, 33].

To progress sports injury prevention, it will be necessary for implementation studies to have a firm theoretical basis. Because of the lack of international implementation research in any aspect of injury prevention or health promotion[1, 4, 34], there is very little information about how best to conduct intervention studies in community sport settings. Whilst some theoretical considerations have been developed specifically for some safety programmes (e.g. safe communities [35]), and others have recently been applied to sports medicine contexts (e.g. knowledge transfer for sport concussion [32]), most of the available examples come from the health promotion or behavioural sciences. Theoretical considerations also have implications for how intervention studies are conducted and reported and there is a need to improve the reporting standards of implementation studies to provide a more comprehensive analysis of the factors affecting intervention uptake and effectiveness[1, 36]. Application of health-promotion frameworks to evaluate the public health impact of interventions could potentially help to better understand contextual and policy influences in this setting.

Despite the availability of injury-prevention interventions, proven through efficacy studies, it is clear that limited research attention has focussed on understanding the intervention-implementation context and processes, including barriers and facilitators to sustainable programmes. Some Australian studies examining the safety policy and practice contexts within grass-roots sports delivery (e.g. through community sports clubs) have shown than most sports have an *ad hoc* approach to safety, with limited adoption of safety policy and little strategic planning or co-ordination of implementation efforts either by administrators or coaches[37–43]. Whilst there is an increasing acceptance of safety policy and risk-management approaches, widespread and consistent adoption of safety interventions is lacking. The reasons for this lack of uptake of scientific evidence are largely unknown but have been stated as an international challenge for researchers[1, 4, 34]. To address this challenge, future sports-safety research aimed at real-world uptake of safety measures research will need to:

- engage relevant sports bodies and other stake-holders in implementation and injury-prevention research from the outset
- continue to partner with these stake-holder groups in further intervention and intervention-delivery developments
- develop multi-faceted and multi-action strategic approaches towards injury prevention in relevant real-world sports settings
- develop and evaluate strategic implementation plans designed to address key barriers and facilitators towards intervention uptake at all levels
- adopt a multi-disciplinary approach that embraces both qualitative and quantitative research methodologies.

The RE-AIM model

Implementation research is broader than just studies of intervention-effectiveness, though the latter are a key component of the broader research goals. The RE-AIM health-promotion frame-work[3, 44] is one health-promotion model with high applicability to sports injury prevention that could underpin much implementation research[2]. This framework has previously been used with individually targeted behavioural change through exercise programmes for elderly falls prevention[45] and people with arthritis[46], lifestyle interventions targeting cardiovascular disease risk factors[47], and other community-based behavioural interventions[48]. The RE-AIM framework can be applied to:

- sports injury preventive initiatives directed at individual sports participants, such as individual behavioural change (e.g. taping ankles or wearing protective equipment)
- interventions delivered by a coach to a whole team of participants (e.g. exercise training programmes)
- higher-order interventions delivered by sports governing bodies (e.g. safety regulations)
- the need of sports safety interventions in community sport settings[2].

The RE-AIM framework has five key dimensions for assessing interventions that are useful for guiding new thinking about the full complexities of the implementation context[3, 44]:

1. Reach – the proportion of the target population that participated in the intervention
2. Effectiveness – the success rate if implemented as intended, defined as positive outcomes minus negative outcomes
3. Adoption – the proportion of people, settings, practices, and plans that adopt the intervention
4. Implementation – the extent to which the intervention is implemented as intended in the real world
5. Maintenance – the extent to which the intervention is sustained over time. This aspect is often categorized according to individual-level and setting-level maintenance.

One study has applied the RE-AIM framework to evaluate a Tai Chi group exercise programme delivered through community health services to prevent falls in community dwelling older people[45]. The model's five dimensions were assessed as:

1. Reach – the number of eligible people; number of people who participated; and the representativeness of target population.

2. Effectiveness – individual participant changes in measure of physical performance; changes in measures of quality of life; and frequency of falls.

3. Adoption – the percent of local community centres that agreed to participate and the percent of local community centres that implemented the programme.

4. Implementation – adherence to the implementation plan provided; maintenance of a 2-week programme schedule; attainment of attendance >74% over 12 weeks; and documentation of >30 mins in-home practice per week.

5. Maintenance – determined through centres' willingness to consider Tai Chi as part of future programmes and the likelihood of continuation of programme after completion of the intervention. For the older people who participated in the programme, maintenance was also assessed as the number of participants continuing Tai Chi practice 12 weeks after the classes had finished.

Care needs to be taken when directly applying the RE-AIM framework to interventions implemented in the community sport setting because the definition for each dimension will depend on the specific level being targeted. Whilst some interventions will be targeted at only one level (usually the individual athlete), implementation of most sports injury interventions is multi-faceted and complex and often needs to be targeted at multiple levels. Table 16.2 shows an adaptation of the RE-AIM framework that explains how each of its dimensions can be assessed across the sports delivery hierarchy to account for delivery-setting complexity and optimize intervention delivery and evaluation[2].

As listed in the article by Finch and Donaldson[2], the factors that could be considered at each level of the sports delivery hierarchy are:

◆ national, state, and regional level – commitment; communication strategies; education and training provided; finance and other resources allocated; formalizing of safety committee

Table 16.2 The RE-AIM Sports Setting Matrix: evaluation dimensions for community-sport-intervention delivery with demonstrable public health benefit

RE-AIM Dimension	Level of assessment/intervention setting or target					
	National sporting organization	State/provincial sporting organization	Regional association or league	Club	Team	Participant
Reach						
Effectiveness						
Adoption						
Implementation						
Maintenance						

This table shows all possible intervention points. The relevance of each point will depend on the nature and target of each intervention.

Reproduced from Finch and Donaldson[2] with permission from BMJ Publishing Group Ltd.

structures and monitoring processes; policies; documented decision processes; and attitudes/ knowledge of key personnel, etc.

- ◆ club level – organizational infrastructure; policy development/implementation/monitoring; training/support for coaches; sports administrative support/monitoring; promotion and communication; and attitudes/knowledge of club officials and key administrators

- ◆ team level – implementation of training guidelines; coach plans/practices and attitudes/ knowledge; documentation; accountability to club; and communication strategies.

- ◆ individual participants level – the proportion (and number) of participants exposed to the intervention; participant awareness/knowledge of interventions; proportion of participants incorporating the intervention into routine activity; and rates of relevant injuries (e.g. per 1 000 participant exposures).

One of the injury-prevention interventions currently receiving considerable attention in the international literature across a range of sports is specially designed exercise training programmes delivered by coaches to prevent lower-limb injuries in their players. Table 16.3 illustrates how the RE-AIM model could be used to guide the implementation and evaluation of such a programme in a community sports setting.

Table 16.3 Application of the RE-AIM Sports Setting Matrix to the evaluation of the implementation of an evidence-based coach-lead lower-limb injury-prevention exercise programme in a community-sports setting

RE-AIM Dimension	Setting/Individual level	Implementation factor*
Reach	National sports body	◆ % of National sports-body relevant administrators aware of the programme
		◆ % of National sports-body relevant administrators think the programme is a good idea
	State or regional sports body	◆ % of State or regional sports-body relevant administrators aware of the programme
		◆ % of State or regional sports-body relevant administrators think the programme is a good idea
	Association/ league	◆ % of association/leagues participating in the programme
		◆ representativeness of participating association/leagues (e.g. size, geographical location, etc.)
		◆ % of association/leagues offering education about the programme
	Club	◆ % of clubs aware of the programme
		◆ representativeness of clubs
	Team	◆ % of coaches aware of the programme
		◆ % of coaches attending education about the programme
		◆ representativeness of coaches
	Participant	◆ % of participants exposed to the programme via educated coaches
		◆ representativeness of participants

Table 16.3 (continued) Application of the RE-AIM Sports Setting Matrix to the evaluation of the implementation of an evidence-based coach-lead lower-limb injury-prevention exercise programme in a community-sports setting

RE-AIM Dimension	Setting/Individual level	Implementation factor*
Effectiveness	National sports body	◆ % reduction in lower-limb injuries in association/leagues implementing programme compared to other association/leagues affiliated with the National sports body
	State or regional sports body	◆ % reduction in lower-limb injuries in association/leagues implementing programme compared to other association/leagues affiliated with the State or regional sports body
	Association/league	◆ % reduction in lower-limb injuries in associations/league implementing programme compared to other clubs affiliated with Association/League
	Club	◆ % reduction in lower-limb injuries in club compared to other seasons
		◆ % clubs believing the programme reduces injury risk in participants
		◆ % clubs believing the programme has other benefits for their participants (e.g. technique or performance gains)
	Team	◆ % coaches believing the programme reduces participant injury risk
		◆ % coaches believing the programme has other benefits for participants (e.g. technique or performance gains)
	Participant	◆ % reduction in lower-limb injury rates compared to previous seasons
		◆ % participants able to perform programme-related exercises appropriately
Adoption	National sports body	◆ extent to which programme is part of National sports body overall safety strategy
	State or regional sports body	◆ extent to which programme is part of State or regional sports body overall safety stratergy
	Association/league	◆ promotion of programme by association/league
		◆ resources invested in programme by association/league
	Club	◆ % of clubs with formal policy about the programme in place
		◆ resources invested in programme by club
	Team	◆ % of coaches who deliver the programme to their participants
	Participant	◆ % of participants participating in the programme-related coach-led activity
Implementation	National sports body	◆ extent to which programme is implemented as planned by National sports body
		◆ investment in programme by National sports body (e.g. infrastructure, documentation, resources)
	State or regional sports body	◆ extent to which programme is implemented as intended by State or regional sports body
		◆ investment in the programme by State or regional sports body

(continued)

Table 16.3 (continued) Application of the RE-AIM Sports Setting Matrix to the evaluation of the implementation of an evidence-based coach-lead lower-limb injury-prevention exercise programme in a community-sports setting

RE-AIM Dimension	Setting/Individual level	Implementation factor*
	Association/league	◆ extent to which programme is implemented as intended by association/league ◆ investment in the programme by association/leagues ◆ % of association/leagues offering programme training to coaches ◆ distribution of programme resources and support material
	Club	◆ % of clubs implementing the programme as intended ◆ % of clubs investing adequately in the programme
	Team	◆ % of coaches delivering the programme as intended ◆ number of programme sessions delivered ◆ % of coaches who modified or adapted the programme
	Participant	◆ % of participants who undertake programme as intended ◆ % of participants who receive promotional and support material
Maintenance	National sports body	◆ National sports body has, or intends to develop, a formal policy on the programme ◆ National sports body has programme integrated into strategic or business plans
	State or regional sports body	◆ State or regional sports body has, or intends to develop, a formal policy on the programme ◆ State or regional sports body has programme integrated into strategic or business plans
	Association/league	◆ % of association/leagues with, or intending to develop, a formal policy on the programme ◆ % of association/leagues with programme integrated into strategic or business plans ◆ % of association/leagues implementing the programme as intended 3 years after introduction
	Club	◆ % of clubs with, or intending to develop, a formal policy/guidelines on the programme ◆ % of clubs implementing the programme as intended 3 years after introduction
	Team	◆ % of coaches implementing the programme as intended 3 years after receiving training ◆ % of coaches intending to implement the programme with participants in the future
	Participant	◆ % of participants doing the exercises contained in the programme 3 years after being introduced to it ◆ % of participants intending to do the exercises contained in the programme on an on-going basis

This table does not provide an exhaustive list of implementation factors that could be assessed.
* Needed to guide both study design and implementation plans.
Reproduced from Finch and Donaldson [2] with permission from BMJ Publishing Group Ltd.

A phased approach towards undertaking an implementation study

The above text has summarized the major issues in the design and conduct of implementation studies and has recommended that a theoretical basis, such as the RE-AIM model, is used to guide future research in this area. In this section, a phased approach to the design of a comprehensive injury-intervention-implementation study is outlined, to provide a guide for those wishing to undertake this sort of research.

The example is generic and broadly applies to any sports injury intervention. It is expected that such a study would need to be conducted over a few successive years and it is assumed that adequate efficacy evidence exists to justify the trialling of the intervention. The context for this specific example is any intervention aimed at sports participants, but delivered through coaches through their interactions with teams of players or training squads. However, the principles apply equally to other types of intervention. The study plan is framed within the RE-AIM framework's extension to community sport [2] so that the major programme-outcomes measures relating to the five RE-AIM domains of reach, effectiveness, adoption, implementation, and maintenance can be determined. The overall study design is that of a randomized controlled ecological trial that assesses an intervention against a usual practice situation (i.e. a control), but it is relatively straightforward to extend this to a comparison of more than one intervention against a control. For ease, the term 'intervention' is used to refer to the direct injury-prevention measure (e.g. a type of protective equipment, or a set of exercises) and the term 'intervention package' refers to the broad dissemination, delivery, and evaluation plan used to guide its implementation.

Phase 1: Developing the evidence-based intervention package

Any safety intervention needs to begin with evidence-based information about what is likely to be effective in reducing injuries. This phase therefore involves the translation of the available scientific evidence for the intervention into formal, practical guidelines for dissemination to the required sport setting. Key research questions that need to be addressed in this phase are:

- What are the specific injury-prevention needs and priorities of the groups being targeted (e.g. community sports clubs, individual members of a tennis club, etc.)?
- How can the evidence of efficacious relevant injury-prevention interventions be summarized for this context?
- What should be the content of the intervention package in this real-world setting?
- What is the preferred format and presentation of the intervention package based on this evidence?
- What is the process for reaching expert consensus on the construct and delivery of sports-safety interventions and how could these processes be improved?

The first three questions can be addressed through a systematic review of both peer-review literature and the 'grey' literature. It is important to not rely solely on RCT evidence, Cochrane reviews or meta analyses, because important cues to implementation factors are likely to be published elsewhere, including in non-peer review sources. This stage should involve the scoping and summarising of the evidence-base for the interventions to prevent the target injury/ies. A summary profile of the rate and factors associated with the causation of the target injuries should be generated from studies previously conducted and other published evidence. Information about the likely intervention-package components can also be determined from a systematic literature review. Because of the importance of involving stake-holder groups in implementation research, this summary information should be collated and presented to a convened (size-constrained) expert group representing key stake-holders to review and then develop a first draft of the intervention guidelines.

The other questions need to be addressed through a qualitative research approach. This would involve wider consultation with a broader group of stake-holders who are purposively selected from those who hold state or national positions with responsibility for the development, design, and implementation of safety intervention programmes across the sport, including at both the high performance and more community-focussed levels of play. One of the best qualitative approaches to use for this research aspect would be a Delphi consultation process [49] involving at least 15 participants and a 3–4-round consensus process. Following a clear explanation of the context and purpose of the intervention package, the first Delphi round should present the draft package and ask the group to provide feedback on its content and focus. Subsequent rounds would then build on the most common responses until a high level of consensus is reached (e.g. >75% of panel members agreeing). Whilst such consensus discussions can be held-face-to-face, with recent advances in electronic surveys, it may be more convenient to conduct this process via online survey. This has an additional advantage of providing a clear record of all stated views and inputs.

The final stage would be for a reconvening of the expert panel to review the intervention package, in light of the Delphi consensus consultations, and agreeing on the content and design of the final package formats. The output from this phase would be an evidence-informed, expert consensus-agreed, intervention package aimed at the target population. Time up to 6 months should be allowed for this phase.

Phase 2: Refining of the intervention package and development of a delivery plan

The next phase of research would involve the development of a delivery plan for the intervention package developed in phase 1. It would also involve obtaining community feedback on the content and format of both. Specific questions to be addressed include:

- To what extent is the developed intervention package able to be fully understood, and likely to be implemented, by the target group?
- How should the package be constructed and marketed to ensure relevance to the target group and contribute to maximal adoption and implementation?
- What other documentation and support (e.g. training, policy, resources) are likely to be needed to disseminate the intervention package guidelines with high reach?

As with much of phase 1, qualitative research approaches are the most appropriate. It would be valuable to link to your own networks and those of your expert panel for access to community sports groups.

To begin with, consultation with community club representatives should be undertaken to obtain feedback on the draft intervention package (in terms of its content, format, language, etc.) and to inform a feasible delivery plan. For efficiency, these consultations could be via focus group discussions [50] involving representatives of the typical target group individuals who make safety decisions and implement interventions. To ensure richness of information, and adequate data saturation, this is likely to require about 6–8 focus groups, each with 10–12 participants representing a mix of key safety actors across the target group (e.g. coaches, administrators, first aid providers, parents, players). Following this, data has been collected and collated, the expert panel should be reconvened to develop a recommended delivery plan in the light of the focus group feedback and to prepare the full intervention package for delivery in the subsequent year/playing season. This phase of research is likely to take a few months.

Phase 3: Implementation and evaluation of the intervention package and its delivery plan

This phase aims to evaluate the delivery of the intervention package in the target group to understand the processes, enablers, and barriers of implementing the new evidence-based safety interventions. It is recommended that a randomized controlled ecological design be used because of its highest level of rigour for implementation- and effectiveness-evaluations of this type. Whilst it is possible to compare different intervention packages or more than one delivery modes, this example considers the evaluation of just one intervention package against usual practice (control) in the target group. At this point, it is worth commenting on the choice of control group. Because effectiveness research is as much about assessing how interventions are delivered and how/why they are adopted, and the expectation is that the intervention package does this better than what is currently available, it is necessary to compare against a randomly selected control group representing normal practice. Unlike many fully controlled efficacy trials, it is neither possible nor ethical to require control groups to not be undertaking any form of preventive action they consider necessary. Of course, the evaluation of process outcomes across both study arms will also monitor the activities of the control group and this can be adjusted statistically for in the comparative analyses. It is recommended that the RE-AIM sports-safety matrix[2], as shown in Table 16.2, be used to underpin the evaluation.

Specific questions that can be addressed in this phase are:

◆ What formal injury-prevention policies and practices do the target and control groups adopt/implement?

◆ Does providing an intervention package change the commitment to, and implementation of, injury-prevention policies and practices in the target group, compared to usual practice?

◆ What factors are most predictive of sustainable intervention implementation, or otherwise?

◆ How does intervention-uptake/adoption/implementation influence injury rates in the target group?

◆ What enables or impedes sustainable intervention-implementation within the real-world sport setting?

◆ What is the optimal process/mix of activities to support target groups to uptake evidence-based safety guidelines?

◆ How can research evidence be successfully translated to target groups through a specific set of evidence-informed guidelines?

Ideally, an ecological RCT should be conducted over more than one year or playing season, with a particular focus on measuring the reach, effectiveness, adoption and implementation in the first year/season and on the same factors plus maintenance/sustainability in the subsequent years/seasons. A cluster-randomization design is optimal for sports-safety studies as it replicates the real-world context of the sports injury-intervention delivery[11, 51, 52]. One good approach would be to randomly select similar sports associations/leagues from each of two (or more) well-defined, but distinct, geographical regions. Importantly both groups should each represent a strong and representative, microcosm of the target sport with comparable standard of play and community-delivery context. Some other factors that should be considered when selecting the associations/leagues include the following:

◆ the geographical location in relation to where the main research team is based;

◆ having a mix of metropolitan, regional, and rural clubs (or some other socio-demographic representation of the setting) as this will impact on local resources, ability to gain assistance, willingness to engage, etc.;

- similar sports-delivery issues to those in other parts of the country where the sport is delivered at the same level, including size of the association/league as this will impact on the number of employees available to support the programme;
- having established links with the research team;
- having large numbers of relevant teams and registered players, across a range of competition levels; and
- level of professionalism of the league and its ability to pay players.

The extent to which any or all of these factors needs to be considered will depend on the availability of project funding and resources, support for the intervention package, and intended reach of the final product.

Each association/league should then be randomly allocated to one of the study arms. Generally, more than one association/league could be allocated to each study arm. If these sampling units are sufficiently large (e.g. a given league with many clubs), it may be necessary to only allocate one to each study arm. Sample size estimates should be adjusted for the likely clustering effect (see Chapter 14). The association/league needs to be the unit of randomization because it represents many clubs/teams participating in it on a regular basis and is an independently contained context for sport-policy development and implementation. It is very unlikely that there will be a large enough sample size if the study is only conducted within one club, though this may be adequate for some pilot studies. Each association/league will also have its own management structure and accountability back to regional, state, and national sports bodies. Within the associations/leagues, all clubs should be invited to participate. Each club is responsible for a number of teams and has its own management structure and sports-safety processes.

The RE-AIM domains should then be evaluated within each tier as shown in Table 16.2. The intervention package effectiveness should largely be assessed directly with the players, as the anticipated injury/health benefits/outcomes will be in individual players within the teams. By allocating all clubs within a specific league to the same intervention study arm, the chances of contamination across clubs/teams will be minimized. Nonetheless, some of the collected data should include information about potential contamination and broader awareness of the intervention package by control clubs. Whilst is it expected that the clubs across the two randomization groups would be similar with regards to key factors, club characteristics will be collected at baseline and can be adjusted for in the analyses, should imbalance exist. Another benefit of the group-level randomization is that by allocating the intervention to associations/leagues rather than clubs, no specific club (within a league) will be advantaged or disadvantaged in terms of performance or injury-prevention benefits. Delivery outcomes and processes associated with the intervention package can then be evaluated by comparing the RE-AIM domains across the two study arms.

All field-based data-collection processes for the injury surveillance, exposure monitoring, and collection of RE-AIM dimensions (such as adoption) should be highly standardized, to remove the potential for measurement error. It will be extremely valuable to formally measure and assess coach, player, and league/club personnel attitudes, knowledge, and behaviours before and after the intervention package delivery, as well as at pre-determined regular intervals during the implementation phase. Within each delivery arm, a dedicated and trained co-ordinator should be appointed collect data for the RE-AIM domains according to rigidly standardized data-collection procedures.

Across both study arms, the five major RE-AIM dimensions of the intervention package then need to be assessed across the sports-setting matrix[2], shown in Table 16.2. Qualitative data should also be collected and content analysed to identify themes and the data categorized according to such themes. The effectiveness of the intervention package can be assessed through injury surveillance and exposure monitoring with statistical modelling used to compare injury rates and their trends across study arms, with adjustment for key factors and potential confounders, including any baseline imbalance.

Phase 4: development and release of a final intervention package

The final step is to take the lessons learnt from phase 3 to develop and implement a wide-scale policy action plan for the prevention of the target injuries. The aim should be to develop a resource that could then be adopted and promoted by peak sports bodies for implementation across all levels of a sport. Specific questions associated with this research phase are:

◆ What should be the content and format of a peak body policy/action plan to support the intervention package?

◆ How could this be best integrated into existing structures to support sport safety delivery at the grass roots?

The intervention package should be refined or modified for peak-body roll-out, according to the outcomes of phase 3. To complete the process, this should be ratified by the same expert panel that participated in phases 1 or 2. The product will be then an intervention package with the highest likelihood of being adopted.

The research team should work closely with the peak sports body and other stake-holders in its formatting and presentation of the final version of the intervention package. For example, a national sports body may like to make the resource available online through their website for the general public and sports groups to download and provide additional feedback on it. A suitable and timely feedback process needs to be established, such as one facilitated by an online survey on the peak-body website. All feedback can then be collated and analysed by the research team and fed back to the peak body and stake-holder groups so that it can be taken into account before its full formal release of the resource.

Translation research

A major goal of all sports injury research is to prevent injuries and so it is important that the research does not stop here. This brings us to translation research, whereby research into the processes for ensuring that the evidence is formally integrated into policy and practice is undertaken. Whilst this is not strictly speaking intervention research, it is worth making some notes about how this could be achieved. There is an emerging body of literature about how such studies could be undertaken and it is beyond the scope of this chapter to discuss this sort of research in detail. However, the interested reader is referred to recent health-promotion and health-policy literature on this topic[53–58].

If the previous research phases are followed, the final product will be a nationally or regionally relevant safety policy/action plan based on procedures for clubs to adopt to prevent injuries and formal release of the final resource. It is expected that multi-agency engagement of all major stake-holders from the outset would enhance the long-term success of the intervention package, in terms of its sustainability. Translation research would include the documenting and analysis of this process to develop an understanding of why, how, and when specific decisions were made.

There may also be scope to extend the intervention package more broadly to other regions, sports injury problems, or sports. Given the sport-specific nature of some intervention, separate consideration should be given to the evidence-informed prevention guidelines and the delivery plan components. Specific questions that could be addressed in the translation research activities include:

- ◆ Which sports are most likely to benefit from (i) adoption of the specific injury intervention and/or (ii) the evaluated intervention package, including delivery plan?
- ◆ What are the key components to delivering evidence-based injury-prevention packages that could be used to inform state/national strategic approaches to implementing other safety or health-promotion interventions in the community sport setting?
- ◆ What unique, but complementary, role could each stake-holder agency play in a future strategic approach to sports safety?

Throughout phases 1–3, it will be useful for the stake-holder groups to each review the delivery of their sports-safety interventions. Researchers can participate in discussions with partner agencies to identify potential roles in any future strategic approaches (which will be determined from results of previous phases). This process should be documented and analysed to develop an understanding of why, how, and when decisions were made. Lessons learnt from the intervention-delivery in the implementation trial should be reviewed and the direct relevance to other sports identified through these researcher and stake-holder consultations.

Active engagement of the stake-holder groups through all aspects of the research will increase the profile of, and acceptance for, sports-safety activities within sport more generally. They will also generate background support for sports safety within the culture of sport and increase knowledge and awareness amongst a range of relevant consumers. These activities will include fostering and encouraging research into the translation of sports-safety evidence and should include dissemination of information through specific scientific sessions at relevant sports medicine conferences and industry forums convened by stake-holder groups to plan and deliver sports safety and injury-risk-management forums for community sport-delivery bodies and participants. Finally, researchers should work with stake-holder agencies to write and publish regular, plain-language articles describing latest advances in sport safety targeted at their members.

References

1. Finch C (2006). A new framework for research leading to sports injury prevention. *J Sci Med Sport*, **9**(1–2), 3–9.
2. Finch C, Donaldson A (2009). A sports setting matrix for understanding the implementation context for community sport. *Brit J Sports Med*, Published online 6 Feb 2009; doi:10.1136/bjsm.2008.056069.
3. Glasgow R, Lichtenstein E, Marcus A (2003). Why don't we see more translation of health promotion research to practice? Rethinking the efficacy-to-effectiveness transition. *Am J Hlth Prom*, **93**(8), 1261–7.
4. van Tiggelen D, Wickes S, Stevens V, Roosen P, Witvrouw E (2008). Effective prevention of sports injuries: a model integrating efficacy, efficiency, compliance and risk taking behaviour. *Brit J Sports Med*, **42**, 648–52.
5. Mallonee S, Fowler C, Istre GR (2006). Bridging the gap between research and practice: a continuing challenge. *Inj Prev*, **12**, 357–9.
6. Glasgow R (2008). What types of evidence are most needed to advance behavioural medicine? *Ann Behav Med*, **35**, 19–25.
7. Kirkwood B (2004). Making public health interventions more evidence based. *BMJ*, **328**(7466), 966–7.
8. Sanson-Fisher R, Boneski B, Green L, D'Este C (2007). Limitations of the randomized controlled trial in evaluating population-based health interventions. *Am J Prev Med*, **33**(2), 155–61.

9. West S, Duan N, Pequegnat W, Gaist P, Des Jarlais D, Holtgrave D, Szapocznik J, Fishbein M, Rapkin B, Clatts M, Mullen PD (2008). Alternatives to the randomized controlled trial. *Am J Pub Hlth*, **98**(8), 1359–66.

10. Armstrong R, Waters E, Moore L, Riggs E, Cuervo LG, Lumbiganon P, Hawe P (2008). Improving the reporting of public health intervention research: advancing TREND and CONSORT. *J Pub Hlth*, **30**(1), 103–9.

11. Finch C, Braham R, McIntosh A, McCrory P, Wolfe R (2005). Should Australian football players wear custom-made mouthguards? Results from a group-randomised controlled trial. *Inj Prev*, **11**, 242–6.

12. Braham R (2004), Finch C. Do community football players wear allocated protective equipment? Descriptive results from a randomised controlled trial. *J Sci Med Sport*, **7**(2), 216–20.

13. Kilding A, Tunstall H, Kuzmic D (2008). Suitabiliity of FIFA's "the 11" training programme for young football players – impact on physical performance. *Clin J Sport Med*, **7**, 320–6.

14. Cook D, Cusimano M, Tator C, Chipman M (2003). Evaluation of the ThinkFirst Canada, Smart Hockey, brain and spinal cord injury prevention video. *Inj Prev*, **9**, 361–6.

15. Eime R, Owen N, Finch C (2004). Protective eyewear promotion: applying principles of behaviour change in the design of a squash injury prevention programme. *Sports Med*, **34**(10), 629–38.

16. Eime E, Finch C, Wolfe R, Owen N, McCarty C (2005). The effectiveness of a squash eyewear promotion strategy. *Brit J Sports Med*, **39**, 681–5.

17. Abbott K, Klarenaar P, Donaldson A, Sherker S (2008). Evaluating SafeClub: can risk management training improve the safety activities of community soccer clubs? *Brit J Sports Med*, **42**, 460–5.

18. Quarrie K, Gianotti S, Chalmers D, Hopkins W (2005). An evaluation of mouthguard requirements and dental injuries in New Zealand rugby union. *Brit J Sports Med*, **39**, 650–4.

19. Gianotti S, Hume P, Hopkins W, Harawira J, Truman R (2008). Interim evaluation of the effect of a new scrum law on neck and back injuries in rugby union. *Brit J Sports Med*, **42**, 427–30.

20. Nilsen P (2004). What makes community based injury prevention work? In search of evidence of effectiveness. *Inj Prev*, **10**, 268–74.

21. Timpka T, Lindqvist K (2001). Evidence based prevention of acute injuries during physical exercise in a WHO safe community. *Brit J Sports Med*, **35**, 20–7.

22. Knapik J, Bullock S, Canada S, Toney E, Wells J, Hoedebecke E, Jones BH (2004). Influence of an injury reduction program on injury and fitness outcomes among soldiers. *Inj Prev*, **10**, 37–42.

23. Ward V, House A, Hamer S (2009). Knowledge brokering: exploring the process of transferring knowledge into action. *BMC Hlth Serv Res*, **9**(12), doi:10.1186/472-6963-9-12.

24. Catford J (2009). Advancing the 'science of delivery' of health promotion: not just the 'science of discovery'. *Hlth Prom Int*, **24**(1), 1–5.

25. Glasgow R, Klesges L, Dzewaltowski D, Bull S, Estabrooks P (2004) The future of health behaviour change research: what is needed to improve translation of research into health promotion practice? *Ann Behav Med*, **27**(1), 3–12.

26. Thompson R, Sacks J (2001). Evaluating an injury intervention or program, in Rivara F, Cummings P, Koepsell T, Grossman D, Maier R (eds). *Injury control: A guide to research and program evaluation*, pp. 196–216. Cambridge University Press Cambridge.

27. Timpka T, Ekstrand J, Svanstrom L (2006). From sports injury prevention to safety promotion in sports. *Sports Med*, **36**(9), 733–45.

28. Christoffel T, Gallagher S (2006). *Injury prevention and public health. Practical knowledge, skills, and strategies.* 2nd edition. Jones and Bartlett Publishers, Sudbury.

29. Robertson L (2007). *Injury epidemiology. Research and control strategies.* 3rd Edition. Oxford University Press, New York.

30. Scott I (2004). Laws and rule-making, in McClure R, Stevenson M, McEvoy S (eds). *The scientific basis of injury prevention and control*, pp. 283–302. IP Communications Pty Ltd., Melbourne.

31. Henley N (2004). Social marketing, in McClure R, Stevenson M, McEvoy S (eds) *The scientific basis of injury prevention and control*, pp. 318–33. IP Communications, Melbourne.

32. Provvidenza C, Johnston K (2009). Knowledge transfer principles as applied to sport concussion education. *Brit J Sports Med*, **43**, i68–-i75.

33. Brussoni M, Towner E, Hayes M (2006). Evidence into practice: combining the art and science of injury prevention. *Inj Prev*, **12**, 373–7.

34. Timpka T, Finch C, Goulet C, Noakes T, Yammine K (2008). Meeting the global demand of sports safety – the role of the science and policy intersection for sports safety. *Sports Med*, **39**(10), 795–805.

35. Nilsen P (2008). The theory of community based health and safety programs: a critical examination. *Inj Prev,* **12**, 140–5.

36. Roen K, Arai L, Roberts H, Popay J (2006). Extending systematic reviews to include evidence on implementation: methodological work on a review of community-based initiative to prevent injuries. *Soc Sci Med*, **63**, 1060–71.

37. Finch C, Hennessy M (2000). The safety practices of sporting clubs/centres in the City of Hume. *J Sci Med Sport*, **3**(1), 9–16.

38. Donaldson A, Forero R, Finch CF, Hill T (2004). A comparison of the sports safety policies and practices of community sports clubs during training and competition in northern Sydney, Australia. *Brit J Sports Med*, **38**(1), 60–3.

39. Donaldson A, Forero R, Finch C (2004). The first aid policies and practices of community sports clubs in northern Sydney, Australia. *Heal Promo J Aus,* **15**, 156–62.

40. Swan P, Otago L, Finch C, Payne W (2009). The policies and practices of sports governing bodies to assessing the safety of sports grounds. *J Sci Med Sport*, **12**(1): 171–6.

41. Zazryn T, Finch C, Garnham A (2004). Is safety a priority for football clubs? *Sport Health*, **21**(4), 19–24.

42. Finch C, Donaldson A, Mahoney M, Otago L (2008). The safety policies and practices of community multi-purpose recreation facilities. *Saf Sci*, doi:10.1016/j.ssci.2009.02.004

43. Twomey D, Finch C, Roediger E, Lloyd D (2009). Preventing lower limb injuries – is the latest evidence being translated into the football field? *J Sci Med Sport*, **12**(4): 452–6.

44. Glasgow R, Vogt T, Boles S (2001). Evaluating the public health impact of health promotion interventions: the RE-AIM framework. *Am J Pub Hlth*, **89**, 1322–7.

45. Li F, Harmer P, Glasgow R, Mack KA, Sleet D, Fisher KJ, Kohn MA, Millet LM, Mead J, Xu J, Lin ML, Yang T, Sutton B, Tompkins Y (2008). Translation of an effective Tai Chi intervention into a community-based falls-prevention program. *Am J Pub Hlth*, **98**(7), 1195–8.

46. Gyurcsik N, Brittain D (2006). Partial examination of the public health impact of the People with Arthritis Can Exercise (PACE) Program: reach, adoption, and maintenance. *Pub Hlth Nurs*, **23**(6), 516–22.

47. Bescculides M, Zaveri H, Hanson C, Farris R, Gregory-Mercado K, Will J (2008). Best practices in implementing lifestyle interventions in the WISEWOMAN program: adaptable strategies for public health programs. *Am J Hlth Prom*, **22**(5), 322–8.

48. Dzewaltowski D, Estabrooks P, Klesges L, Bull S, Glasgow R (2004). Behavior change intervention research in community settings: how generalizable are the results? *Hlth Prom Int,* **19**(2), 235–45.

49. Hasson F, Keeney S, McKenna HR (2000). Research guidelines for the Delphi survey technique. *J Adv Nursing*, **32**(4), 1008–15.

50. Krueger R, Casey M (2000). *Focus groups: a practical guide for applied research*. 3rd edition. Sage, Thousand Oaks.

51. Emery C (2007). Considering cluster analysis in sport medicine and injury prevention research. *Clin J Sport Med*, **17**(3), 211–14.

52. Hayen A (2006). Clustered data in sports research. *J Sci Med Sport*, **9**, 165–8.

53. Buse K, Mays N, Walt G (2005). *Making health policy*. Open University Press, Berkshire.

54. Bowen S, Zwi A (2005). Pathways to "evidence-informed" policy and practice: A framework for action. *PLoS Medicine*, **2**(7), e166.

55. Tran N, Hyder A, Kulanthayan S, Singh S, Umar R (2009). Engaging policy makers in road safety research in Malaysia: a theoretical and contextual analysis. *Hlth Policy*, **90**, 58–65.

56. Choi B, Gupta A, Ward B (2009). Good thinking: six ways to bridge the gap between scientists and policy makers. *J Epidem Comm Health*, **63**, 179–80.

57. Morandi L (2009). Essential nexus. How to use research to inform and evaluate public policy. *Am J Prev Med*, **36**(2S), S53–S4.

58. Mitton C, MacNab Y, Smith N, Foster L (2008). Transferring injury data to decision makers in British Columbia. *Int J Inj Control & Saf Prom*, **15**(1), 41–3.

Index

2X2 table 22–3, 24, 25, 28, 189
Academy for Physical Education Teachers Education
      (ALO) 164
active approaches 144, 147–8
administrative data 63
adoption:
   of the intervention 159, 163–4
   see also RE-AIM
adverse events 176
Aerobics Center Longitudinal Study 64
aetiological studies and statistics 125–33
   covariates in multiple regression 129–31
   mediating effects determination through multiple
         regression 131–3
   patterns of injury 125–7
   rates of injury 128
aetiological time zero 105–6
allocation concealment 174
alpha-numeric coding systems 49
alternate explanations, consideration of 111
American College of Sports Medicine 141
analysis, unity of 214
anatomical location 50
arithmetic mean 202
Attitude-Social influence-self-Efficacy (ASE)
      model 162

back-transformation 71, 78
background information 86
baseline assessment 175
behavioural approach (intervention mapping) 157–66
   adoption, implementation and sustainability of the
         intervention 159, 163–4
   evaluation plan 159, 164–5
   intervention components and materials 159, 162–3
   matrices of change objectives 159, 160–1
   needs assessment 158–60
   theory-based methods and practical strategies 159,
         161–2
benefit versus harm 106
bias 10
   accidental 174
   aetiological studies 129, 130, 132, 133
   confounding 131
   cost-effectiveness studies 207, 208–9
   evaluation studies 171, 177
   interviewer 16
   measurement 176
   misclassification 57
   observation 10
   specification 57
   see also selection bias
billing data 63
binary variable 69, 71
binomial sampling distribution 73, 76

biomechanical experiments and injury 119
blinding 12
Boolean operators 88
bootstrapping 75, 78, 126–7, 128, 203–5, 206
bottom-up interventions 150–1
buckle transducers 119
burden of injury 69, 77–8

cadaveric studies 119–20
career ending injury 48, 49
case-control studies 15–17
causal contrast 100
causal effects, indirect 131–2
causal inferences 129
causality in epidemiology 99–101, 109–11
causation of inury 50–2
CEAC 206–7, 208
ceiling ratios 204, 206
Centers for Disease Control and Prevention 62, 64
Centre for Allied Health Evidence: Critical Appraisal
      Tools 91
change objectives 161
CHEC-list 208–9
chi-square test 22–4, 25, 27–8, 33, 36
   aetiological studies 126
   effect studies 186, 190, 191
   evaluation studies 178
   Pearson 23
classification of injury 49–50
clinical equipoise (ethics) 11
clinical error rates 80
clinical records data 63
clinical studies 117
clinical trials 11–14, 15
club level 224
clustering 178–80
   aetiological studies 128
   effect studies 191, 193
   evaluation studies 173–4
   inter-cluster 179
   intra-cluster 178, 179–81, 193, 194
   see also random-effects modelling; randomized
         controlled trial
co-ordination 140–1
Cochrane Collaboration 92
Cochrane Library 85
coefficient of variation 194–5
Cohen's kappa 92, 113
coherence 111
cohort studies 14–15
communication 140–1
company's perspective 198
comparison population 14
complementary log-log link function 76
complementary log-log transformation 77

concerns 142–4
conditional association 130
confidence interval 20–1, 24, 25, 27, 36, 93
   aetiological studies 125, 127, 128
   cost-effectiveness studies 203
   descriptive studies 60, 70–1, 75, 78, 79
   effect studies 185–6, 187–90, 191, 192
   evaluation studies 172–3, 175, 178–9
confounding 10, 16, 21, 37–9
   aetiological studies 131
   definition 105–6
   and effect modification 37–9
   effect studies 188, 189, 190, 193
   evaluation studies 174
   multi-causality of injury 101
consistency 110
CONSORT diagram 90
CONSORT Statement 178
constant 25
consultation 140–1
contamination 174, 176
contexts, importance of 141–42
continuous determinant 28
control groups 11, 16, 229
correlation coefficients 114–15
cost of illness study 197
cost prices, appropriate 201–2
cost-benefit analysis 198–9
cost-diaries 201
cost-effectiveness studies 197–209
   analysis of costs 202–3
   control treatment, choice of 198–9
   cost-effectiveness curve 206, 207
   cost-effectiveness plane 204, 206, 207, 208
   costs, identification, measurement and valuation
      of 200–202
   economic valuation, critical assessment of 208–9
   economic valuation, definition of 197–8
   economic valuation, design of 198
   effects, identification, measurement and valuation
      of 199–200
   incremental cost-effectiveness ratio 203–5
   missing data 207
   net-benefit approach 206–7
   perspective 198
   piggy-back economic evaluation 198
   sensitivity analysis 207–8
   statistical analysis 202
   uncertainty 204–5
cost-minimization 197–8
cost-outcome description 197
cost-utility 197, 199
costs 203
count and count ratios 74
counterfactual theory 129
Cox regression analysis 34–7, 39, 76–7, 220
critical appraisal of study quality 91
cross-sectional studies 17, 25, 60
cumulative complementary log-log 74

data:
   extraction and analysis 91–4
   missing 207

   sources for descriptive studies 61–5
databases 85, 87–8
decision-model 198
decomposition analysis 131–3
defining a research question 3–7
   methodology 4–7
      common mistakes and problems in question
         construction 6–7
      mechanics of question 5–6
   purpose of research 3–4
delivery plan 228, 229–31
Delphi method 208, 228
descriptive studies 17
descriptive studies, research designs for 55–65
   cross-sectional studies 58–60
   data sources 61–5
   ecologic studies 55–8, 59
   epidemiology studies 60–1
descriptive studies, statistics used in 69–81
   count and count ratios 74
   hazard, time to injury and their ratios 75–7
   magnitude thresholds for injury outcomes 79–81
   odds, odds ratio and generalized linear
      modelling 71–4
   rate and rate ratios 74–5
   risk, risk difference and risk ratio 69–71
   severity and burden of injury 77–8
design effect 193
determinant definition 105–6
dichotomous outcome 19–20, 28
Differential Variable Reluctance Transducer 119
direct effect 131–3
directed acyclic graph (DAG) 129–32
disease-specific instruments 199
dose-response relationship 110
drop-out 175
dummy studies 119–20
dynamic, recursive model of aetiology in injury 103

early recurrences 45
ecological approach 55–8, 59, 148, 151–52, 229
economic evaluation *see* cost-effectiveness studies
effect studies, statistics used in 183–95
   clustering 191
   coefficient of variation 194–5
   confounding 188
   examples 183–4
   generalized estimating equations 192
   incidence rates 185–6
   intra-cluster correlation coefficient 193
   Mantel-Haenszel methods 188–90
   multilevel models and random-effects models 192–3
   Poisson regression 190–1
   rate ratio 186, 187–8
   sample size, implications for 193–4
   standard error, robust 191–2
effect-modifiers 37–9, 105
effectiveness 170, 213–14, 215–16, 217
   see also cost-effectiveness; RE-AIM
efficacy studies 170, 213–14, 215–16, 221
eligible papers, selection of 88–9
endnotes 95
environmental causes 157

environmental conditions 160–1
environmental measures 152
epidemiological criteria for causation 109–11
error:
    rates, statistical 80
    systematic 115
    Type I and II 179
    see also standard error
evaluation plan 159, 164–5
evaluation studies, research designs for 169–80
    analysis, considerations for 177–8
    baseline assessment 175
    cluster analysis 178–80
    intervention 175–6
    outcome measurement 176–7
    randomization 174–5
    research design 170–73
    research question 169–70
    study population and sampling methods 173–4
event time phase 143, 145, 152
evidence, levels of 89–91
evidence synthesis 83, 84
evidence-based interventions 144, 227–8
exacerbations 46
exclusion criteria and reviews 87
experiment 111
experimental design 9
exposure 10, 14, 105
    aetiological studies 128, 129
    descriptive studies 57, 58, 59, 60–1
    effect studies 185, 186, 193

factorial designs 170
fatal injury 48
Fédération Internationale de Football Association
    (FIFA) 146
fibreoptic sensors 119
Fisher exact test 23, 25
five-step approach to preventive measures
    development 140–4
fixed-effects modelling 127
Fleiss' kappa 113
flow-charts 94
focus group discussions 228
footnotes 95
forest plot 93
Friction Cost Approach 202
function of literature reviews 83–4

g-estimation 130
general (traditional) reviews 84
generalized estimating equations 71, 130,
    178, 192
generalized linear modelling 71–4, 75, 76, 77, 190
government databases 61–2
gradual-onset injury (overuse) 50–2
graphs 94
GRONORUN trial 13

Haddon's hierarchy of 10
    countermeasure strategies 148–50
Haddon's matrix 143, 145, 152–3
Hawthorne effect 175

hazard ratio 35–6, 70, 72–3, 74, 75–7, 79–80, 81
    see also incidence density ratio
health-care costs 200–1
health-care insurer's perspective 198
health-care provider's perspective 198
health-care system as data source 62–3
health-care utilization 200–202
health-promotion services 151
heterogeneity 20
    see also standard deviation
hierarchical modelling see random-effects modelling
High School Reporting Information Online (RIO)
    study 63
historical cohorts 171
host-agent-environment relationship 151–3
Human Capital Approach 202

impact of injury 59
implementation:
    of the intervention 159, 163–4
    see also RE-AIM
implementation of studies into real life 213–32
    effectiveness versus efficacy 213–14
    evidence-based intervention package, development
        of 227–8
    examples of implementation studies 214–21
        controlled pre-, post- and follow-up evaluation of
            risk-management training programme aimed
            at soccer clubs 219
        interrupted time-series analysis of population level
            impact of mouth-guard regulation on dental
            injuries 219
        pre-post evaluation of responses to brain and
            spinal cord injury-prevention video aimed at
            ice hockey players 218
        quasi-experimental evaluation of a multifaceted
            injury-prevention programme using historical
            controls 220–1
        quasi-experimental non-randomized
            evaluation of a safe community
            programme 220
        randomized controlled trial of FIFA's 'The 11'
            training programme 217–18
        randomized controlled trial of soft-shell
            headgear and custom-fitted
            mouth-guards in Australian football
            216–17
        randomized ecological evaluation of
            squash eye-wear promotion strategy 218–19
        time-series analysis comparison of observed and
            predicted population-level injury-claim
            numbers 220
    intervention package, development and release
        of 231
    intervention package, implementation and
        evaluation of and its delivery plan 229–31
    intervention package, refining of and development
        of delivery plan 228
    intervention-implementation study designs 314
    RE-AIM health-promotion framework 222–6
    theoretical basis 221–22
    translation research 231–32
in vivo strain/force measurements 119

incidence 78
  density 29, 35, 73
  rate ratio *see* rate ratio
  see also in particular descriptive studies
inclusion criteria and reviews 87
incremental cost-effectiveness ratio
  (ICER) 206
index injury 45–6
index population 105–6
individual participants level 224
inflation factor 178, 179, 193
Injury Control and Risk Study 64
injury definitions 43–52
  case, definition of in injury surveillance
    studies 44–6
  causation of inury 50–2
  classification of injury 49–50
  definition of injury 43–4
  impact of on study outcomes 52
  pathology 50
  severity of injury 46–9
injury-surveillance studies 50
insurance data 63
intention 162
  to treat analysis 177, 179
inter-cluster variation 179
interaction term 39
intercept 25
Intercooled Stata 171
International Classification of Diseases 44,
  49–50, 61–2
International Rugby Board 220
interrupted time-series analysis 214
intervention delivery, unit of 214
intervention/intervention 175–6
  components and materials, production of
    159, 162–3
  effect 37–8
  –implementation study designs 314
  –level dimension 146–50
  mapping *see* behavioural approach
  package 228, 229–31
  process, direction of 150–1
  study 20
interviews 115–17, 201
intra-cluster correlation 178, 179–81, 193, 194

Joanna Briggs Institute 91
joint probability of agreement 113

Kaplan-Meier survival curves 29–34, 77
kappa statistics 91, 92, 113–14

laboratory motion analysis 118–19
limits of agreement 115
linear model 78
linear regression analysis 25, 26
link function 71
log rank test 30, 32–3, 34–5
log transformation 78
log-log link function, complementary 76
log-log transformation, complementary 77
logistic regression analysis 25–8, 37, 71, 72

logit link function 73
logit transformation 71

macro/community level 146
magnitude thresholds for injury outcomes 79–81
maintenance *see* RE-AIM
Mann-Whitney U-test 203
Mantel-Haenszel methods 188–90, 191
marginal models *see* generalized estimating equations
masking 12
matching 16, 174
matrices of change objectives, preparation of 159,
  160–1
mean deviation 78
mechanism of no injury (MONI) 104
mechanisms of injury *see* risk factors and mechanisms,
  investigation of
mediating effects determination through multiple
  regression 131–3
medical records data 63
medication 48
MeSH 88
meso/groups and organizations level 146
meta-analysis 92–3
meta-synthesis 93
micro/individual level 146
minimum severity 46
missed-match injury (time-loss) 49
missing at random (MAR) 207
missing completely at random (MCAR) 207
missing not at random (MNAR) 207
mixed-modelling *see* random-effects modelling
Monte Carlo simulations 208
multi-causality of injury – current concepts 99–107
  causality in epidemiology 99–101
  models of injury prevention 99
  object of study 104–5
  outcome, determinant and confounder
    definitions 105–6
  sport and recreational injuries 101–4
  taking action 106–7
Multi-Centre Orthopaedics Outcomes Network
  (MOON) 14–15
multi-disciplinary approach 140–1
multi-factorial model of injury 101–2
multi-level modelling *see* random-effects modelling
multinomial distribution 74
multiple imputation techniques 207
multiple regression 129–33, 178
multivariate analysis 177
Multivariate Imputation by Chained Equations
  (MICE) algorithm 207

National Ambulatory Medical Care Survey 62
National Basketball Association 63
National Center for Catastrophic Sport Injury
  Research 64
National Collegiate Athletic Association Injury
  Surveillance System 61, 63
National Electronic Injury Surveillance
  System 56, 59, 62
National Federation of State High School
  Associations 56, 59, 62

National Health & Medical Research Council
(Australia) 90
National Health Interview Survey 60, 62
National Hospital Ambulatory Medical Care
Survey 62
National Hospital Discharge Survey 62
national level 223–4
National Public Health Partnership Planning
Framework 140
National Registry of Sudden Death in Athletes 64
natural logarithmic scale 185
necessary cause 100
needs assessment 158–60, 162
negative likelihood ratio 114
negative predictive value 113, 114
negative-binomial 74
net monetary benefit 206–7
net-benefit approach 206–7
New South Wales Sport and Recreation Sport Rage
Program 146
New Zealand Football 'Soccer Smart' Program 144
non-experimental studies 104
non-fatal catastrophic injury 48, 49
non-health-care costs 200, 201
non-independence of data *see* clustering
non-probability sampling 173
non-randomized controlled trial 172
null-hypothesis 22–3, 32, 33
number of injuries 185
numerator-only data 125

observational studies 9, 129, 171
Occupational Injury and Illness Classification 44, 49
odds/odds ratio 24–5, 27–8, 38, 60–1, 70,
71–4, 93, 129
operational model 102–3
Orchard Sports Injury Classification System
(OSICS) 50–1, 52
outcome 10
case-control studies 16
cohort studies 14
definition 105–6
descriptive studies 57, 58, 59, 60–1
magnitude thresholds 79–81
measurement and evaluation studies 176–7
multi-causality of injury 101, 104
primary 199, 200
secondary 200
statistic and descriptive studies 75
variable 38
outliers 177–8
'outside' agencies 150
over-dispersion 128

p-value 22–3, 24, 25, 27, 30, 33, 36, 39
effect studies 187–8, 190, 191
evaluation studies 178, 179
pain tolerance 48
participation *see* exposure
passive approaches 147–8
patterns of injury 125–7
Pearson chi-square test 23
Pearson correlation 114–15

PECOT 86, 87
performance objectives 160–1, 163, 164
person characteristics 56
PICO 86, 87
place characteristics 56
planning, long-term 144
plausibility 111
point estimates 125, 175
Poisson distribution/regression 190–1
aetiological studies 128
descriptive studies 72, 74, 75
effect studies 185–6, 189, 191–92
evaluation studies 179
two-level 193
positive likelihood ratio 114
positive predictive value 113, 114
post hoc analysis (data-dredging or fishing) 177
post-event time phase 143, 145, 152
pragmatic approach 139–53
five-step approach to preventive measures
development 140–4
host-agent-environment relationship 151–3
intervention process, direction of 150–1
intervention-level dimension 146–50
time dimension 144–6
pre-event time phase 99, 143, 145, 152
PRECEDE-PROCEED model 158
prevalence studies 28, 76
preventive measures 107, 140–4
prices, appropriate 200–1
primary data collection 158
primary prevention 99, 145
primary research 84
primary restraints 119
priorities 144
probability 69
distribution 22–3
sampling 173
productivity-loss 201–2
programme design 162–3
proportion 69
proportional-hazards regression 73, 76–7
prospective studies 11, 15, 25
publication of reviews 95
PubMed 85, 88
purpose of research 3–4

qualitative data 228, 230–1
quality of life 199, 200
quality-adjusted life-years 197, 199
quasi-experimental designs 171–72, 214
questionnaires 201

random error 10–11, 115
random-effects modelling 127, 171, 192–3
randomization 12, 174–5
randomized controlled trial 129, 229
cluster 178, 179, 191, 194
cost-effectiveness studies 107, 197, 198, 199, 207
effect studies 188, 193
effectiveness versus efficacy 213
evaluation studies 170–73, 176
four-arm 216

randomized controlled trial *(cont'd)*
  intervention-implementation study designs 214
  multi-causality of injury 104
  three-armed 170
  two-armed 170
rank-transformation 78
rate difference 128
rate ratios 74–5, 128, 169, 185–6, 187–90, 191, 192, 193
rates 74–5
  comparison 186
  difference 187
  of injury 128, 189
RE-AIM model 163, 222–6, 227, 229, 230
re-injuries 46
reach *see* RE-AIM
recall 16
recurrrent injury 45–6
recursive model approach 130, 175
reference population 105–6
references to studies 94–5
regional level 223–4
registries as data sources 63–4
regression analysis 33, 187
  multiple 129–33, 178
  see also linear; logistic
regression coefficient 27, 35, 37–9
relative risk 20–1, 22–4, 25, 27, 29, 35–6, 72
reliability 113–15, 176–7
  inter-rater 113, 176
  intra-rater 113, 176
repeated measures designs 170
research designs *see* descriptive studies, research
    designs for
retrospective studies 15, 25
return to fitness criteria 46
Review Manager 92
reviews 83–95
  background information 86
  critical appraisal of study quality 91
  data extraction and analysis 91–4
  definitions and classifications 83
  function of literature reviews 84
  inclusion and exclusion criteria 87
  levels of evidence 89–91
  objectives linked to review question 86–7
  publication 95
  references to studies 94–5
  search strategies for databases 87–8
  selection of eligible papers 88–9
  setting an explicit review question 86
  statistical synthesis 94
  synthesizing research studies 83–4
  types of 84–5
  writing systematic review protocol and conducting
      the review 85–6
risk 69–71, 140–2
  compensation 106–7
  difference 19, 20–1, 22–4, 25, 27, 29, 72, 79–80
  factors 70, 101–2, 104, 174–5
  identified 144
  ratio 72
  see also relative risk; risk factors and mechanisms
risk factors and mechanisms, investigation of 109–21

epidemiological criteria for causation 109–11
mechanisms of injury 115–20
  biomechanical experiments and injury 119
  cadaveric and dummy studies 119–20
  clinical studies 117
  interviews 115–17
  laboratory motion analysis 118–19
  mathematical modelling 120
  video analysis 117–18
  in vivo strain/force measurements 119
reliability 113–15
risk factors 111–12
validity 112–13, 114
Royal Association of Teachers of Physical Education
    (KVLO) 164

safety issues 142–4
sample size 20, 193–4, 230
  descriptive studies 80–1
  evaluation studies 173, 178
  random 173, 174
sampling 173–4
  consecutive 173
  convenience 173
  cumulative 72, 73
  distribution, binomial 73, 76
  non-probability 173
  snowball 173
  see also sample size
scenario analysis, extreme 208
schools/sport organizations as data sources 63
search strategies for databases 87–8
secondary data collection 158
secondary evidence production 84
secondary prevention 145
secondary restraints 119
selection bias 10, 12, 16, 118, 131, 171, 175
self-report 201
sensitivity analysis 93, 114, 207–8
severe functional disability 48
severity of injury 46–9, 77–8
slopes 72
snapshot time period 58–9
societal perspective 146, 198, 200, 201
Spearman correlations 114
special studies as data sources 64–5
specialty clinics data 63
specificity 111, 114
Sporting Goods Manufacturers Association 62
Sports Medicine Australia 141
Sports Medicine Diagnostic Coding System
    (SMDCS) 50
SPSS statistical package 126
standard deviation 72, 78, 80
standard error 21, 27, 36, 128, 171
  effect studies 185, 187–8, 189, 190–92
Standards Australia Guidelines for Managing Risk in
    Sport and Recreation 140
state level 223–4
statistical analysis software (SAS) 190
statistical error rates 80
statistical methods, basic 19–39, 202
  adding time at risk to the analysis 28–9

confidence intervals around risk difference and
relative risk 20–1
confounding and effect modification 37–9
Cox regression analysis 34–7
dichotomous outcome variables 19–20
Kaplan-Meier survival curves 29–34
logistic regression analysis 25–8
odds ratio 24–5
risk difference and relative risk, testing of 22–4
statistical packages 126
statistical synthesis 94
statistical tests 22–3
statistics *see* aetiological studies and statistics;
descriptive studies, statistics used in; effect studies,
statistics used in; kappa
Statview 126
stratification 12, 177
strength (epidemiological criteria) 109–10
structure, type of 50
study designs 9–18
bias 10
case-control studies 15–17
clinical trials 11–14
cohort studies 14–15
confounding 10
descriptive studies 17
random error 10–11
study population 14, 173–4
sub-group analysis 177
sufficient cause 100–1
summary profile 227–6
summary statistic 92, 93
surveillance studies 48
surveys 59–60
survival:
analysis 28
Kaplan-Meier survival curves 29–34, 77
plot 77
probabilities 30
sustainability of the intervention 159, 163–4
systematic reviews 84, 95

t-statistic 71, 78
t-test 74, 202–3

tables 94
see also 2X2 table
team level 224
temporality 100, 109
tertiary prevention 145
test statistic 33
test-re-test 113
theory-based methods and practical strategies 144,
159, 161–2
Three E's (Education, Engineering and
Enforcement) 146, 151–2
time:
adding at risk to the analysis 28–9
characteristics 57
–dependent variables 104
dimension 144–6
elapsed 45
to injury 35–6, 75–7
see also temporality
top-down interventions 150–1
translation research 231–2
traumatic injury 50–1
trip or run logs 62–3
TRIPP framework (Translating Research into Injury
Prevention Practice) 3–4, 5, 6, 213

uncertainty 20–1, 125–7, 128, 204–7
see also standard error

validity 112–13, 114, 115, 176–7
value criteria 152–3
Vancouver referencing style 94
video analysis 117–18

Wald statistic 27, 36
Wald-test 190
withdrawals (from analysis) 177
Women's National Basketball Association 63
World Health Organization 48, 49

Youth Risk Behavior Survey 62

z-statistic 187–8